> ### 'There are no short cuts to success.'
>
> You have to be self-motivated, dedicated, committed, focused, and persistent — day after day, week after week, month after month, year after year.
>
> When it comes time to test yourself — when you stand on the starting line — if you know in your heart that you have done everything possible to be the best you can be on the day, then you will succeed, regardless of the outcome.
>
> You can't ask anymore of yourself if you've given everything you've got.
>
> ### Life requires of you to 'give your best' and be happy in the attempt.

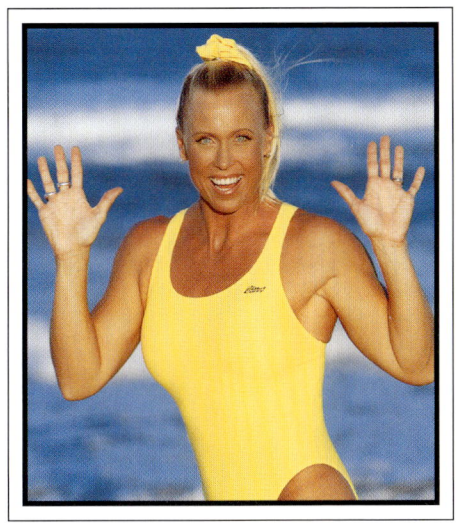

LISA CURRY
Get UP & GO!

with Mark McKean *Dip.T, PhD Candidate*

HarperSports
An imprint of HarperCollins*Publishers*

A Note from the Publisher

All reasonable care, diligence and attention has been taken in the preparation of material for this book. It is not intended that the information and suggestions made in this book, including but not limited to matters concerning diet, health, exercise and treatment, are to be used by the reader as a substitute for appropriate professional attention and proper medical advice.

The Reader should first consult his or her own doctor before beginning any exercise, dietary or other program, including any such programs suggested in this book, and the reader should not rely on any such information and suggestions in this book without first seeking appropriate medical consultation. The Publisher, author, co-author, consultants and editors, or their respective employees and agents, shall not accept responsibility for any injury, loss or damage caused to any person acting or failing to act arising from the material in this book whether or not any such injury, loss or damage is caused by any negligent act, or omission, default or breach of duty by the Publisher, the Editor, or their respective employees or agents, except as provided by the operation of law.

Acknowledgements

Co-author: Mark McKean **Consultants:** Diana Barr, Peter Webb, Dr Alan Hadley.
Editors: Ali Orman, Jesse Fink, John Campbell, Robyn Flemming.
Design/Illustration: Melanie Calabretta, Russell Jeffery, Clare Watson.
Photography: All photographs by Ian Golding, except page ix above right, 28, 112, 136–138 (Sue Neil); 4 (Australian Picture Library); 18, 30 (Ross Easom); 58–59, 66, 73, 76 (HarperCollins); 105, 163 (Duane Hart); 122 (Harvie Allison); 144 (Robert Coella); and 194 (Uncle Toby's).
Steps to Healthy Eating: (page 84) Adapted from the Australian Nutrition Foundation Inc. Healthy Eating Pyramid.

Get Up & Go: 1/12 Newspaper Place Maroochydore Qld 4558

Harper*Sports*
An imprint of HarperCollins*Publishers*, Australia

First published in Australia in 1998
by HarperCollins*Publishers* Pty Limited
ACN 009 913 517
A member of the HarperCollins*Publishers* (Australia) Pty Limited Group
http://www.harpercollins.com.au

Text copyright © Lisa Curry 1998
Illustrations copyright © Clare Watson 1998

This book is copyright.
Apart from any fair dealing for the purposes of private study, research, criticism or review, as permitted under the Copyright Act, no part may be reproduced by any process without written permission.
Inquiries should be addressed to the publishers.

HarperCollins*Publishers*
25 Ryde Road, Pymble, Sydney, NSW 2073, Australia
31 View Road, Glenfield, Auckland 10, New Zealand
77-85 Fulham Palace Road, London W6 8JB, United Kingdom
Hazelton Lanes, 55 Avenue Road, Suite 2900, Toronto, Ontario M5R 3L2
and 1995 Markham Road, Scarborough, Ontario M1B 5M8, Canada
10 East 53rd Street, New York NY 10032, USA

National Library of Australia Cataloguing-in-Publication data:

Curry, Lisa, 1962–
Get up & go!.
Includes index.
ISBN 0 7322 5877 4.
1. Physical fitness. 2. Exercise. 3. Diet. I. Title
613.7

Printed in Australia by Griffin Press Pty Ltd, Adelaide, on 115gsm Matt Art

5 4 3 2 1   98 99 00 01

Dedication

This book is written to educate, inform and inspire the reader
to challenge themselves to reach the greatness that is in all of us.
I have been inspired by many people, and my career, hard work and
experiences are wasted if I can not use them to help and inspire others.

I would like to dedicate *Get Up & Go!* to all the people
who are prepared and willing to make a change to their lives,
so that they can experience the wonderful benefits of being fit and healthy.

To my friends and team-mates in all the sports I participate in.
By helping each other, we help ourselves. We've all had great
fun and success and will continue to do so.

To my competitors — without you, I wouldn't have anything to strive for.
If there's a way to beat you — I'll find it!

To my personal trainer, Mark McKean — a constant inspiration to
strive for new challenges and always someone who keeps
my feet firmly on the ground!

To my great family who have had to put up with my late nights,
early mornings, long days, and days away, to make this book happen.

To my dear coach Mr King who passed away at the age of 86.
He was always my hero, and I miss him dearly.

Mark and I are happy to share our training ideas with you.
If one person changes their life because of this book, then the
two years it has taken to put it together has been worthwhile.

Have Fun!

Contents

Lisa Curry — Page viii-ix
Mark McKean — Page x
Consultant Profiles — Page x-xi
Introduction — Page xii-xiii

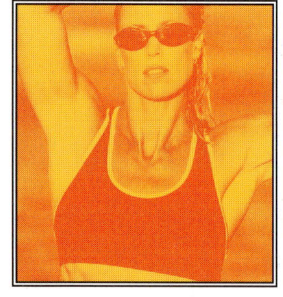

Getting Started
Success: What Does It Mean? — Page 3
Setting Goals You Can Achieve — Page 9
Managing Your Life — Page 17

Your Body
Understanding Your Body — Page 35
How Your Body Works — Page 40

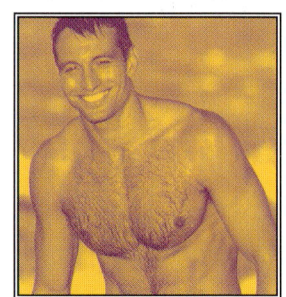

Food & Nutrition

Food for Life — Page 61
You & Your Diet — Page 82
Food for an Active Lifestyle — Page 91

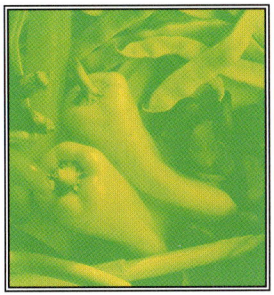

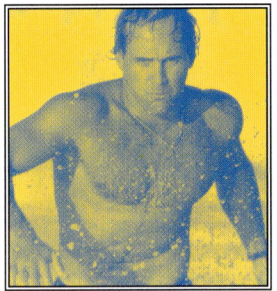

Training & Fitness

Preparing to Train — Page 111
Test Your Fitness — Page 124
Smart Training — Page 143

Training Manual

Introduction — Page 162
Training for Fat Loss — Page 168
Training for Aerobic Fitness — Page 183
Training for Increased Muscle Size — Page 192
Training for Muscle Definition — Page 202
Training for Shape — Page 207

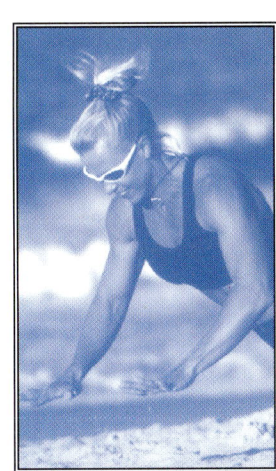

Appendix — Page 217
Index — Page 241

Lisa Curry

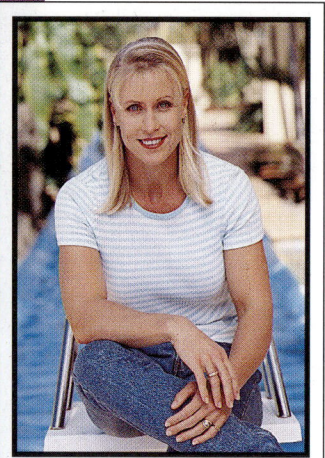

Lisa Curry is undoubtedly one of Australia's most popular personalities, a woman who has transcended her well-deserved place in the annals of Australian swimming to become a highly respected author, commentator, public speaker and promotional presenter. But Lisa is much more than that — she defines the true essence of health and fitness.

Swimming was the theatre for Lisa's early achievements. She started swimming in 1975, at the age of 12, and trained under coach Harry Gallagher for two years before moving to the Leander Swimming Club with master coach Joe King. At that time, Lisa was ranked as one of the fastest 12-year-olds in the world with a personal best of 28.3 seconds in the 50 metre freestyle.

In 1977, at age 15, Lisa entered her first international competition and was ranked number five in the world for the 100 metre breaststroke.

It was an auspicious beginning to a wonderful career. Lisa went on to win 30 medals in international competition, including 15 gold, seven silver and eight bronze medals and competed in two World Championships (1978 in Berlin and 1982 in Guayaquil), three Commonwealth Games (1978 in Edmonton, 1982 in Brisbane and 1990 in Auckland) and three Olympic Games (Moscow in 1980, Los Angeles in 1984 and Barcelona in 1992).

Lisa married ironman champion Grant Kenny in 1986 and soon afterwards gave birth to their first child, daughter Jaimi.

Four years later, Lisa rejoined the ranks of Australian swimming after watching 33-year-old American swimmer Sandy Nelson-Ball eclipse all before her in the pool. Lisa made the national swimming team for the 1990 Auckland Commonwealth Games and won a career-best four gold and one silver in competition. She was the toast of the swimming world. A different training program — half swimming, half weight training, complemented by regular massage and a high-quality nutritious diet — was instrumental in her comeback.

In 1990, at age 27 and with one child, Lisa was ranked third in the world in the 50 metre freestyle, fifth in the 100 metre butterfly and tenth in the 100 metre freestyle.

Working towards the Olympic trials in 1992, Lisa embarked yet again on a strength program under the National Strength and Conditioning Director of Australia, Ian King. At the Olympic trials she won the

50 metre butterfly and 50 metre freestyle, came in second in the 100 metre butterfly and fourth in the 100 metre freestyle — thus qualifying for four events at the Barcelona Olympics. Her results were outstanding!

At age 30 and the mother of two children, Lisa won the consolation (B) final of the 50 metre freestyle in Barcelona in 25.87 seconds — just seven one-hundredths of a second outside the Commonwealth record! She anchored both the freestyle and medley relay teams with personal best splits and the best-ever by any Australian relay member anywhere in the world with 55.61 and 55.48 seconds!

Lisa is the only Australian swimmer to have held Commonwealth and Australian records in such a variety of events, and in every stroke except backstroke:

- 50 metre freestyle
- 50 metre butterfly
- 100 metre breaststroke
- 100 metre freestyle
- 100 metre butterfly
- 200 metre breaststroke
- 200 metre individual medley
- 400 metre individual medley
- 4 x 100 metre freestyle relay
- 4 x 100 metre medley relay

Attesting to her reputation for healthy, clean living, Lisa has been the face of Uncle Toby's Muesli Bars for 15 years — the longest association between an elite Australian athlete and a company — and juggles a high-profile media career with speaking commitments and public promotions for Fernwood Fitness Centres, designing swim, gym and active wear for her fashion label Hot Curry and putting together her best-selling books and videos. After she's finished doing all of that, she likes nothing more than spending time with family and friends, exercising and training, and coaching and competing in surfboat rowing and outrigger canoe racing competitions.

After only five months of learning and training her surfboat rowing team, Lisa led her team to victory in the Queensland State Surf Lifesaving Championships. She has competed in five Molokai to Oahu outrigger canoe races — the World Championships of outrigger canoe racing — and in 1997, her team won the race, making them the first-ever Australian team to achieve such a feat.

Lisa continues to train and to learn to be 'the best I can be.' Her motto will always be: 'The fire inside still burns and it's the fire that takes you to success.'

Get Up & Go! is Lisa's third book, following *Total Health & Fitness* and *Pregnancy & Fitness*. She lives on the Sunshine Coast with her husband Grant and their three children, Jaimi, Morgan and Jett.

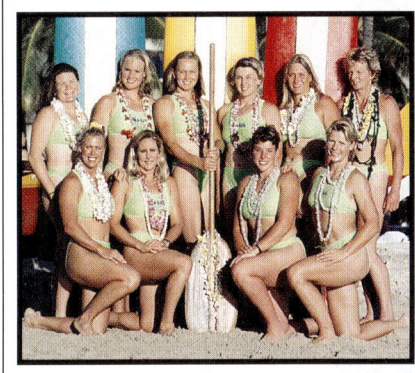

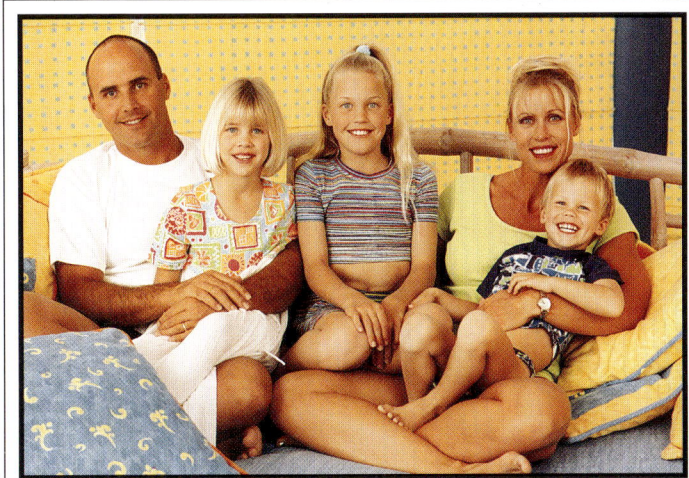

Co-author:
Mark McKean

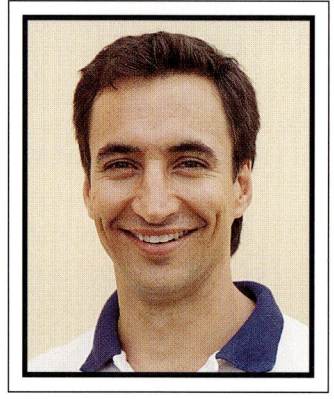

Mark has been teaching, training and coaching people and world-class athletes for over 15 years. A highly respected fitness consultant, Mark has a burgeoning list of private, sporting, educational and corporate clients and has worked in both the print and electronic media as a presenter and columnist.

Working with Lisa, Mark says, has been one of his career highlights and likens the relationship to maintaining a Rolls Royce automobile. With Mark's expert guidance, Lisa has been able to train less but achieve more than ever before.

Mark is presently completing his PhD at Sunshine Coast University. His current research is based on athletic performance and the influence of training at different ages and how this affects long-term performances. Mark and his wife Ros have two daughters, Sophie and Eliza.

Consultant:
Peter Webb

Peter is an Australian registered psychologist and naturopathic physician with over 16 years experience in private practice. He claims being both a psychologist and naturopath earns him the right to be called a psychopath!

Peter is a popular speaker and lecturer throughout Australia and New Zealand and is currently technical consultant to Metagenics (Health World Limited). He lives in Brisbane with his wife Michelle and their four children.

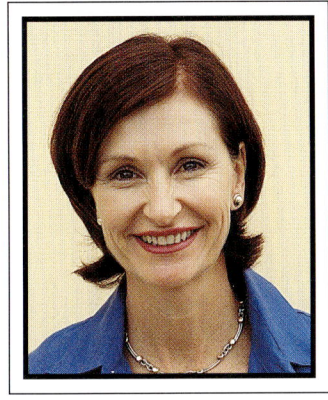

Consultant:
Di Barr

Di is a respected dietitian with a special interest in sports nutrition. She trained at Sydney University and has over 15 years experience working in major hospitals and private practices both in Australia and overseas.

She is a consultant to several sporting clubs and fitness centres on the Sunshine Coast, Queensland, and regularly talks to sporting groups, community groups and schools.

Di has been involved in competitive sport for most of her life. Her husband, Brian, is a world-class triathlete in his age group, and their four children regularly compete in triathlons and other sporting activities.

One of Di's greatest achievements has been to juggle work and family while still preparing delicious and nutritious meals at home. She follows the basics of a well-balanced diet in feeding her family, and in *Get Up & Go!*, she shares some of her secrets.

Consultant:
Dr Alan Hadley

Alan is a leader in the field of applied nutritional therapeutics. He diversified his general practice into a complementary medical clinic over 10 years ago. His wealth of experience and success in integrating dietary and natural medicines with conventional medicine has made him a highly sought after speaker both in Australia and internationally.

If your 'get up and go' has got up and gone...

Then it's time — right now — to make some decisions about what you want out of life.

Most people don't really live life, they just exist. You know that if you made a little more effort with your diet, made time available for some moderate exercise and changed certain lifestyle habits, your life could be better. So, why don't you make those changes?

It's too hard — or, that's what you think.

Life can be complicated — trying to juggle busy work schedules with family responsibilities, money worries, rearing children, trying to establish some security for the future — just trying to get by. But stop right now and consider how much better your life could be.

There's no point spending all your waking hours making more money if you're too sick to enjoy it, or don't have family and friends to spend it with — or, worse still, if you burn out at a young age from stress and a poor-quality lifestyle. You're only cheating yourself and everyone around you if you operate in 'existence' mode and don't really live your life to the full. You have to have a balanced life. Work, rest and play.

If you were even just a bit healthier in mind and body, your life would be a lot better — you could cope better with minor problems and irritations, work more productively, enjoy your sport and recreation more, you wouldn't be so tired or feel so sick all the time, your concentration would improve, and you'd have more fun and energy playing with the kids or your partner.

You probably agree with all of the above. But this doesn't alter the fact that, despite having it pointed out, it still seems too hard to make the sacrifices. I can hear you saying, 'Who is she to lecture us, anyway? She's a sports freak, an Olympian, she's super-fit.' Right — and wrong! These days I'm a working mother of three with a job, a husband, a mortgage, and my share of health and lifestyle problems. I constantly need to reinforce to myself the need to maintain a balanced lifestyle. I have to try to stay calm when the kids need me and I'm snowed under at work; and it takes effort to grab just an hour a day for a bit of exercise. It's hard to stay motivated — it takes constant work — but it's worth it.

I do understand how overwhelming life can be at times, and how hard it is to make those necessary changes for a better life, and harder still to maintain those changes, to make them part of your life — part of what you do every day. But it can be done. Plenty of people do it, and I want you to be part of that group.

And that's what this book is all about — to help make it easier. To make it achievable, exciting and enjoyable to get the life you want; to look and feel your best; to give you the very best chance to be happy and successful. It's not going to be a piece of cake, but it's going to be a lot easier than you think because we're going to do things gradually, to suit you. No throwing you in at the deep end. No huge upheavals. No drastic diets. No gut-busting exercise regimes.

Regardless of your age, your physical shape and condition, and the demands of your job and your family, this book will help you to change your life so that you can achieve your ambitions, hopes and dreams.

Get Up & Go! will help you to:

■ Establish how healthy you are at present to give you a starting point for improving your life.

■ Understand what's going on in your body and your mind so that it's easier to grasp what you have to do, how you are going to do it and why.

■ Start thinking positively about the exciting adventure you're going to take — this will create a mindset that will get you motivated and keep you motivated.

■ Set some goals — short-term, medium-term, long-term and lifetime goals — so you know exactly what you're working for. To be better than you are, you must be willing and prepared to change.

■ Establish your very own exercise regime — one that you can fit into your busy schedule and that you will enjoy and maintain for life.

■ Create your very own food plan that's easy to set up and to maintain, cleanses your body and that tastes good, too!

And, through goal-setting, we're going to show you how to gauge your progress so that you can enjoy your achievements: your new feeling of wellbeing, your new energies, your new self-confidence.

Get Up & Go! is divided into four main sections: Getting Started, Your Body, Food & Nutrition, and Training & Fitness, with a supplementary Training Manual and Appendix. Use it in the order that suits your needs — read it from cover to cover, or just delve into the bits that best relate to your needs right now. Remember that designing your life is a personal choice. You decide what you want. You take full responsibility for your actions. You reap the rewards.

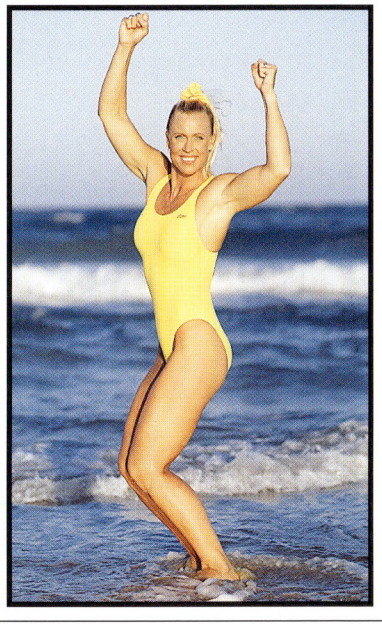

Don't be one of those people who wish they had the opportunity to do this or that — stop wishing and go out and do it! It's never too late to start. At any given moment you can change. It's your life, so make it a good one! Don't be afraid — in any new venture there is always a risk, but you have to step outside your comfort zone and go where you haven't been before. There is great personal satisfaction when you achieve what you didn't think you could.

Know what you want and know that you deserve the best. Know that when people try to put you down (and they will), and when times get tough (as they do), you can count on yourself to do the job you set out to do. I hope that, through this book, you'll come to understand the importance of self-management and self-responsibility. You, and only you, are responsible for making your life happen.

Don't just exist. Live your life. Have fun and do all the things you want to do. Are you ready for the challenge?

Enjoy!

Lisa

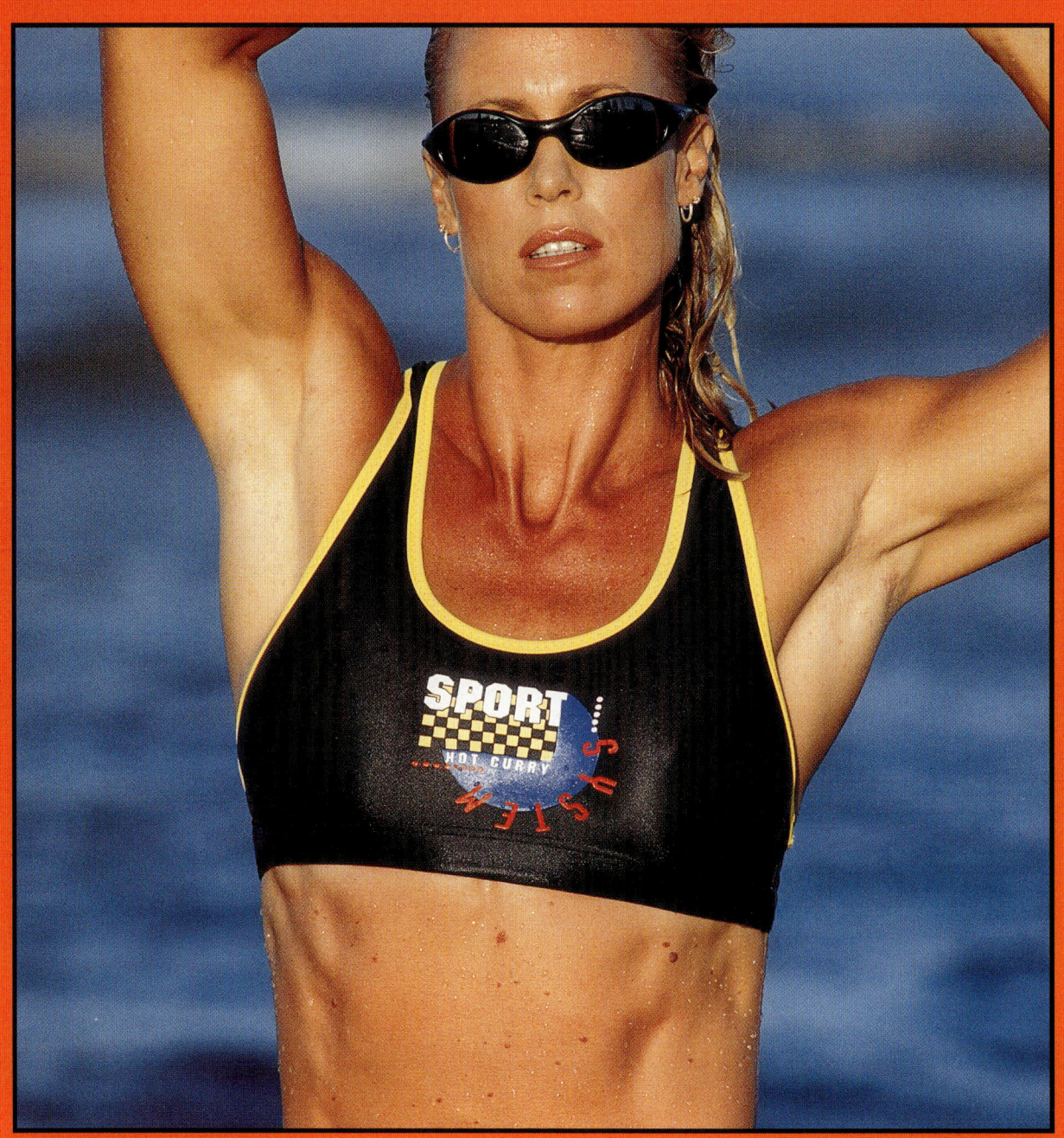

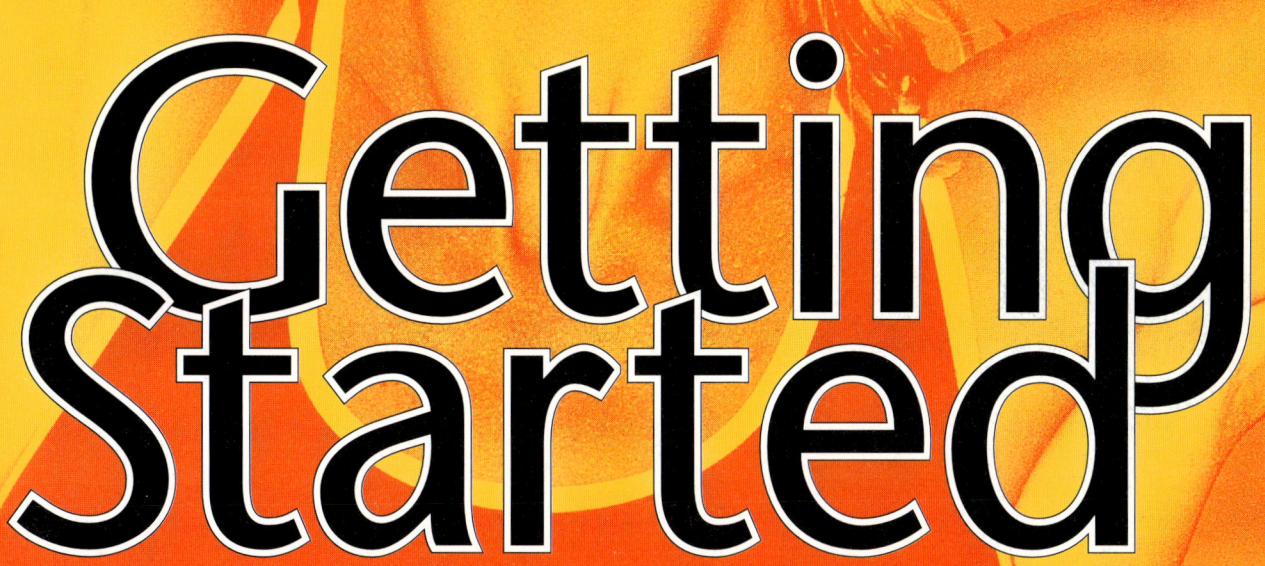

Getting Started

'Taking the first step to making it happen, is an affirmation of your willingness to have it all.'

Success: What Does it Mean?

Establishing the motivation to change your life is vital, but sustaining that motivation is just as important. You need to think about what success means to you and what you are aiming for in life. Committing yourself to change is a big step. This chapter sets out what you can expect — both the good and the bad.

[Commit Yourself to Change]

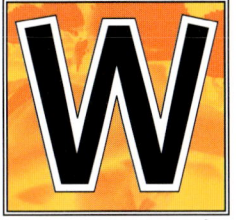

What does it take to be the best? What does it take to be *your* best? Why do some people make it, while others don't quite get there? What do champions do differently that separates them from the rest?

Most people aiming to achieve their goals have a plan, but actually applying all the necessary ingredients — day in, day out; week after week; month after month; year after year — is what makes the difference. What is required is an absolute and consistent commitment to your goals. It's the extra five per cent you give every day. It's going out and working as smart as you can even when you don't feel like it. It's sticking to your guns when people say you can't, won't or shouldn't. It's hanging in there when the going gets tough. It's getting up each time you fall down. It's realising that in every failure or loss, there's an opportunity to learn.

Deciding to change the way you live will have great benefits for your health and longevity. But permanent changes don't happen overnight. A lot of people are motivated to eat well and exercise for a particular event. How many brides do you know who have gone on crash diets the month before their wedding? How many people do you know who start rigid running programs only a short period of time before a fun run? Optimal health, ideal fitness and effective habits happen over time and with a long-term commitment.

Success: What Does it Mean?

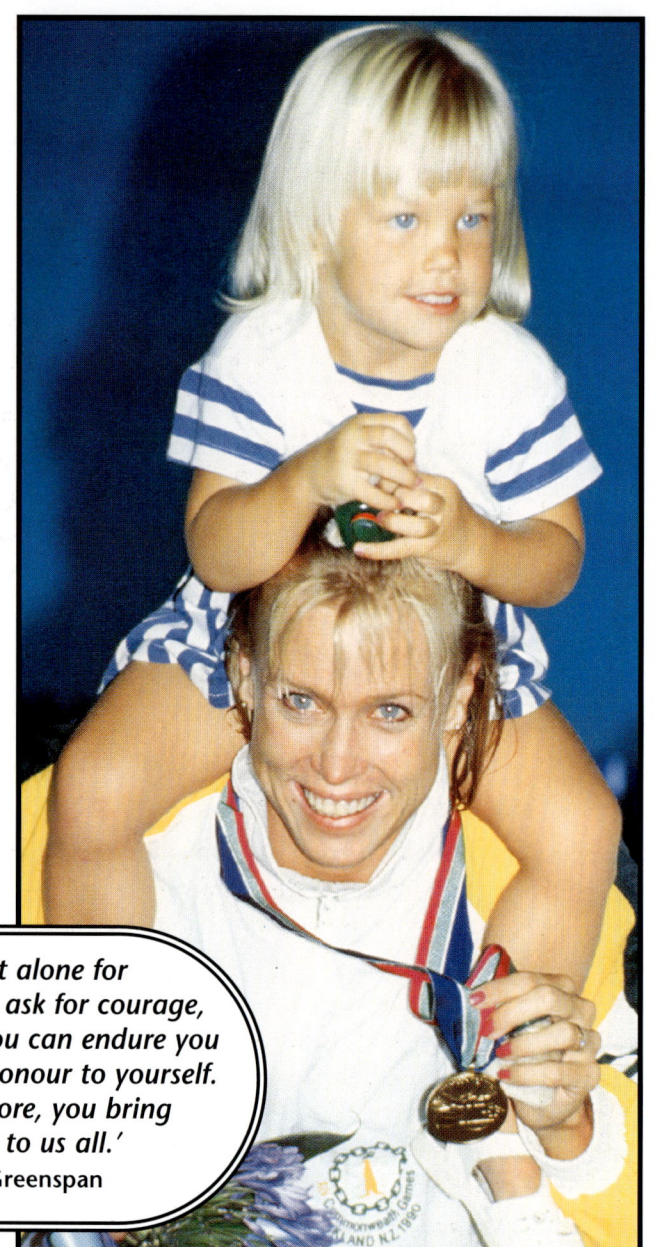

'Ask not alone for victory, ask for courage, for if you can endure you bring honour to yourself. Even more, you bring honour to us all.'
— Bud Greenspan

After winning four gold medals at the 1990 Auckland Commonwealth Games. Many people thought a 27-year-old mother shouldn't, couldn't or wouldn't achieve what I did. I said, 'Mothers can achieve anything they want'.

Give Yourself Some Inspiration

The sun doesn't shine everyday, some days are good, some days aren't so good. But as they say — everyday above the ground is a good one! When you hear or see something that gives you goose bumps, it has special significance to you. There is a direct link between your emotions and your body.

Learning from people who have 'made it' can help you to formulate your own ideas on how *you* can 'make it' too. Take a little bit from here, a little bit from there, a lot from one person, not much from another, heaps from your own experience — and you're well and truly on your way to knowing what you need to 'have it all'. Talk to these people, soak up all the information you can. Read their stories. Apply what you learn to yourself and your situation.

Successful people *know* what they want, and they know *how* to get it. Associate with people who possess the qualities that you admire. The more time you spend with them, the more you start to become like them. Watch events that inspire you. Try something new. Be adventurous. Take control.

Have the Courage to Succeed

I sometimes wonder why people bother putting their every effort into something when they're not having fun along the way. They usually end up being disappointed. If you're not enjoying what you do, then find something you do enjoy. Have the courage to stand out and be different. It may mean doing what you do differently, or changing what you do altogether. It takes courage to do this, as there could be risks, and it's scary being outside 'the comfort zone'. Many times I've put myself in situations where I was under intense pressure, anxious and scared. But sometimes you just have to try it. Remember that every record, every great feat, was once thought impossible.

My training for the 1990 Commonwealth Games in Auckland at age 27 with one child, and the 1992 Olympic Games in Barcelona at age 30 with two children, was very different, much less, and smarter, because with family and business responsibilities, I didn't have the time I used to have when I was younger and single.

My coach Joe King and I planned a program that we knew would work, but also fitted into my lifestyle. It wasn't conventional, but it suited me. I had chosen a different course that I was prepared to take responsibility for. Everything I did was planned right down to the finest detail. Anyone can achieve what they want — just *know* what you want, be *organised* and work *smarter* than your competition. As it turned out, those competitions were two of the greatest times of my life. I made it happen.

Think Positively — It Works!

Our minds are awesome machines which continue to defy a complete understanding and analysis. We all at one time tap into hidden abilities that are inexplicable and, for most of us, unrepeatable — at least, we can't keep summoning these abilities at will.

If we can believe that our minds are capable of just about anything, and we then put our minds to it, it follows that we are similarly capable of doing — of achieving — just about anything.

What we have to do is educate ourselves to have a realistic understanding of the importance of health and fitness in everyday life. An understanding that you must take control of your life today — don't procrastinate or put it off until times are less stressful. It's important to develop this knowledge sooner rather than later when it will have most influence on your life. Don't allow yourself to wallow in the comfort zone.

No matter how bad your life might be right now — how complicated, busy, frustrating or whatever — you have to seize this opportunity to change your life for the better, because it could save you from disaster. Some people have to become seriously injured or sick to realise that they have to make changes to their lives. When a loved one dies, it makes you realise how important it is to make the most of your life. Don't wait until it's too late — do what you can while you can.

> 'You will always be rich if your desires are simple.'
> — E. James Rohn

Dare to be Extraordinary

Ordinary people can do extraordinary things. You see it every day. *You* can do extraordinary things, too. You can achieve any dream or goal you set for yourself so long as you:

- know what you want
- believe in yourself and your dreams
- become organised, plan, work smart and take responsibility

Make the decision to take action right now. Say it out loud: 'I will change my life.' Write it down in capital letters and stick it on your bathroom mirror. Read it and remind yourself of your commitment every day.

Tell yourself you deserve to achieve your goals. Tell yourself you are good. Look yourself straight in the

Success: What Does it Mean?

eye and *tell* yourself you are going to succeed. Say these things to yourself constantly:

'I know I can do this.'

'I will do this.'

'There are plenty of people who have changed their lives. I'm going to be one of them.'

'I'm going to make a difference to this world and to myself.'

'I'm going to be the best I can be!'

The Importance of Success

Success is important, perhaps the most important thing in life. But exactly what does this word 'success' mean? What is more important: to be successful or to feel successful?

To some people the measure of success is money and material possessions. To others it means achievement in sport, art or other endeavours where the monetary rewards are secondary. Success can mean achieving happiness and balance in life — a loving, functional family, a settled mind, good friends. Some of the happiest people I know are not wealthy, but they give love and they receive love. If that's not being successful in life, then I don't know what is!

When your family and friends are cheering for you when you are coming last in a race, that's success. When you finish last and you still have a smile on your face, that's success.

Ask a few of your friends, workmates or children what success means to them — I bet you'll get a different answer from everyone. Success to me means being the best I can be, at whatever I attempt, taking advantage of opportunities as they present themselves, and being happy along the way.

Success is doing what you want, when you want, with the people you love. If it means that you have to work a 60-hour or 80-hour week to do that, then so be it. But be happy doing this, and don't complain. Remember, it's *your* choice. You must be responsible for your own decisions. You can't go around blaming everyone and everything else for your life.

Write this down on a piece of paper: For me to feel successful I must . . .

Whatever success means to you — and it could be a combination of the things I've already mentioned, or something else altogether — you'll be much closer to achieving your success goals if you have a fit and healthy mind and body.

These are My Strategies For Success —

1. Be healthy and have lots of energy — be aware of what you are putting into your mouth.

2. Exercise at least once a day, for at least an hour.

3. Get out in the fresh air and sunshine often, and appreciate what is around you.

4. Have a list of goals, prioritise them, and stick them in a prominent place. Look at them daily, add to them, or delete from them as you achieve and improve. Make a commitment and plan your attack. Write it down. Make sure it's realistic.

5. Know how to relax and take time out. Learn how to say 'no'. Control your own stress and pressure.

This book will help you to become fit and healthy in both mind and body. Committing yourself to the ideals and practices that you'll learn here and following them through will be a major success in itself. You'll have achieved something extremely worthwhile. If you can do it once, you can be successful over and over again. You can be what you want to be, you can get the things you want out of life, whatever they might be.

Know What to Expect

Any kind of success requires hard work and dedication. Good health and fitness won't come instantaneously and you will, more than likely, feel worse before you feel better. It's important for you to be aware of what's going to happen to your mind and your body as we progress.

You might feel worse before you feel better.

When you start to eat better, and do a little exercise, you might feel lousy for a few days. Your body will be getting rid of all those toxins that you've pumped into it over the years — you might even get headaches, feel nauseous, get a sore throat or a runny nose. Don't panic. This is your body reacting to change. It is getting rid of what it doesn't need or want. Ride it out.

How long you feel lousy will depend on how long you've been abusing your body, and just how 'clogged up' you've let it become. I find that the first week of any new health and fitness regime is the hardest — I once started my first week three times — then it will just click, and you'll find yourself thinking: 'It's not so hard, this is okay.'

After about 10 days of eating well, things will start to improve markedly. You'll feel lighter, you'll have more energy, and you'll want to keep eating those healthier foods that you thought were making you sick in the first place. Remember, though, that everyone is different, everyone has different levels of toxins in their body, everyone started the new regime from a different diet base and with a different fitness level. So, it might take *you* a few more days until you've turned the corner, or it might take less time, or you mightn't feel sick at all. Whatever happens, don't despair. Keep going until the benefits start to kick in.

Your muscles will ache and you'll be sore and tired.

What can I tell you? You're going to be working your way to a new body, and the old body isn't going to like it very much. But, you're going to plan your

6. **Purchase the appropriate equipment to help you reach your goals.**

7. **Explain your goals to your closest friends and family — they are now your support group. There will be people who will say things can't be done. It doesn't matter what others think — do what you know you can.**

8. **Educate yourself. There is knowledge all around. If you don't know about something, go and find out. Read the books, talk to people you admire, watch events that stimulate and motivate you. Learn all you can. Listen to the experts. Then, from all you know, draw your own conclusions.**

9. **Go out and apply what you know. Don't talk about it, just do it!**

10. **Enjoy what you do. This is the most important element. When you are happy, it's easy to achieve.**

training program so that you progress slowly and carefully, with a minimum amount of discomfort and a maximum amount of pride and pleasure in your achievements. And there is a kind of pleasure in nursing an ache from a 'worked' muscle in contrast to an 'overworked' muscle.

You won't get fit and healthy overnight.

We're talking about a *lifetime* commitment. I'm not asking you to drop everything and change your life dramatically, to get super-fit in six weeks and stress yourself in the process. The changes you make will be progressive and manageable. While you won't get fit and healthy overnight, changes will start happening quickly enough for you to see small improvements in your mind, body and general feeling of wellbeing so that you'll be encouraged to go on. Things will only get better and better.

You'll have to change a few things.

Bad habits such as smoking and drinking will slow your progress down. If you can't give up cigarettes, try to cut down on them a bit as part of the 'new you'. Any reduction of the habit can only be a good thing, and eventually you might even manage to give them up altogether. As for drinking, well, I like a drink as much as the next person, but everything in moderation, as they say. Drink sensibly, cut back as much as you can, and never binge drink. Use your common sense.

You're going to be anxious.

When you first start exercising, you're going to experience some anxiety — an increased heart rate, a fluttering of the stomach muscles, you might even break out in a sweat.

I remember when I first went snow skiing. I stood at the top of the mountain with a few lessons in my head, my heart in my mouth and wondered how on earth I was ever going to get all the way down. Finally, in a mild panic, I got up the courage to push myself off and down I went, slipping and sliding and skiing all the way to the bottom. I looked back up to where I had come from and wondered what I'd been worrying about. I couldn't wait to get back on that ski lift and have another go. And, of course, it was much easier the next time.

The more you practise something the easier and more enjoyable it becomes. If it doesn't happen right the first time, keep trying until you make it. Having a go is what takes intestinal fortitude, whether or not you make it all the way up or down!

■ ■ ■

If you experience any of the above changes, be patient and hang in there. Focus on what you are trying to achieve. In time, your hard work and dedication will be rewarded. When I make a decision to work on a new goal, I have a relentless commitment to follow through until the job is done. How many people stop halfway because it's too hard? Being better at something is not always easy. It's hard work, but when you enjoy what you do, that's what makes hard work seem easy.

In the next chapter you will be setting your goals for success. You really have to want something very badly if you're to have the strength to get through the tough days. And remember, you have to have those tough days — they help you to appreciate the good days even more!

The next time you see someone out jogging, know that they started off just like you. At some time in their life they decided that the benefits of a healthy and active lifestyle were worthwhile. If you've never felt fit and healthy, you don't know what you're missing. It is *so* good to have energy to expend on whatever you want.

Setting Goals You Can Achieve

You are committed to becoming fitter, healthier and having more energy. Now you must plan your path so that the changes you want to make are achievable and manageable. This chapter will determine why you need to establish goals for the immediate future, as well as long-term ambitions. Your goals will give you something to work towards and help you to gauge your success. The feeling you get when you accomplish your goals will give you the strength and motivation to strive to achieve even more in life.

The Importance of Goals

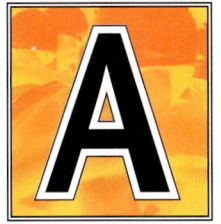

A life without goals is a life going nowhere: a life without direction, a life lived in confusion. This is how most people live — going around in circles, confused, unfocused and lost. You simply can't achieve more in life if you don't know what you want.

In order to achieve anything in life, you first have to be able to visualise what you want. Having a goal that you can see in your mind makes it so much easier to get out of bed when it's cold, dark and raining! Your health and fitness goals should inspire you so much that you will do 'whatever it takes' to achieve them. Doing whatever it takes means sacrifices, hard work, tired muscles and smart planning. It also means you will have to learn from all the mistakes you make. Often it is the learning experience that gives you more insight into what life, success and self-satisfaction is all about.

Setting Goals You Can Achieve

Guidelines for Goal-setting

For the purposes of this book, your main goal is to be fitter, healthier and happier with your life and yourself. But stating it like this is not setting a goal — it's simply making a wish!

For your goals to be meaningful, they must be:

Measurable. Measurable goals give you feedback and reinforce what you have achieved. Feeling good can't be measured, but body fat, heart rate, weight, cholesterol level etc, can. If you can't measure your goals, how will you know if you have improved? You need to be able to track your progression so that you can reassess what you are trying to achieve if things aren't quite going to plan, or if you are ahead of schedule and want to make your goals more ambitious.

Written. You need to write down your goals for reference and reinforcement. It will also make you think more seriously about what you hope to achieve. Having written goals also lets others see what you are working towards — when others are aware of what you are trying to achieve, you tend to commit yourself to them even more. Reading over your objectives on a daily basis will also remind you what you have set out to do.

Specific. Your goals must be specific to those areas you want to improve in. If you set obscure short-term goals, then be prepared to fall short of achieving your long-term goals. For example, if your long-term goal is to reduce body fat, then make sure your short-term goals allow for some kind of progressive fat loss.

Structured. Prioritise your goals. Set your long-term goals first and then use medium- and short-term goals to build the bridge to your long-term aspirations. Find out what you need to be able to do in order for you to achieve your longer-term goals, then set up ways to achieve your short-term goals before you aim for the big one. This may not give you an immediate reward, but it will make your long-term goals far more attainable. For example, if you really want to swim 1.5 kilometres for a team event in a triathlon, it may be more important to get physically stronger and take some lessons in stroke correction before you start training to cover the distance. These short-term goals may not enable you to swim 1.5 kilometres straightaway, but eventually they will allow you to swim the distance faster and more efficiently.

Realistic and achievable. Having goals that are unrealistic requires more time to achieve them and makes the possibility of dropping out far more likely. Small, achievable goals will eventually lead you to bigger and better things.

Most people drop out of sport or fitness programs, or a healthy way of life, because they really didn't want to do it in the first place. But what if your life depended on it? When we have a good enough reason, it's easier to stick to a plan, no matter how difficult it is. If someone offered you a lot of money to stick with a plan for three or six months, would you do it? Of course you would, because money is a great motivator!

I can't stress too strongly the need for you to work out what your personal goals are and your motivation for having these goals. Write down your goals and work towards achieving them — day by day, week by week, month by month, year by year. In order to achieve your goals, you will have to ask yourself: What are the real reasons I want to achieve these goals? Are they really what I want, or are they what I think I should do?

Understanding Goal-setting

If you truly believe you can achieve your goals in the time frame you set, then you will. The most difficult aspect of goal-setting is being realistic. If you set goals you are capable of achieving, then you will always have success. By building on this success you will make progress every time you train, every time you eat a nutritious meal, and every time you take some time off and spend it with your family. This builds confidence and self-esteem, two very important aspects of personal happiness.

We can gain a better understanding of goals if they are broken down into three main categories: long term, medium term and short term. In a nutshell:
- Long-term goals are what you are aiming to achieve over the next one to five years.
- Medium-term goals are those that will take between three months and a year to achieve. They are 'bits' of your long-term goals.
- Short-term goals are those goals you hope to achieve in the next one to three months. Again, they are smaller bits of the medium-term goals. Breaking your goals into smaller bits makes them more achievable, and each small goal achieved goes towards fulfilling your long-term goals.

You may have a general long-term goal along the lines of: To be healthier, fitter and happier. That's great, but you also need to be specific. For example, I'll know if I'm fitter in two years if I can:
- comfortably run 5 kilometres every morning;
- swim 25 laps every day;
- walk my golf buggy around 18 holes without fatigue;
- work a productive eight-hour day; or
- you name it!

Let's assume your long-term goal is to be able to run 5 kilometres comfortably every morning in two years' time. You're starting from scratch: you're unfit, you don't eat properly, you have trouble finding the time for exercise, and who knows what else stands in your way.

After establishing this long-term goal, you will need to break it down. The next step is to map out your short-term goals that will enable you to achieve your long-term goal. You could break the first month down as follows:

Week 1

- Have a physical check-up to see what restrictions there might be on changing your diet or performing your chosen training program.
- Plan a new eating program that takes in breakfast, lunch, dinner and nutritious snacks for the next month.

Setting Goals You Can Achieve

■ Purchase the food you'll need to get your eating plan started.

■ Make sure you've got the right gear for your chosen exercise — goggles to protect your eyes from chlorine if you'll be spending time in the pool, an exercise bike, weights, etc. In this case, you will need comfortable, supportive running or walking shoes, a comfortable pair of shorts and a top, or a tracksuit.

■ Tell your friends and family what you'll be doing from now on — to solicit their support or encouragement, or just to warn them that things will be different in your life. Are they with you?

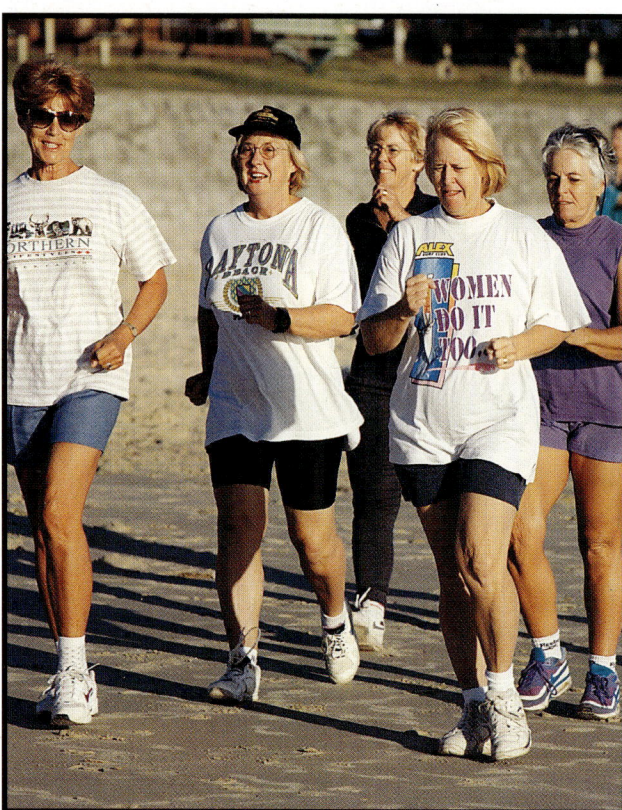

Joining a group or enlisting friends to join you in your fitness program will help you remain motivated and committed to your goals.

■ Enlist the help of a friend. Doing it together keeps motivation high.

■ Work out how you're going to find the time, if necessary, to:

— prepare your meals; and

— exercise for around 40 minutes a day three to five times a week for the first three months.

This might mean getting up an hour earlier in the morning, or doing some food preparation at night and refrigerating it a day or two in advance, or getting someone to look after the kids while you exercise — or all three! You will have to make changes, but it won't take long before you stop regarding these new activities as difficult or inconvenient. With the right mental attitude they'll soon become part of your life.

Weeks 2 to 4

Let's say that, by the end of the month, you want to be running 1 kilometre a day. In week 2, when you really start into it, your goal might simply be to warm-up for five minutes with a few stretches and then run around the block twice. In week 3 you might try running a little further, until, by the end of the month, you're running your 1 kilometre without overexerting yourself. But remember, you need to set yourself distance and time goals for every achievement: 'Week 3, I'll run around the block three times in 15 minutes.'

After the first month or two you will need to look at your medium-term goals. At this point, you'll probably need to adjust your eating program. If you want to achieve your two-year plan of being able to run, comfortably, 5 kilometres a day, simple mathematics tells us you'll have to be running 2.5 kilometres comfortably by the end of year 1. But after achieving your short-term goals you'll probably find you're getting so fit, and feeling so good, that you

Setting Goals You Can Achieve

can go back to your original long-term plan and double it to 10 kilometres and move everything else up a notch or two. You might want to add some weight training, or swimming, or aerobics to your exercise regime. Or, now that you're feeling fitter and healthier, perhaps you can take up a leisure activity and/or sport that you've been thinking about for a while, such as tennis, golf or horse riding. As you start to become fitter and more confident about your ability to achieve, revisit your goals and adjust them. One success leads to other, bigger successes.

Goal-setting Activities

Let's get started on your goal-setting by doing a needs analysis to find out how you want to improve your body and what you need to start putting in place to achieve your aims.

Activity 1

Strip down completely, look at yourself in the mirror and write down *what you see*. Be specific, but also be objective. Write down every detail that you notice about your shape, your posture, your body fat and your muscular build. Make some notes about the state of your hair, your skin, your eyes and your complexion. This will give you a very clear picture of the way you are now and help you to establish what you have to work on to get to the way you want to be.

Activity 2

Now, write down *what you would like to see*. How would you like to look if you could improve those things you see in the mirror? Include comments on all those areas mentioned in activity 1.

Keep a Diary

Throughout the book, there will be numerous activities for you to do. You might like to think about keeping a diary. A diary is a great place to write down all your goals and record how you are going with your health and fitness goals. It's also great for inspiration. When you have days where you don't feel like you are achieving anything, or you haven't achieved a goal you previously set, or you just feel like giving up, referring to your diary will remind you of what you are trying to achieve and why. If you have already achieved some goals, reading what you wrote when you experienced success can help you to renew your commitment and remain motivated.

When you do so, be realistic about your shape. Write down only those things you can be positive about; don't reflect on things such as your lack of height, your general shape or the fact that you have knocked knees. These things are out of your control so there is no point in worrying about them.

Activity 3

Once you have a list of physical points that you want to improve, add to this the ways you would like to change your lifestyle. This will include points about your general fitness, eating patterns, recreation, leisure time, social activities, family time, and so on — how you want your life to be and how you want to feel within yourself.

Setting Goals You Can Achieve

Having Your Cake . . .

During one particular stage of my training in 1996, I was finding it difficult to reach the target body-fat levels that I had set with my trainer, Mark. We both felt my goal was achievable, but for some reason I was having trouble getting there. At the time, I had a fetish for Mexican food (I still do) and would rush off to my favourite Mexican restaurant every chance I could get. So, what Mark and I did was set goals that included the number of times I could have Mexican food and what I could eat when I went out. We both knew the cook and together we planned my menus. After six weeks of this, I achieved my target. And I still got to eat my Mexican food — beans, rice and vegetables with enchilada sauce is a special low-fat favourite. The secret here is not to stop doing something you enjoy, but controlling how you do it. Sure, in this case I was lucky enough to know the chef, but you can work out your own menu. Eat at your favourite restaurants — you've got to enjoy life — but just be aware of what you are putting into your mouth.

When setting your goals, try to make them not only realistic, but also enjoyable.

'You build a successful life a day at a time.'
— Lou Holtz

Setting Your Own Goals

After completing your needs analysis, you should have a list of points from which you can start setting your goals. This list is the crucial starting point for making long-term, positive changes to your life.

Spend some time writing down your long-term, medium-term and short-term goals for each of the following areas of your life. Adapt the goal sheet on page 15 to your own needs and address the areas of your life that you want to change.

Don't try to change everything at the same time. Pick one thing and work on it until it is comfortable and a habit, then slowly introduce others.

Reward Yourself

One of the best things about having goals is the feeling you get when you achieve them. When you reach a goal, reward yourself.

Everyone sees rewards differently depending on their attitudes, values and beliefs. There are a number of strategies that will encourage you to be motivated and stick to your health and fitness plan.

Rewards can come in three ways:

1. Feedback on results. Keeping track of your fitness level, girth measurements, body-fat level, heart rate etc, will provide you with the incentive to improve these areas. Measuring these results will let you know how successful you've been.

2. Social reinforcement. This is how your self-esteem is built. When other people tell you how well you have done or how good you look, it makes you feel that you have actually achieved something. Accept the compliment and say thank you.

Setting Goals You Can Achieve

My Goals

When setting your goals you may like to consider these areas:
Health ■ Family ■ Fitness ■ Career ■ Financial ■ Leisure ■ Travel ■ Self

Short term (1–3 months)

_____   _____   _____
_____   _____   _____
_____   _____   _____
_____   _____   _____
_____   _____   _____
_____   _____   _____

Medium term (3–12 months)

_____   _____   _____
_____   _____   _____
_____   _____   _____
_____   _____   _____
_____   _____   _____
_____   _____   _____

Long term (1–5 years)

_____   _____   _____
_____   _____   _____
_____   _____   _____
_____   _____   _____
_____   _____   _____
_____   _____   _____

Getting Started

Setting Goals You Can Achieve

3. Material gain. This may be in the form of promising yourself a new set of golf clubs, a facial or a dinner out, when you reach a set level of body fat or fitness. Evaluate your goals often, and compare your progress to what you hoped to achieve. Reward yourself when you have achieved each level of each goal. Material rewards are the easiest, but positive reinforcement from your family and friends will mean much more. Rewarding yourself for achieving a goal is one way of getting good results. However, be careful not to promise yourself a reward that is worth more than the effort it will take to achieve your goal. Don't promise yourself a car if you can lose a certain amount of weight; the new car could be more important to you than losing the weight. After you've lost the weight and bought the car, your health and fitness would probably decline drastically!

> 'When you sit, sit. When you stand, stand. Whatever you do, don't wobble. Once you make your choice, do it with all your spirit.'
> — Dan Millman

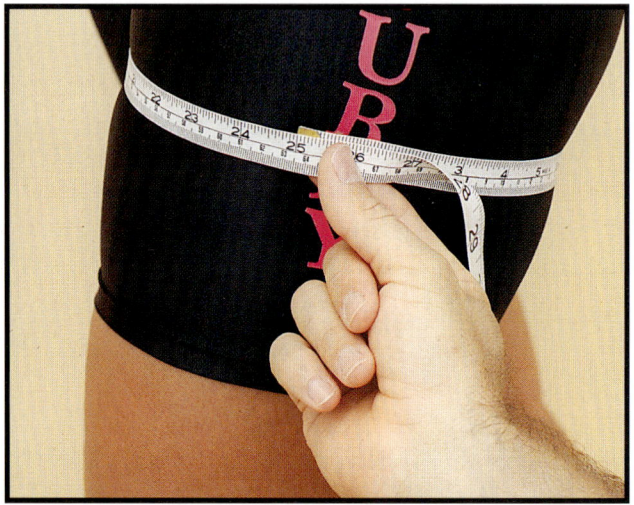

Measuring results will show you how much you have achieved and how far you have to go.

Why Many People Who Set Goals Still Don't Achieve Success

I see so many people who go to the gym every day and work out really hard and yet, at the end of the month, they still look the same and they wonder why nothing has changed.

Every time you walk into the gym or go for a walk or a run, you should have a goal in mind for that session. Every training session I do has a set goal. It might be to squat 80 kilograms, do 12 chin-ups, swim 3 kilometres, or keep my heart rate below 120 beats per minute in recovery. There's a plan for everything I do, and it has to be this way with you, too.

Remember this: *Failing to plan means planning to fail.* If each and every thing you do doesn't match up with your goals, then you simply won't get ahead. Know what you should be doing and where your health and fitness should be every month, every week and every day. To get results, don't just go out and aimlessly exercise. Go out and train according to your program.

■ ■ ■

Not everyone is successful at everything they do for the first time. Achieving your goals is great fun, but even more challenging is the constant persistence and dedication needed to get the job done. You should now know exactly what your goals are and feel committed to achieving them. As we move on through the book, you can keep coming back and adding to your goals, and to the tasks you need to complete to achieve them.

The next step is to ensure that you are able to manage your life properly so that you can make the time you need to achieve your goals.

Managing Your Life

Learning to manage your time effectively is the first step in managing your life. Every day, small annoyances crop up and rob you of precious and productive time — careful planning and organisation will help you to deal with these interruptions. This chapter will give you suggestions on how to find the extra time you need to achieve your health and fitness goals and to organise your life. You will also learn how to face stress head on: how to recognise it, cope with it and prevent it.

[The Importance of Planning]

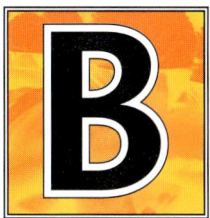

Being fit, alert and healthy makes it so much easier to cope with the stress of everyday living. Running a household, a business and your life requires absolute time management and the ability to prioritise. But, the good news is, it can be done! With careful planning and a commitment to become more organised, you will be able to make time to improve your health and fitness which, in turn, will enable you to manage everything else in your life a lot better.

Think about how carefully and precisely you would plan for your wedding, a deadline at work, a proposal for a new job, or a raise. Nothing gets swept under the mat in these instances, and if things did go wrong, you would desperately work out ways to fix them on time. If you applied the same strategies, enthusiasm, motivation, discipline, persistence and commitment to all the things you do, your life would be very different. Effective planning is the reason why *some* people achieve, while others don't get the same results.

People continually ask me: 'How do you fit it all in? How do you stay so motivated?' Well, the simple answer is that I know what my priorities are, and I have a plan — for my life and my family. To make the most of life, you really need to take time to:

Managing Your Life

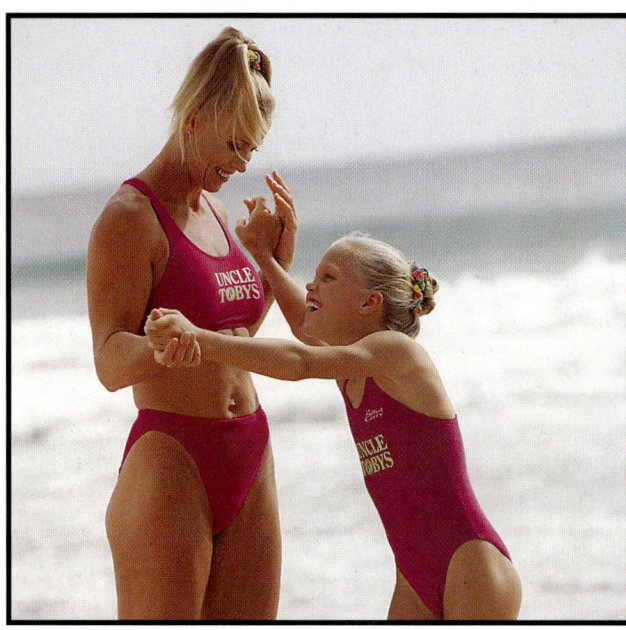

Make the effort to spend quality — and fun — time with your family.

love what you do. I've continued to compete at a high level for all these years because sport is so satisfying and challenging to me. Yes, my life is busy — often hectic — but that's my choice. I might whinge about it every now and then, but if I wasn't enjoying myself, there's no way that I would continue to do everything I do. I could slow down, but when you're on a roll one opportunity seems to lead to another.

I once sat down and wrote a list of all the things I wanted to do in my life — some of them were pretty unrealistic, I admit, but not completely out of reach — and I was amazed at how many things I really wanted to do. I had a list of 53 goals!

People can give you all the excuses in the world as to why they can't find the time to keep themselves fit and healthy; they need to find a reason to motivate themselves.

Well, there really is a good reason. Being fit and healthy will help you to live a fun and energy-filled life.

Anyone can find the time, but you have to *want* to.

- look after your health through proper nutrition, exercise, relaxation and fresh air;
- spend quality and fun time with your family and friends;
- be on your own and enjoy some peace and quiet; and
- budget the household income to reduce financial stress.

Essentially, I prioritise my time so that I can fit everything in. I do what's necessary and important, and I make time to look after myself. I know that if I'm happy and well, everyone else in my life benefits from what I have to give.

Another question I'm frequently asked is: 'Why do you do all the things you do?' Again, the answer is simple: because life is for living and it's full of opportunities.

It's easy to be motivated and enthusiastic when you

'When you love what you do, you'll never have to work a day in your life.'
— Steve Ackerie

Procrastination — A Thief of Time

Procrastination is a bad but easy habit to fall into. You need to be able to recognise this habit and do something about it. How many people will step over the same thing half-a-dozen times before they pick it up? If that's you, then start getting into the habit of picking it up — because it needs to be done by *someone* — just do it! How many days does the dry-cleaning sit in the back seat of your car before you eventually drop it off? Just do it!

When you hear yourself saying 'I must do that one day', stop and do it immediately if it's at all possible. Get into the habit of writing daily and weekly 'to do' lists. Allocate all your running around to one day, or plan to do it on the way to an appointment, leaving enough time (by being organised) to do it.

Managing Your Life

When you have phone calls that you've been putting off, just grit your teeth and make them. Afterwards, you'll wonder why you didn't do it before and you'll feel great satisfaction and relief from being able to cross another thing off your list.

Can you walk from one end of the house to the other and do numerous things along the way? Do your eyes scan the hallways and bedrooms as you work out what needs to be done? If this simple 'skill' could be mastered by everyone in the house, imagine how much extra time you would all have. Help yourself, and everyone else in your household, by doing your share around the house. If, in the workplace, your promotion depended on you doing small things to impress your boss, I bet you wouldn't think twice! It's all a matter of priorities.

Time Management Charts: A Key to Organising Your Life

To keep organised, I fill in a time management chart — for the entire family — every week.

I get my husband to fill in his appointments and to add any that come up during the week. When your partner, or anyone else in your household, leads a busy life it's essential to know each others' commitments so that you can plan around them. I then fill in my commitments — school activities, the kids' sports activities, my training and work. I also ensure that I include leisure time, a night out for dinner or the movies, or both. I even schedule in time where I don't have to do anything specific, time where I can choose to lie around, read, sleep, shop, or go and have lunch and a good laugh!

TIMES	MON	TUE	WED	THURS	FRI	SAT	SUN
5.30 - 7.00	Grant trains	Lisa paddle		Lisa/Grant paddle		Lisa paddle	Grant trains
7.00 - 9.00	Kids school	→	GK to SYD →	→	→	Netball	Nippers
9.00 - 12.00	W O	Lisa Gym	W O	W O	Swimming lessons Lisa swim		
12.00 - 3.00	R K		R K	R K		Birthday Party	
3.00 - 6.00	Kids activities Swim while kids at swim club	→	→	Gymnastics Netball Run while kids practising	Ballet stretch while kids at ballet		
6.00 - 8.00		Movies Dinner	Mums Dinner	pick-up Grant airport 7.05pm	Grant paddle	Family Dinner	Family BBQ
8.00 - 10.00							

This simple chart makes my life organised!

Get **UP&GO!**

Managing Your Life

Everyone should make time for this every so often, and make sure you don't feel guilty or let anyone else make you feel guilty for it. When you are really busy, you appreciate these days.

Create your own time management chart and use it to plan your time effectively.

Personal Organisation and Self-discipline

You have to be self-disciplined to be organised. Being organised is an ingrained habit, and being *disorganised* is also an ingrained habit. You can have all the good intentions in the world, but if you're not organised your plans will fly straight out the window.

It seems as though there are *always* a million things you need to get done. But, by sorting out your priorities — making your daily, weekly and yearly plans, being assertive, and working out strategies to eliminate wasted time — you could save around two hours a day. When you consider that to increase your fitness level and control your weight requires a minimum of 40 minutes, 4-5 times a week, you can see how managing your time effectively could enable you to start making all those changes you've been putting off or making excuses about. Be prepared to take control of your life and to take responsibility for your own wellbeing.

Tips for Personal Organisation

■ Put things in their rightful place so you will always know where they are. Teach your children to put their things where they belong — when they can't find their school shoes in the last-minute rush to get out the door, they'll know where to look.

■ Make a list of the things you need to accomplish within a certain time frame. Get your partner to make a list also. Together, make a list for your children. When they are older, get them to make their own lists.

■ Keep up to date with the washing and ironing. If you beat procrastination and do it as it needs to be done, you will keep on top of it. I have a wonderful dryer that takes a big load of clothes and, when they're dry, hardly anything is crinkled. Isn't it better to take everything out and fold it straightaway, than leave it for a couple of days and have to iron everything?

■ Every Sunday, I ask my family what they want for dinner during the week. Then, I do one 'big shop'. This saves trying to guess what everyone wants and from having to stop at the supermarket every day — so it also saves you time.

■ Always get your clothes ready for the following day the night before.

■ If you're in the family car without the kids, fill up with petrol. It's much easier than having to unload the tribe and try to get them back in the car without them wanting chips and chocolates from the shop. (This one will save you time *and* money!)

■ When the alarm goes off, get up. How many times do you reset it for 'just another five minutes'? If you've made a commitment to get up — get up and get going!

When you decide to take control over your self-organisational skills, it won't be long before they become firmly embedded in your lifestyle. Do it for your own peace of mind. It's worth it.

Managing Your Life

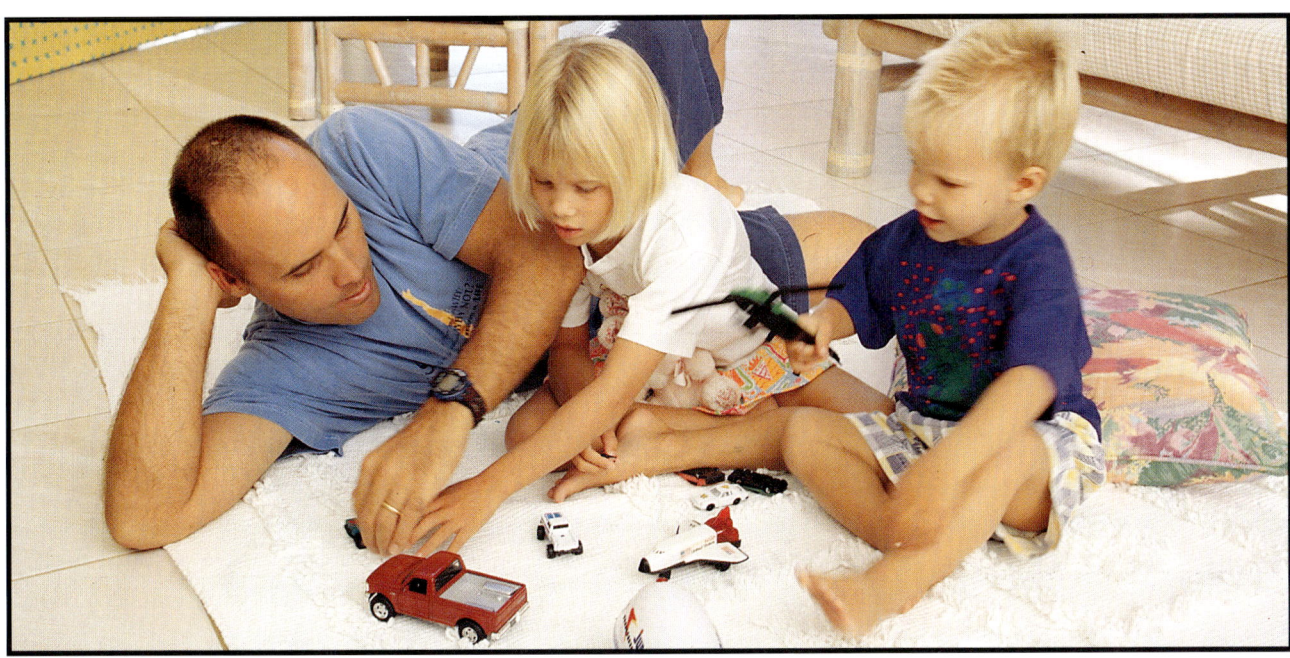

Spending time with your children should be a priority — enjoy the time you do spend with them.

Make Time for Your Children

When you have more than one child, it's sometimes hard to spend one-on-one time with them. Take one child to do the grocery shopping or banking, or let them run errands with you. Driving children to different activities gives you a chance to talk about their day. Kick a ball with them, have a dance, play their favourite sport, go fishing, play cards or hide and seek — anything that's fun for them and that you can do together.

Leaving somewhere early, or not attending an important meeting, because you have to go to your child's school swimming carnival isn't being irresponsible — it's just the opposite. Enjoy being with your children on their big days. It certainly means a lot to them, so don't ever feel guilty about it. If you know in advance what activities you need to go to, then you can plan them into your working days.

At the beginning of each year, I take my husband's diary and fill in all the school holidays, birthdays, competition dates and work commitments. I also fill in holiday breaks, which usually fall after a competition or a conference somewhere away from home. Every month, I fill in any new work or school commitments that I feel my husband should be a part of. Obviously, we don't do everything together, but there are some things that I think we *should* do together. School sports days, and drama and music nights are always occasions when kids love to see their mums and dads in the audience.

It only takes a little time to watch, but just being there can mean a lot to your children. Leave the mobile in the car, and try to be totally absorbed for the short time you're there. If you really can't be there, promise to make it up to them in some other way.

'No success can compensate for failure in the home.'
— David O. McRay

Get UP&GO!   21

Managing Your Life

Shiftworkers

If you are a shiftworker — that is, anyone who works outside the regular 9–5 routine — you need to take extra care of your nutritional, exercise, sleep and relaxation needs. Both your family and social life can suffer if you aren't really organised.

One of the biggest problems with shift work is that your sleep pattern is disturbed. By the time you get used to working at night and sleeping during the day, it's usually time to change back to working a day shift. Many accidents, both in the workplace and on the way home, are caused by fatigue. Your level of alertness and reaction time can be decreased to the point where usually simple tasks are fraught with danger. You will benefit greatly if you can teach yourself relaxation methods and learn how to take short naps when you can. You might like to schedule in relaxation time on your time management chart. A 20-minute relaxed nap can be equivalent to an hour's sleep. When you get up, have a five-minute full body stretch to get your circulation going and wake up properly. If you're having sleeping problems, try a herbal relaxant. Also, try to eat a protein and carbohydrate snack, such as a cheese or grilled chicken sandwich, about 20 minutes before you leave work. This will help to increase your energy and level of alertness.

Be organised: plan your meals ahead and take them to work with you. Don't rely on anyone else to provide your meals, make your own decisions to manage yourself well. Vending machines look enticing and are convenient, but try not to be tempted. Pack small, easy-to-eat snacks such as low-fat yoghurt, dried or fresh fruit, muffins, scones and jam, a cheese sandwich, grilled chicken, tinned spaghetti, and fruit juices. Remember to drink plenty of water and fluids throughout your shift. Dehydration is common in shiftworkers and can affect your bowel habits.

On your breaks (and this also applies to those who work under fluorescent lights all day), make sure you get some fresh air if you can. Try doing some deep breathing exercises, eat your snack, and then have a walk and a stretch — you'll feel a lot better than if you sit in an airconditioned room eating biscuits and drinking coffee or soft drinks. Be aware that healthy food choices will make a significant difference to your energy levels, so it's worth taking the time to plan your meals.

If your job requires you to be on call at any time of the day or night — say, if you're a doctor, member of the emergency services, pilot or police officer — make sure you've always got a food box ready to pick up on your way out the door. Fill it with highly nutritious food to keep your energy and concentration levels up. It does take a bit of organisation, but you'll really appreciate the difference.

Continually changing rosters makes it difficult to commit to any form of consistent exercise and, in particular, team sports. Exercise when you feel freshest — only *you* will know when that is. If you are feeling particularly tired, rest. Sometimes you will really have to push yourself to do some sort of exercise, but you will feel better; your self-esteem and motivation will also improve. Regular exercise

Managing Your Life

will also help to prevent varicose veins, a sore back and bad posture.

Do the right thing by your family and yourself — formulate a plan that allows you to spend quality time with them while still leaving you enough time to exercise and take some time out for quiet relaxation.

Manage your time carefully to keep your body in tip-top condition. Being healthy and fit will help you to work effectively and with ease, and will give you the energy to enjoy your after-work time.

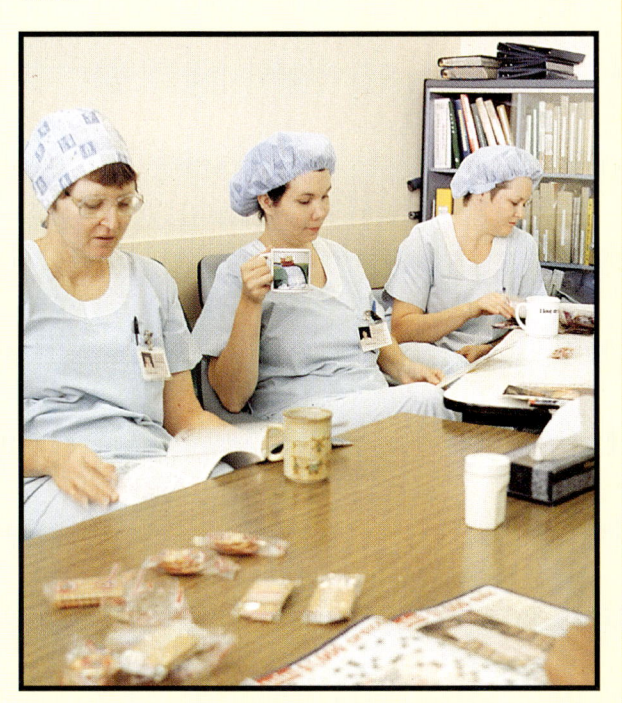

Shiftworkers need to make a conscious decision to manage their lives well. Don't spend your entire break inside, get some fresh air and exercise — you'll feel a lot better when you do.

Paperwork — Deal with it Now

There is always a pile of paperwork on my desk, on the kitchen bench, or shoved into drawers in the hope that it will disappear. Every now and then, I get to the stage where I just can't work efficiently because of the amount of paperwork I have accumulated.

Don't avoid it any longer. On your next free day, get a big paper bag or a bin and buy some folders, or some sort of filing system. Then, sit on the floor and take *everything* out of your drawers and off your desk. Each time you pick up a piece of paper, deal with it then and there. Put it into the appropriate pile. Get into the habit of deciding its priority of treatment:

- Should you deal with it immediately?
- Do you need to file it?
- Can you throw it into the recycling bin?

Only leave on your desk what you absolutely need. The rest can be filed away in drawers. Don't keep anything that you won't use; the more clutter you can get rid of in your life, the better.

How many people store things in cupboards because there is a cupboard? When did you use it last? Do you really need it? Do you really want it? Don't horde. Live by the motto: do it, defer it, delegate it or dump it.

If you have children, don't forget to take care of their paperwork, too. My husband and I got into a habit of filing each of our kids' paperwork in a different folder — notes and newsletters from school, ballet, gymnastics, swimming, Nippers, music; party invites; special drawings, that sort of thing — so everyone knows where the information is and where to put new information.

Get UP&GO!

Managing Your Life

Effective Communication

When talking to someone, keep your story clear, simple and concise. Don't waffle, repeat yourself over and over, or tell someone what you think they want to hear. Tell them what you want to tell them so there can be no misunderstandings. Most people only half listen, so if you want your message to get across, be enthusiastic about what you say and how you say it. It makes it easier to listen to.

Consider which form of communication will be most time efficient for both you and the person you are dealing with. Do you really need to have a meeting (which can involve travelling and waiting time) or could you communicate via the telephone, fax, e-mail or send an associate to a meeting?

Learn to say 'no' — this is one of the hardest things to do, but once you learn how to do it, your life will become less hectic. There are ways for you to communicate 'no' without offending people. Being assertive isn't rude, you are simply establishing priorities and taking care of them — that is, managing your life around your needs. To have more time for yourself and the people you love, sometimes you really do have to say: 'No. I realise what you need is important, but I can't do that for you right now.'

Using Travel Time to Your Advantage

Travelling is a great opportunity to utilise time. When I'm in the car with my children, we talk, sing and enjoy each other's company. If I'm by myself, I use the time to catch up on phone calls, listen to the news, listen to my favourite music or inspirational tape, or record notes onto my dictaphone.

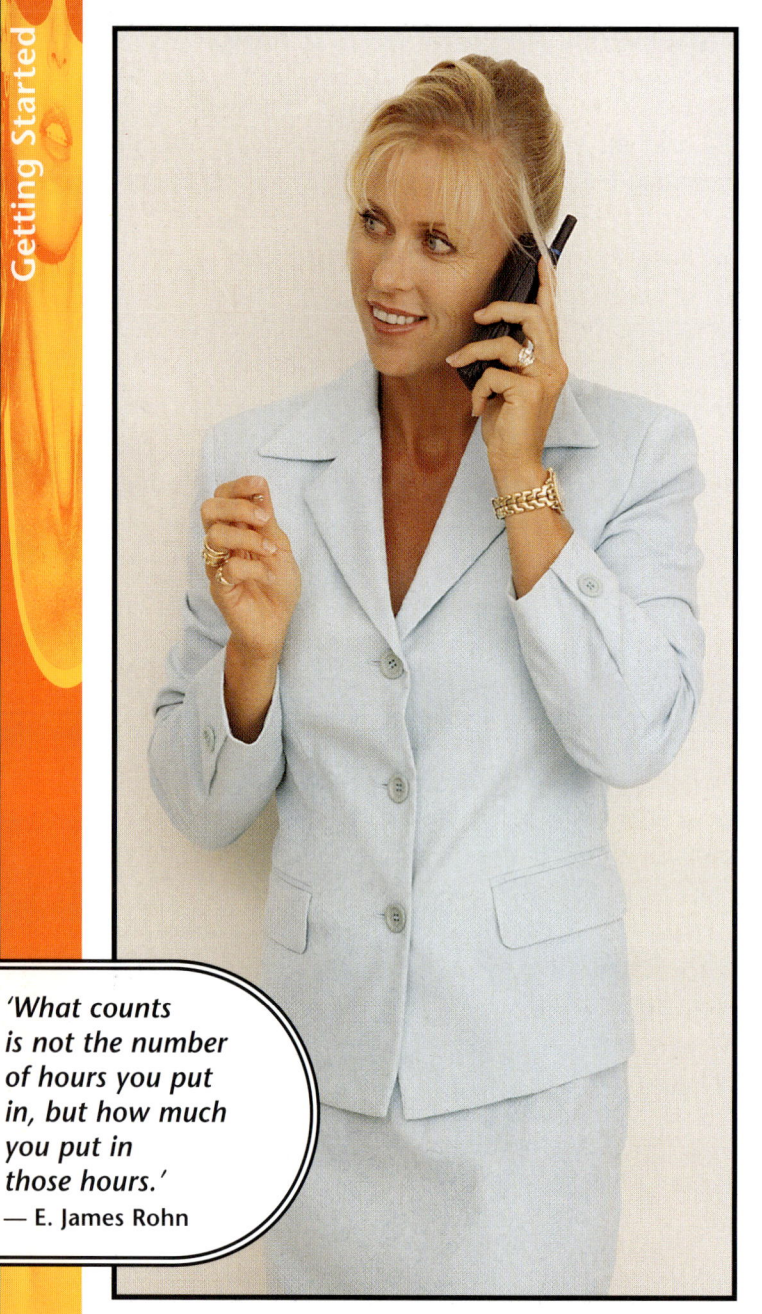

'What counts is not the number of hours you put in, but how much you put in those hours.'
— E. James Rohn

With my busy life, I have to be organised. My mobile phone is a handy way to keep in touch with the office while I'm at meetings or on the road.

Getting Started

Get **UP&GO!**

Managing Your Life

If I'm in a car and someone else is driving, then I catch up on phone calls, read, make notes about things I have to do, or use the time to relax.

Travelling by plane can be a great time to do what you want — read, work or relax. I can get a lot of work done on a flight, as there are no interruptions. If I'm not driving or working at the other end, I'll enjoy a glass of wine (but I make sure I drink plenty of water, too).

Utilise travel time in any way you can: write or dictate letters, plan your weekly/monthly/yearly goals, listen to tapes that interest you, or just relax and enjoy the ride.

I used to drive to and from the airport frequently and, like a lot of people, I would sit just over the speed limit — just enough to get me there one minute earlier, and just enough to make me stressed about whether I would cause an accident or get caught for speeding! One day I simply decided to relax and enjoy the experience of driving, and not worry about getting there one minute earlier. You can't believe how much anxiety it takes away. Try it, for your own peace of mind, for your own safety, and for the safety of others.

Most people are late because they are not organised. Don't blame your lateness on red lights, bad traffic or roadworks — be organised, start getting ready earlier, and take responsibility.

Stress — How to Cope

A key component in managing your life well is learning how to cope with stress. Many people are constantly 'stressed out'. Stress is an inevitable but controllable part of life. Too much stress can break you. Too little stress can make life dull and boring. If no stress is applied, nothing changes, so a certain amount of stress can be healthy. We need to have

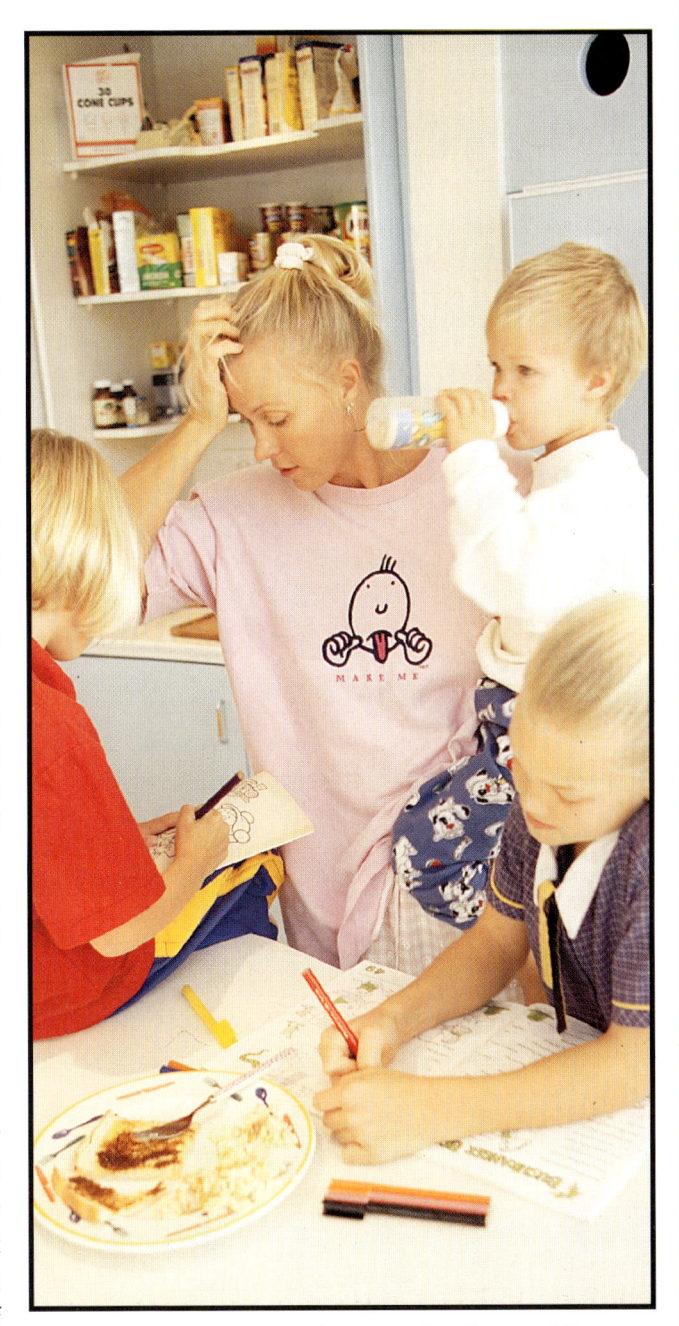

No-one is immune to stress and everyone handles it in different ways. Try to understand the causes and symptoms of the stress in your life and take responsibility for dealing with it.

Managing Your Life

pressure put onto us, otherwise we would consider average abilities to be acceptable, but how we handle these situations depends on our level of understanding of stress.

No one is immune to stress; however, what one person sees as stressful, another will see as challenging. It is up to you to understand the causes and symptoms of stress and be ready to deal with them in a way that is beneficial to you and the people around you. Stress not only affects you, it also affects your family and friends, your training and your work. Stressed-out people send out vibes that are negative and tiring.

Remember, there is no use even trying to start something new if you can't handle what you have on your plate already.

Ten Habits to Adopt for Beating Stress

1. **Be organised. Prioritise your time. What's important to you? Create a 'To do' list for each day.**
2. **Include moderate exercise in your daily routine. Try walking, swimming, cycling, hiking, or anything else that interests you.**
3. **Start a nutritious eating plan, with plenty of fresh fruit and vegetables, moderate amounts of lean meat, and lots of nutritious carbohydrates.**
4. **Drink plenty of water, at least six to eight glasses a day.**

What is Stress?

The three major types of stress are:

1. Necessary stress. This is the stress that gets us going, and is often used as natural motivation for us to get things done — even simple things such as making an appointment to get your hair cut or to get a medical check-up. Appointment times force us into organising ourselves so as to make the most of our time. Other examples of necessary stress include exercise, work deadlines and commitments, and relationships.

2. Unavoidable stress. These stresses include dealing with traffic, waiting in line to be served, work start times, and so on. They are an inevitable part of our everyday life, so we just have to learn how to deal with this type of stress better. If you're organised and allow time for the extra traffic that may be on the road, you can sit in your car happily listening to music and be glad that you allowed that extra five minutes to get to work on time. You can't avoid stress such as traffic, so organise yourself to make it as bearable as possible.

3. Avoidable stress. This is the kind of stress that we know causes us problems, but we just keep bumping our heads against the wall instead of controlling the situation more, and working out how to avoid it. It's often the most frustrating kind of stress. You know you should have done a job differently, or that every time you break for lunch at 12.30 the queue at your canteen or local sandwich shop is enormous, but you just keep doing it day in and day out because it's too much effort to change your routine. Why not get organised? For example, try bringing your own lunch and spend your break outside in the fresh air instead

Managing Your Life

5. Cut out or cut down on caffeine and alcohol.
6. Control your intake of cheese, cream, sour cream, butter, margarine and milk.
7. Cut out refined and processed foods, such as sugars, cakes, chips, soft drinks, etc.
8. Go to bed earlier for a couple of nights, but get up at the same time.
9. Reassess your goals: are they realistic?
10. Look after yourself! If *you* function properly, then the things around you will as well!

of waiting in line, or take your lunchbreak at a later time. You could use the time you save to get more work done so that you don't need to work back as late. Follow your time management chart, pay your bills on time, plan ahead! You should do everything possible to organise your life so that you can eliminated avoidable stress.

How Your Body Reacts to Stress

When your body is stressed it instantly switches to its 'fight or flight' response, which enables you to run from the impending danger or to defend yourself. These responses are built into your system, and will happen every time you become stressed.

The brain receives the stimulus of danger from your eyes and ears and responds by immediately releasing hormones into your body, while at the same time sending out signals to cause adrenaline, noradrenaline and cortisone to be released. You become mentally alert — all your senses are activated, and you well and truly know what's going on.

Instantly, your blood pressure increases, your breathing rate speeds up, and your heart beats very hard and very quickly, pumping blood away from your skin and internal organs and into the muscles you need in your fight or flight mode. Your muscle fibres become tense, ready for your legs to run or your arms to defend you.

Your liver releases fatty acids, sugar and cholesterol into your bloodstream, quickly providing energy for the muscles. You start to sweat, and you can lose control of your bladder and bowel.

Blood-clotting abilities increase, to prepare you for possible injury, and your immunity responses decrease. When the crisis is over, all these responses are reversed. However, if you constantly feel stressed, this continual lowering of your immunity can become extremely harmful to your health.

Over time, if you are constantly stressed and angry, you're not eating well, and you're not getting regular exercise, fresh air and sunshine, your body will remain in a chronic state of fight or flight. Your organs will begin to wear down, resulting in high blood pressure, digestive problems, muscular pain and the possible onset of disease. Cancer and heart disease have a definite correlation to stress. At the least you can get very sick and, as your organs

> 'If we continue to develop a lifestyle based on stress, poor nutrition and low fitness, we will evolve into a weak race of people with poor health and short, stressed life spans.'
> — Mark McKean

Managing Your Life

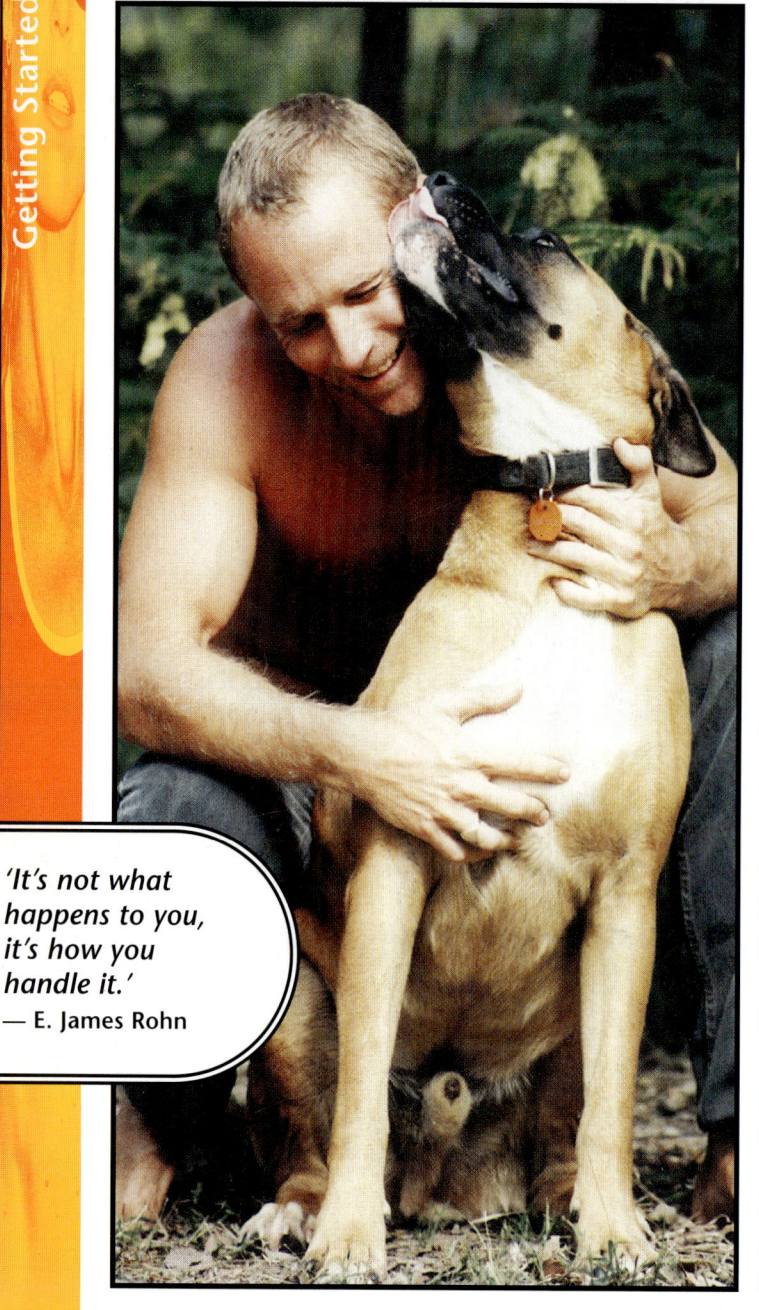

When you're feeling stressed, take time out and get away. Clear your head and relax.

> 'It's not what happens to you, it's how you handle it.'
> — E. James Rohn

continue to wear down, stress can even kill you. Your immediate attention is needed.

If you haven't been managing your stress very well lately, the next time something very small makes you snap, sit down and have a good think about your stress-release options. Usually you snap because little things have been building up over a period of time to the point where you feel you just can't cope any longer. Learn to recognise the causes and symptoms, and work on preventing them from happening again.

Common Causes of Stress

There are an abundance of reasons why people become stressed. Below are some of the most common causes. Do any of these apply to you?

- unrealistic workload: at work, home, school, training;
- lack of quality sleep;
- eating poorly balanced meals;
- not talking openly about concerns or problems, or overexaggerating concerns;
- lack of exercise;
- lack of personal space;
- not enough time for rest, recuperation and leisure activities;
- fighting or constantly arguing with your partner or family members;
- financial concerns;
- generally not knowing how to manage yourself and your time;
- changing jobs;
- moving house;
- major life events such as: marriage, death of a loved one, pregnancy, retirement, separation or divorce.

Symptoms of Stress

When you are experiencing stress, your body and mind react in various ways which can include:
- feeling as if no-one cares;
- headaches;
- inability to fall asleep easily;
- general fatigue;
- loss of patience, especially with people who are close to you;
- forgetfulness;
- procrastination;
- rashes;
- back ache, neck ache, a general feeling of being tired and sore all over for no apparent reason;
- increased or decreased appetite, both leading to poor decisions about the type of food you eat;
- depression;
- anger, especially at small things that usually wouldn't bother you;
- loss of confidence;
- self-doubt;
- worry over unnecessary things;
- general feeling of not being able to cope;
- wanting to get away from life for awhile.

After considering these causes and symptoms, you're probably feeling pretty stressed, because now you know you're stressed! Am I right? Take heart — now that you are aware of your situation, you can do something about it.

You can treat symptoms of stress in a variety of ways. Medication — relaxants and anti-depressants — is a common treatment; however, it usually only provides temporary relief and it doesn't deal with the *cause* of your stress. You need to explore various alternatives and take immediate action to release and alleviate the stress, pressure or tension that you are experiencing.

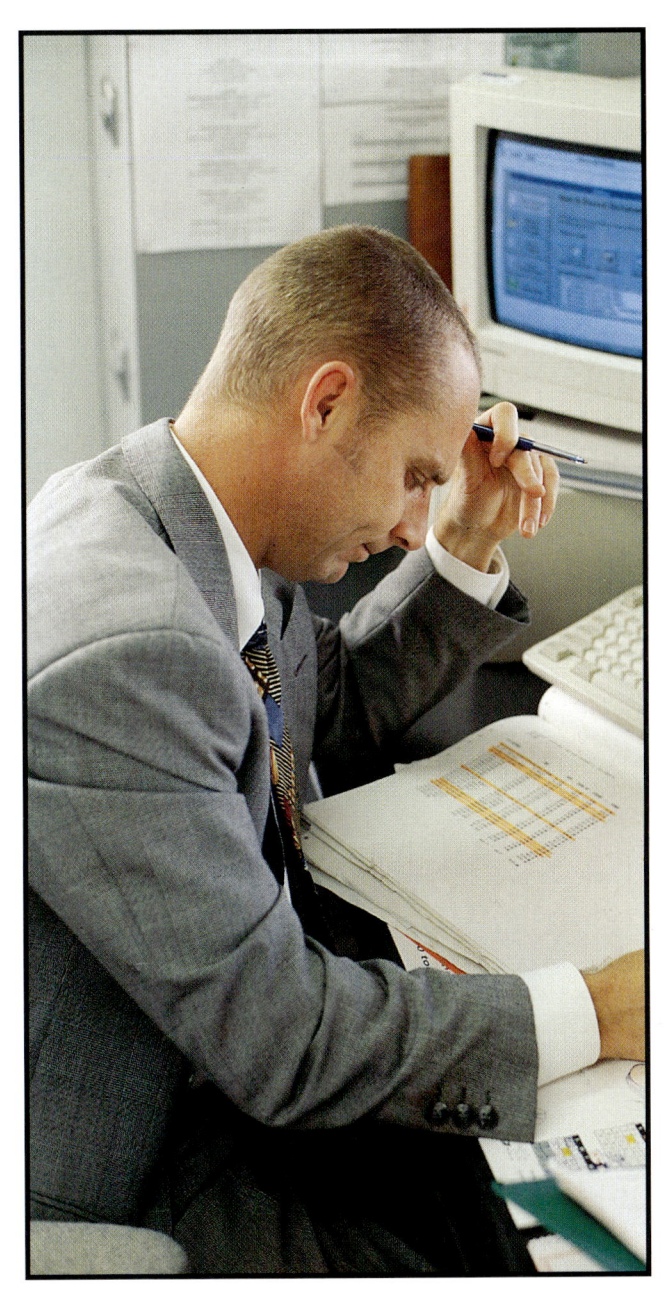

Know what your limits are. When you feel things starting to get on top of you – take a break, go for a five-minute walk, take 10 deep breaths, clear your head, and have a nutritious snack to keep you going.

Managing Your Life

Things to Do Immediately

The first thing you need to do is find about 30–60 minutes to go for a walk to a really nice place — a park, a beach, or anywhere where you can get away from the hustle and bustle of everyday life. Get some clean air into your lungs. First thing in the morning is a good time to clear your head, when you're fresh and alert.

Walk for five minutes, then stop and do a little stretching and take ten really deep breaths. Breathe in through your nose for four seconds, hold for ten seconds, and then let it all go through your mouth. Walk and let your mind wander. As you walk, continue to breathe deeply and take in your surroundings — look at plants, cloud formations, interesting buildings, kids playing, birds flying. Most times you will realise very quickly how fortunate you are, and that there are many people worse off than you. This in itself will make you feel much more relaxed. If you really can't spare the time for a long walk, just get out of the office, or whatever other stressful environment you may be in, and take a five- to ten-minute walk to clear your head.

Whenever you feel a stress attack coming on, take ten deep breaths. Breathe deeply through your nose, right down to your belly, hold it there, then blow it out through your mouth. This will relax your body.

If you can, discuss your concerns with someone else as soon as you can. When you can get problems off your chest, you will feel significantly better. A problem shared is a problem spared.

If you are in a position where you can delegate, then do so! Try to delegate *before* your workload gets out of control.

> 'The world is really made up of three types of people — the people who make things happen, the people who watch things happen and the people who ask "what happened".'
> — Ron Barassi

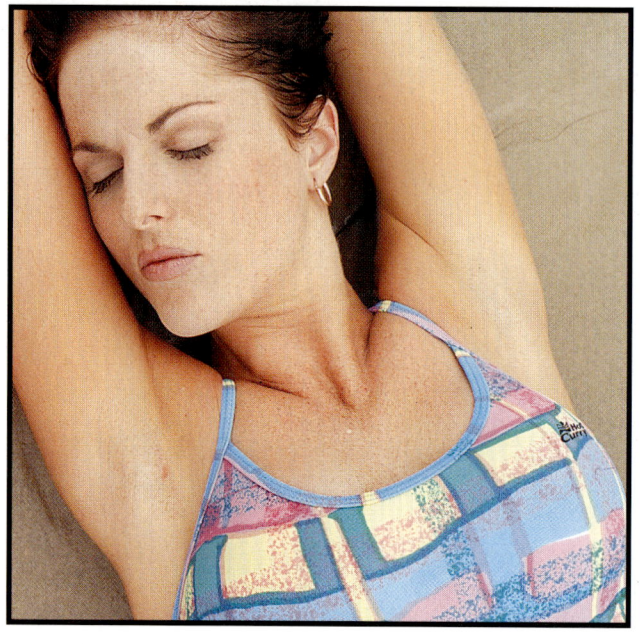

20–30 minutes of rest during the day can do wonders for you. Learn to relax and unwind.

Be Good to Yourself

Once you know the causes and symptoms of your stress, and how to treat it, you are a lot better placed to manage your life effectively. Reducing stress will improve your body's immune system, speed your recovery from illness and help prevent an illness from recurring.

It is also important for you to work out ways to prevent stress. As I keep emphasising, managing yourself and your time carefully plays an important role. So, too, does being good to yourself. Remember to take a break! Take some time to gather your thoughts, gather your strength and gather yourself. Take time to regain your energy, enthusiasm and optimism.

Managing Your Life

Highly motivated people usually keep on going until they drop; *smart*, highly motivated people recognise when they need time out to take a break, regain their energy and regroup their thoughts. Then they get going again.

Feeling calm and relaxed is the key to being productive. When you feel like you are losing control, you must stop, clear your head, eat better, get out and move. Get off the merry-go-round for a while and relax. Use this time to learn about how you respond to stress. Rethink what is important to you. Analyse your feelings, and ask yourself the right questions: Why do I feel like this? Is it really worth being this angry? What will I achieve if I let it get to me?

If there is nothing you can do about a stressful situation, then just let it go. Think about how babies deal with stress. They go all red in the face, cry and scream until they get what they want. Then they are fine. They don't remind themselves about it later, or torture themselves with guilt as adults do. Just let it go.

Control your life. Undertake stress-free activities — paint, garden, walk, cook, stretch, or simply relax tight muscles. Listening to your favourite music can work wonders. Have a massage. Wrestle with your dog. Exercise — participate in a sport you really enjoy. Feel free, run, jump, swim — do what you please. Exercise is a great stress release. The list is endless, but you must continue doing stress-releasing activities your whole life. Plan these activities into your timetable.

■ ■ ■

By now you should have a clear idea of what your health and fitness goals are and how you can manage your life differently to make the time to achieve your goals. In the next section we take an in-depth look at the body, so you'll know exactly what's happening inside.

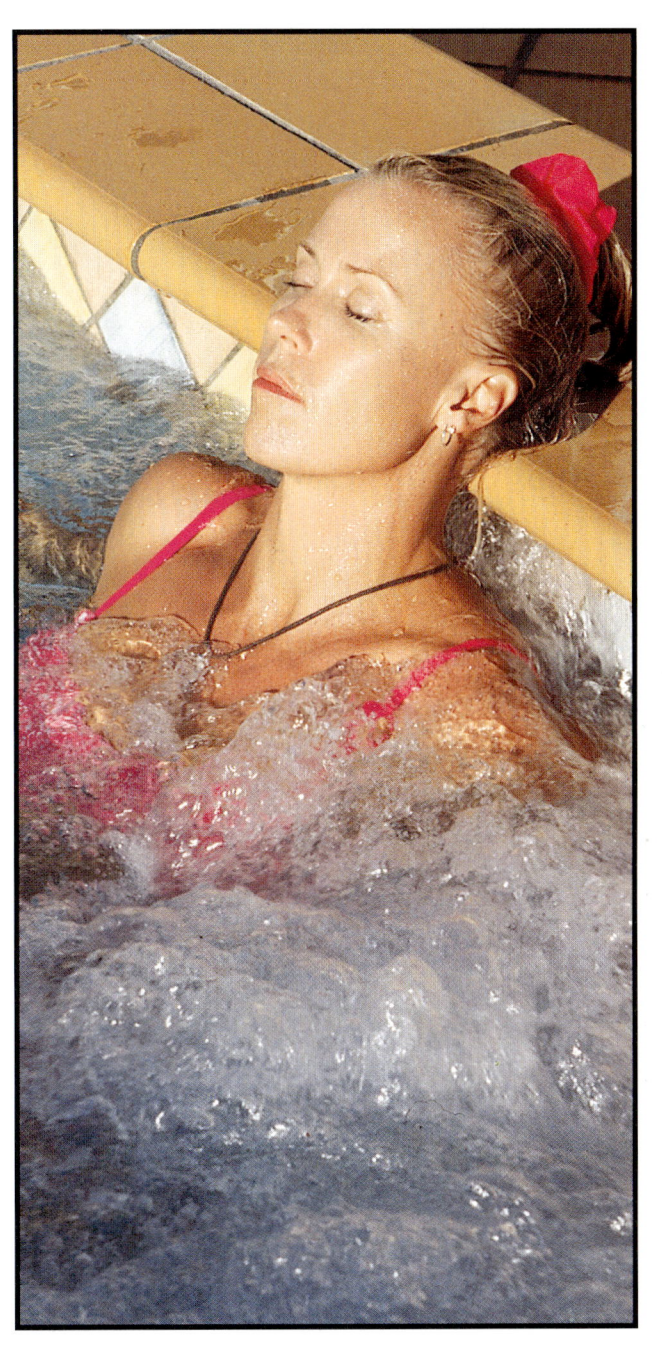

Being good to yourself is an essential part of effective life management.

Get UP&GO!

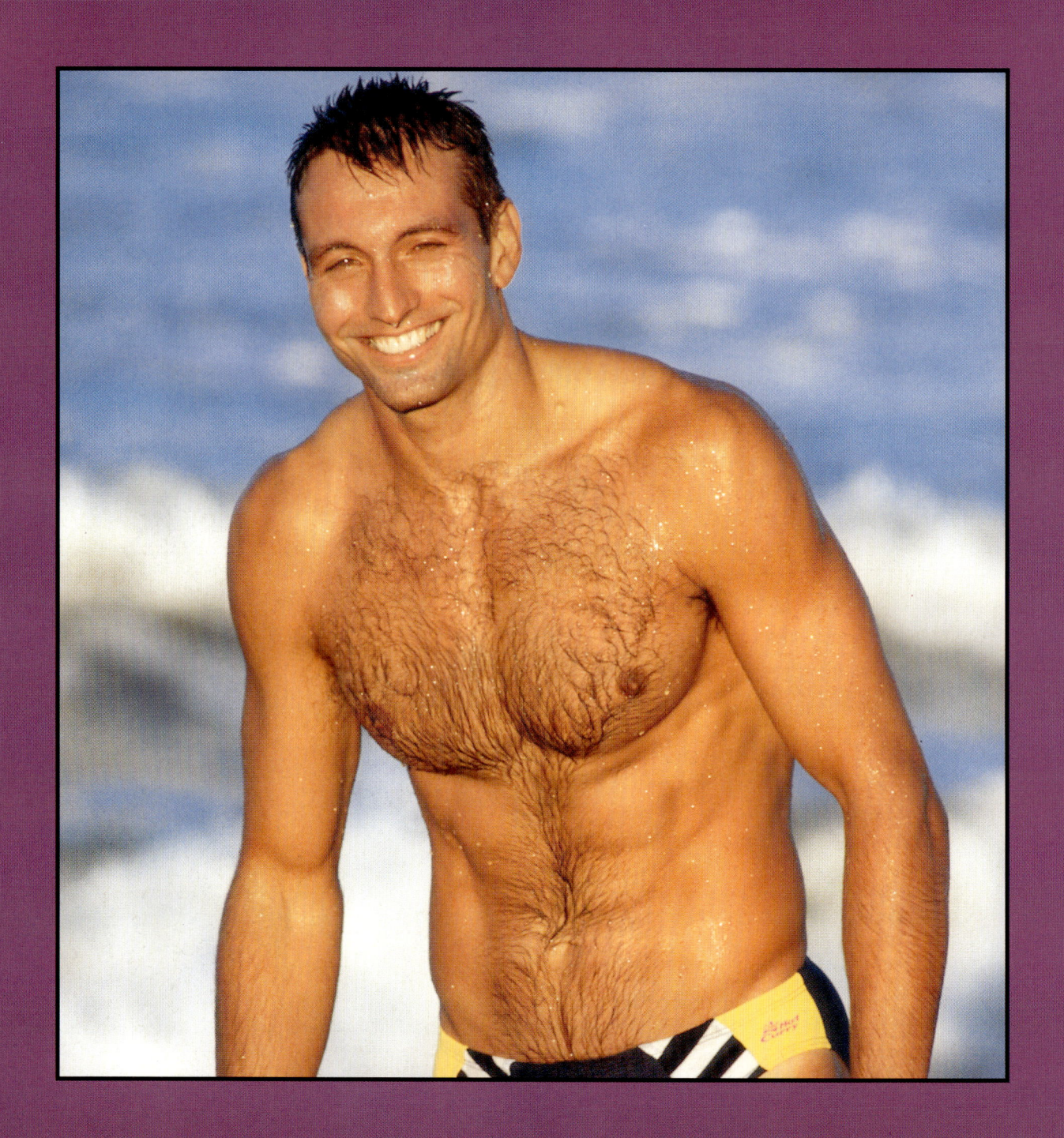

Your Body

'Success is sweet, but it usually has the scent of sweat about it.'

Understanding Your Body

If you want to improve your body, you have to understand it. In this chapter you will learn why you need to understand your body — why you are the way you are. You will also learn how to recognise your body type and to accept what you can and can't change about it.

[Regular Maintenance]

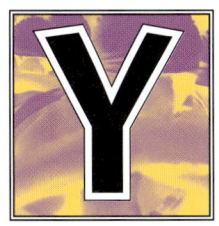

Your body is like a machine — it requires constant maintenance if you want to keep it in peak condition. To do that, you must understand how it works, its capabilities and its weaknesses. If you neglect to take care of your body, it will not perform to its potential and may fall into disrepair. But give it the time and attention it deserves and it will run smoothly — so long as you keep working at it. It doesn't need *much* attention, but it *does* need it constantly — it's all about regular maintenance. Maintaining your body is an ongoing task, not just something you decide to spend a week or two working on. Good health and fitness are long-term habits.

It's not just your external body that needs regular conditioning either. Your internal health is an intrinsic part of your total wellbeing. Physical appearances can be deceiving — you may look and feel healthy enough on the outside, but what kind of shape are you in on the *inside*? After all, it's our internal fitness, not our external, that determines just how 'healthy' we really are. How many people on the verge of a major illness or a nervous breakdown appear to be healthy? How many so-called fit and healthy people die of coronary heart disease?

Once you're in good shape both inside and out, you can enjoy everything you love without guilt, as long as it's in moderation!

Understanding Your Body

Why You Are What You Are

All too often people start exercising with the aim of trying to look like someone they admire — for example, a supermodel or a professional athlete — rather than setting realistic goals. You probably have an ideal shape and figure in mind that you desire. Eliminate all such visions for the moment and absorb the next two sentences before you continue reading.

We are what we are. We can only be the best we can be with what we have been given.

Accept this fact, and you'll have cleared the first hurdle. Everyone can change the way they look, feel or perform, but you can't change genetics. You can't be waif-slim if you have a heavy frame, and you can't be Michael Jordan if you are only 160 centimetres tall. Although you may be able to play basketball as well as him, you simply won't grow as tall.

> '*Do what you can with what you have where you are.*'
> — Anonymous

Why You Need to Understand Your Body

If you know how your body responds to exercise you'll be able to measure your responses and change your activities to get the best results.

If you understand how nutrition influences your bodily functions you'll be more likely to

Certain qualities given to us when we were born decide the final outcome of our shape, health, fitness and wellbeing. We can modify those qualities within certain boundaries but, generally, we have to be happy with what we've got and make the most of it.

Most people waste a lot of time working on the areas where little change is possible. Smart training is about concentrating on the areas where a small amount of effort will make a big difference to you.

Let's Look at Your Body Type

It is the unique combination of muscles, skin, hair and bones that gives us our particular shape and appearance. Everyone's body and metabolism is individual. Understanding this will enable you to accept your body more readily, and then work on making it look as good as you possibly can.

Generally speaking, there are three main body types:

Body type 1

You can eat all day, often poorly; you exercise randomly or not at all, and yet you manage to stay thin.

What you can't change	What you can change <u>a little</u> with effort	What you can change <u>a lot</u> with effort
■ Your height	■ Your muscle shape and bulk	■ Your muscle definition
■ Your frame or skeletal structure (i.e. your bone shape and size)	■ Your body shape	■ Your body-fat levels
■ Your muscle type	■ Your maximal speed	■ Your fitness levels ■ Your strength ■ Your power

Get UP&GO!

Understanding Your Body

make better choices about your daily food intake. If you know what should be happening in your body you can look for early warning signs which may indicate a problem such as overtraining or a change in health.

You may have low body-fat levels and low lean muscle mass levels. You may have difficulty putting on muscle or gaining weight. You may be on the thin side rather than the muscular or fat side. You can eat a variety of food types with little or no effect on your weight or body fat. You have a high metabolism and your body uses all the energy you consume. You need very little exercise and you seem to be naturally fit; yet you do no, or very little, training. You tend to be suited to longer events in sport and you enjoy the *amount* of exercise, rather than the *intensity*. You may find it difficult to increase your strength.

If this is you and you are not an athlete, you should eat a more balanced diet, and include foods that will help you to sustain energy. (Refer to 'Building Up', on page 98.) Some of this excess energy can go to building your muscles and changing your shape.

If this is you and you are an athlete, and you need to get stronger or bigger, a change in training is necessary so that you can reduce your energy output from the volume of training and allow some extra energy to be put into strength or bulk training. You may need to stop your aerobic training for a short period so that your body can get the most out of other aspects of exercise, such as strength training.

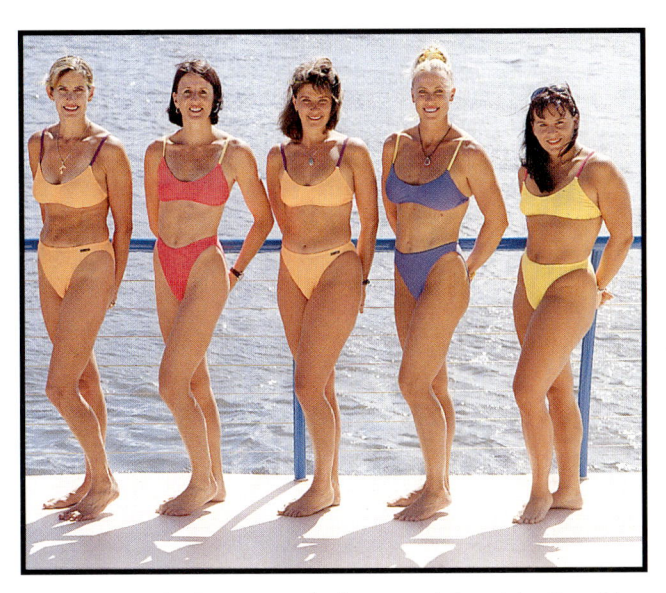

Three different body types on display. From left to right: Fran (2), Sue (1), Ann-Maree (2), Lisa (3) and Michelle (2).

The distribution of fat is different for everyone. You can have a solid build, but have the same skinfold as that of a smaller build, eg. compare Sue and Michelle. Age is no barrier to low levels of body fat, like Fran who has a total of 84.

Fran's thigh measurements are similar to mine, but her abdominal site is nearly three times higher.

Ann-Maree's and Michelle's abdominals are similar, but thigh measurements are quite different.

Because of these differences in body fat distribution, you need to have all eight sites tested and recorded instead of only two or three.

Left to Right	Fran age 42	Sue age 29	Ann-Maree age 31	Lisa age 35	Michelle age 25
Tricep	14.6	14.6	18.9	10.6	15.6
Bicep	6.6	6.8	7.7	3.4	7.6
Axilla	6.4	7.1	9.2	5.6	10.7
Scapula	7.4	10.2	11.9	6.9	7.6
Iliac	8.0	8.6	10.2	3.3	9.2
Abdominal	11.8	12.2	18.4	4.5	16.2
Thigh	19.4	23.2	34.6	17.2	20.3
Calf	10.2	14.8	16.7	11.9	9.6
Total	84.4	97.5	127.6	63.4	96.8

Understanding Your Body

Body type 2

You always have trouble with your weight and often talk about your need to lose a few kilograms. You may also have difficulty maintaining your weight, which often fluctuates by a few kilograms each week. You have low muscle mass with poor muscle definition, and higher than ideal body fat. You may have difficulty maintaining a proper eating plan for any length of time, you'll binge-eat for a few hours, days or weeks before returning to a more balanced eating plan. Exercise appears to have little influence on your fat levels, and you may often have to work very hard to achieve a small success. You may have difficulty losing body fat, as if your body has forgotten how to use fat as an energy source. Your daily eating plan is often irregular. You either miss meals or eat poor-quality food between meals. Your energy levels fluctuate daily: sometimes you feel great and other days you feel flat.

Your biggest problem revolves around your body-fat control. You need to do very low-intensity aerobic exercise for an extended time to teach your body how to use its fat stores. You will need to be very disciplined in your eating plan *for the rest of your life*, but you can reward yourself with your favourite foods once you've been maintaining your eating plan. When you've taught your body to use its fat stores (after four to six weeks), you can add resistance training to your program to increase quality lean muscle mass.

Extra muscle mass will help to consume more energy to maintain your muscles while burning into your fat reserves. For example, if there are two people doing similar exercises, the more muscular of the two will burn more calories.

A healthy low-fat, high-carbohydrate eating plan, mixed with fat burning-type training, will even up your daily energy levels and bring some control to your eating and fluctuating weight.

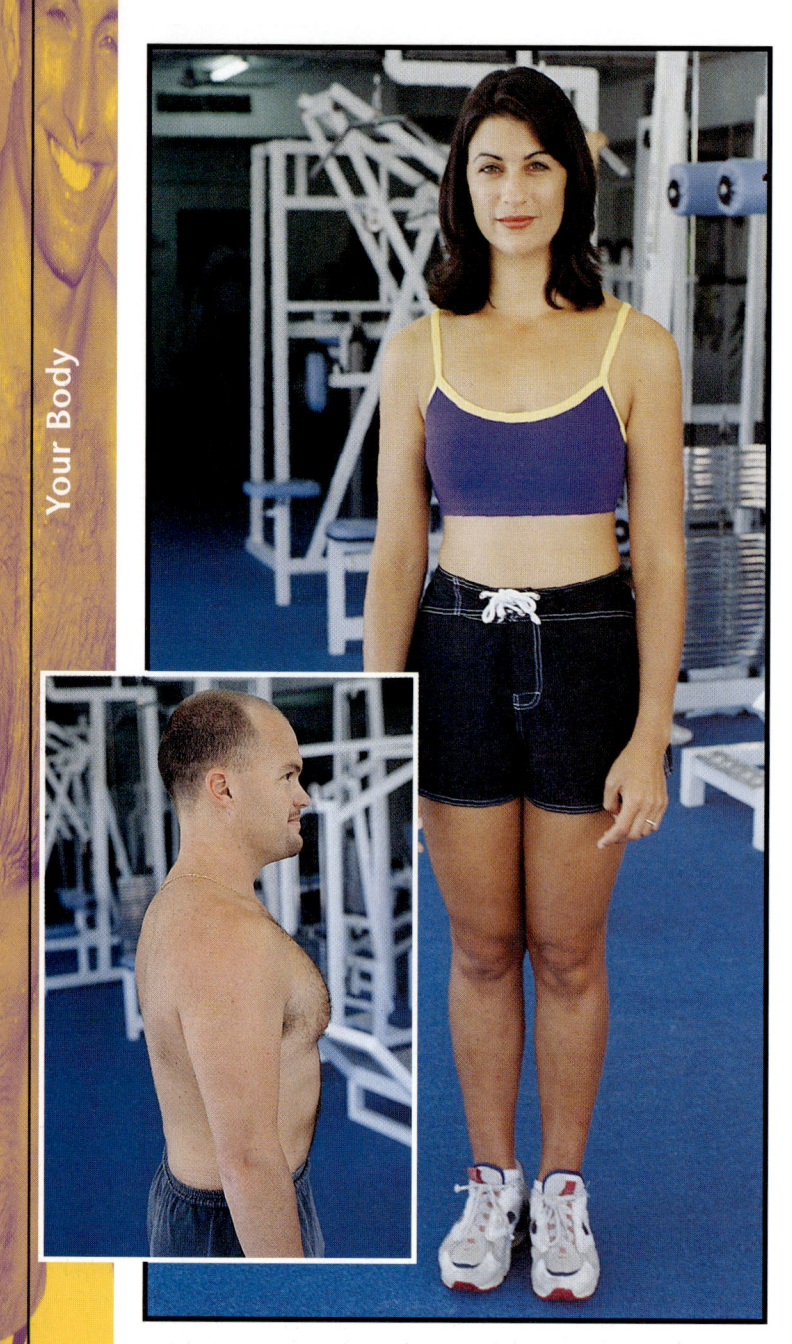

The biggest problem for Body type 2 is controlling body fat. Regular low-intensity aerobic exercise can help reduce these fat stores.

Get UP&GO!

Understanding Your Body

Body type 3

You are the sort we all tend to admire. You have good but not excessive muscle mass, and you appear to do very little to maintain low levels of body fat and a well-muscled frame. You have the ability to increase muscle mass easily. You can drop or gain body fat easily and control it quickly if it changes. It takes very little training to make you look fit and athletic. You can sustain a good shape and a fit-looking body for longer than most with little training. You generally eat well and have a regular routine with eating, sleeping and working — even when you occasionally break your routine, your health isn't influenced too much. You can increase your strength very quickly and you have a very responsible approach to your own wellbeing.

If this is you, you should aim to be more conscious of the sort of training that gives you the best results. With this body type, it's very easy to be a little remiss with training and exercise. Understanding what sort of training gives you the best results will make it easier for you to keep your shape and give you more time to do other things. Taking your body for granted is your biggest concern. Be careful! It may not always be this way.

■ ■ ■

Obviously, not everyone will fit these three categories, but you have probably found that you can relate to one of these body types to a certain extent and that you can identify with some of the associated characteristics. Treat your body individually. Find out what works for you and what doesn't. Accept what you can't change about your body and put all your energies into working on areas that you can improve. When you have chosen a routine, stick with it. Reward yourself often. What you are doing now is what you want to be able to maintain for as long as you live — so it has to be enjoyable.

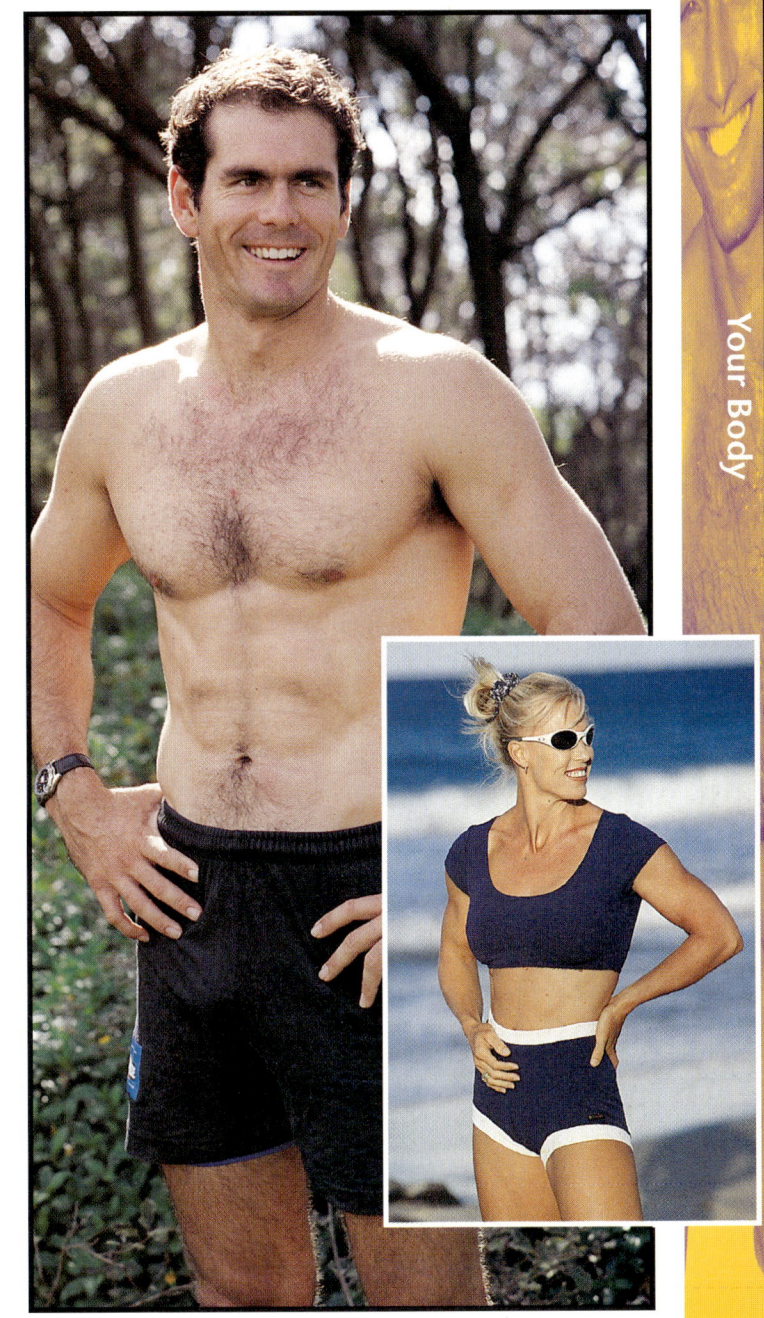

Body type 3 is a perfect balance of low body fat and strong muscle definition.

How Your Body Works

Improving your health and fitness is based on enhancing the way your body functions, but how many of us really understand our body's functions? In this chapter, we will take an inside look at your body's systems — how they work, why they work the way they do, the effect of exercise on each system and how they all fit together.

Your Body's Systems

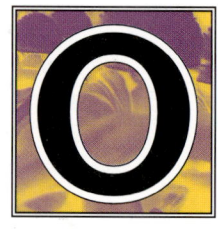

Obtaining good health and fitness involves improving the way each and every cell in the tissue of every organ works. Every five minutes your body produces more than one billion cells to replace those that have died. These cells make up levels of tissue; tissue, in certain forms, makes up organs; organs working in conjunction with each other make up systems; and a number of systems make up the whole body.

All your body's systems are essential to good health and wellbeing. In this chapter, we're going to look at:

- the cardiovascular (heart and blood vessels) and respiratory (air passages and lungs) systems;
- the digestive system (stomach, small intestine and large intestine);
- the musculoskeletal system (muscles, ligaments, tendons and bones);
- the nervous system (brain, spinal chord and nerves);
- the energy systems.

We'll also take a look at how your metabolic rate works.

How Your Body Works

The Cardiovascular and Respiratory Systems

An efficient heart–lung system is the basis of all fitness. When you breathe, oxygen in the air you inhale is drawn through the walls of tiny sacs (alveoli) in your lungs into the blood which is passing by in tiny tubes (capillaries). This oxygen is then transported by the blood throughout your body and absorbed by tissues and organs as required. This includes the brain, digestive system and muscles, just to name a few.

During exercise, the brain assesses the need for oxygen in the many different parts of your body and can send more oxygen to muscles and less to other organs until the demand changes.

Heart and blood vessels

Your heart is a pump that transports oxygen-rich blood out to your organs and other areas of need through your arteries. It also transports oxygen-poor blood through your veins and back to your lungs to be re-oxygenated, releasing the carbon dioxide back into your lungs to be breathed out into the atmosphere. A high-fat diet can create fatty deposits in the arteries, which may lead to clogged arteries and, eventually, circulation problems, such as angina, stroke, or even heart failure.

At rest, your heart beats about 72 times per minute, circulating 4–5 litres of blood per minute. When you exercise, this may increase to 180 beats per minute and 20 litres of blood circulating per minute.

As your heart beats, it alternates between phases of contraction and relaxation. During the contraction, the pressure of the blood forced into the arteries increases, similar to turning up the pressure on a hose. After the muscle contracts, there is a period of relaxation, and the pressure in the heart muscle drops.

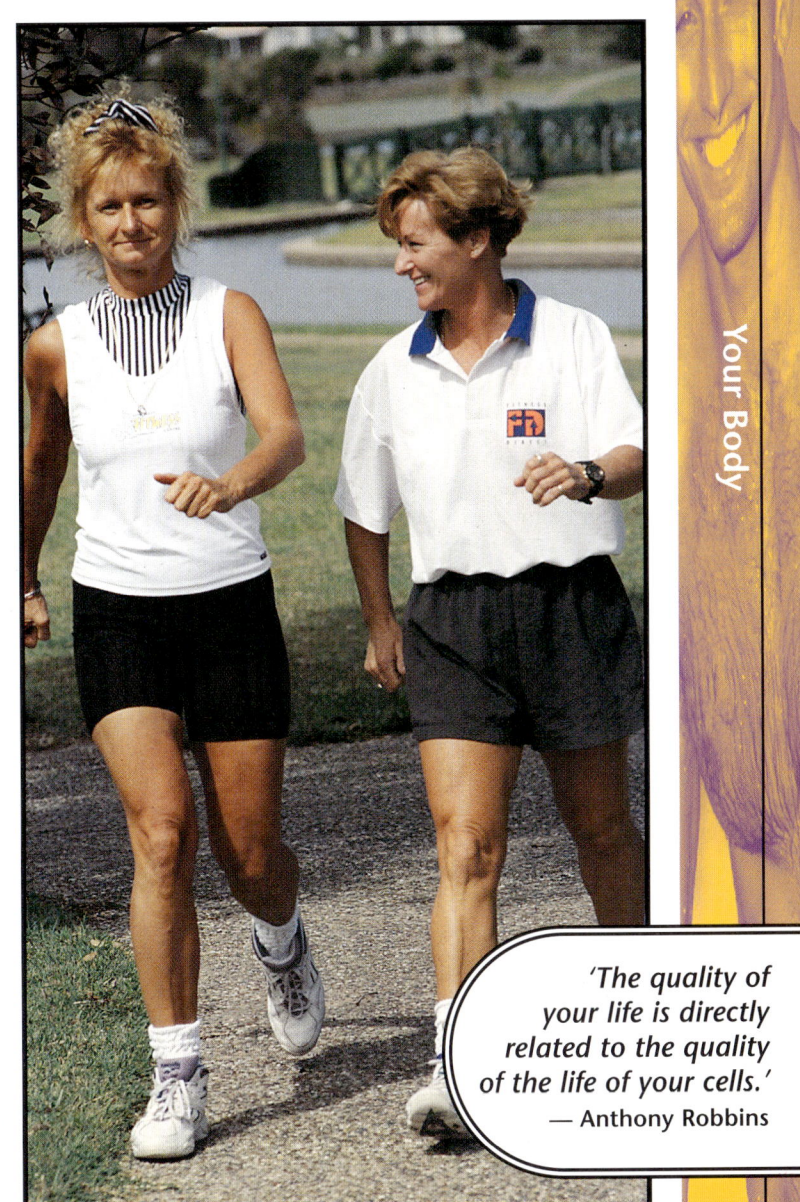

'The quality of your life is directly related to the quality of the life of your cells.'
— Anthony Robbins

Two people can be training at the same speed, but they will each have different heart rates, due to the different demands placed on each body and their different levels of fitness. Although they are doing the same exercise, their bodies will respond to it differently. To get the most out of training, you have to test your own fitness and follow specific programs for your own needs.

Your Body

Get UP&GO!

How Your Body Works

The difference between this maximal pressure and minimal pressure is known as your blood pressure.

Blood pressure is measured by a sphygmomanometer as the height in millimetres of a column containing mercury (mmHg). The first pressure (or higher reading) obtained is the systolic pressure, which shows the pressure as the heart is contracting or pumping. The second (or lower reading) is the diastolic, which shows the pressure as the heart is relaxing or filling.

Your blood pressure is given as a measurement — for example, 110/70 (that is, a maximum pressure of 110 and a minimum pressure of 70). Acceptable measurements are a systolic reading of less than 140 mmHg and a diastolic of less than 90 mmHg.

The average measurement is 120/80. High readings tend to indicate hypertension or high levels of apprehension. During exercise, your maximal pressure can increase to over 200. Check your normal blood pressure reading with your doctor or trainer. Consistently high blood pressure is dangerous to your health.

A strong heart is more efficient because it has the ability to pump out more blood in fewer beats per minute. This is normally indicated by a lower resting heart rate or pulse. As your fitness improves, so too does the fitness of your heart. With regular exercise your resting heart rate will slowly come down. It will also return to normal more quickly after each exercise session.

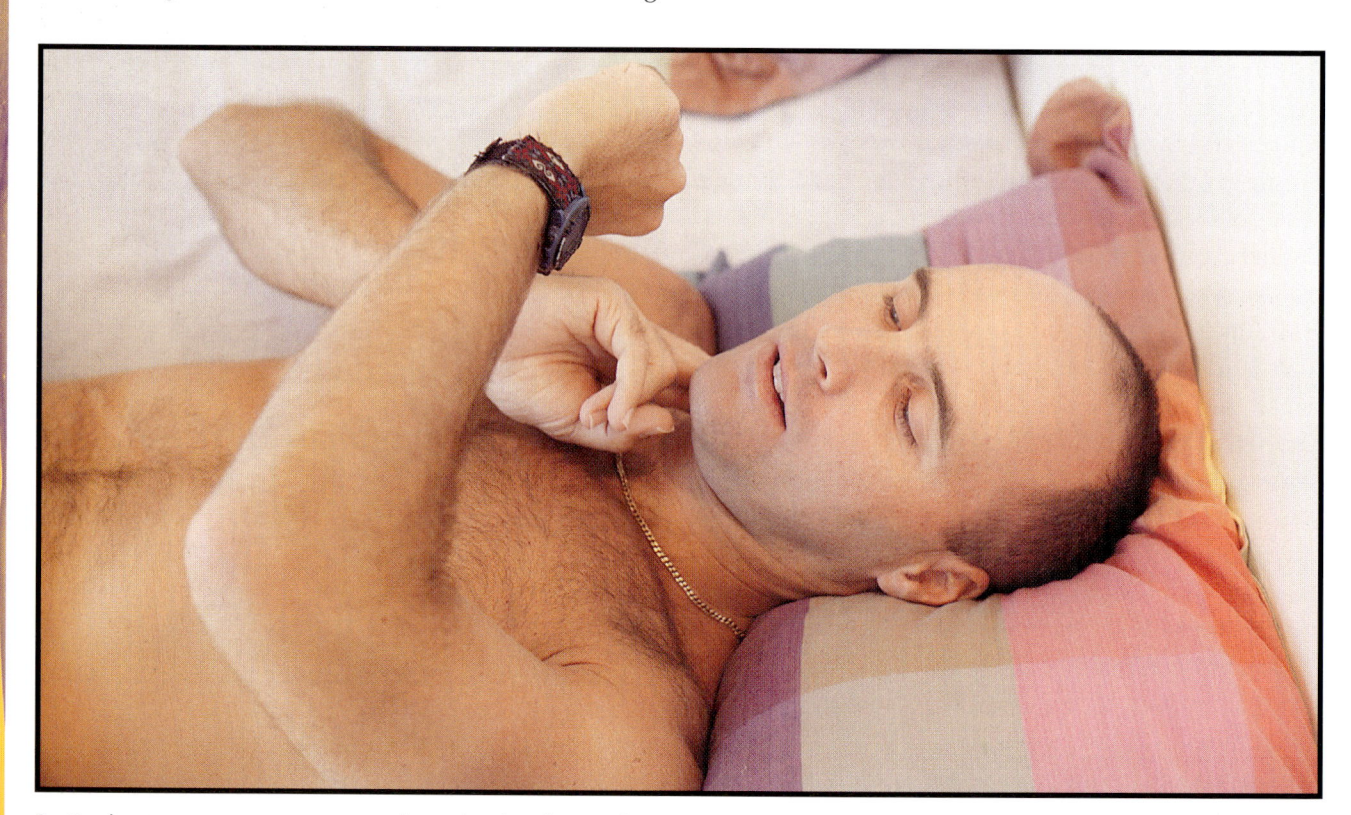

Resting heart rates are most accurate when taken first thing in the morning. Resting heart rates can also be used to measure recovery after training.

How Your Body Works

Air passages and lungs

Your air passages are the cavities from your mouth and nose that go through your windpipe (trachea) and into your lungs. The lungs occupy most of the space inside your rib cage (thoracic cavity). Your lungs sit on top of your diaphragm, which moves up and down as you breathe to fill your lungs with air and release it again. The tissue in your lungs is a very light, spongy, porous material which, if folded out, would cover about half a tennis court. There are approximately 600 million alveoli which fill with air and allow oxygen to pass through and into the blood, and carbon dioxide to pass back into the lungs to be breathed out.

At rest, you might breathe 12–16 times per minute. For children and women the rate is higher because of their smaller lung capacity. When you exercise, you may take upwards of 60 breaths per minute.

There are many muscles in your rib-cage area that assist your breathing. Weak respiratory muscles can cause poor lung efficiency. When training, you can choose activities that will improve the strength of your respiratory muscles — for example, breathing exercises in activities such as yoga and meditation, as well as breathing drills in running and swimming.

Poor posture or bad exercise techniques can restrict your airflow which, in turn, can affect your ability to move, think and react. For example, if you've been sitting at work all day, hunched over a desk in front of a computer, you could have a reduced lung cavity and shallower breathing. This reduces your oxygen intake, which may cause you to have slower-than-usual response times. If you drive home, your ability to respond quickly on the road may be impaired. This could be because you were comfortable in a specific environment at work with little or no external stimulation, and driving requires you to observe and respond to many changing things every second you are in the car. Lower oxygen levels mean slower brain function. So before you drive home after a long day at work, go for a short walk, do some stretches and take some deep breaths to get your circulation going and freshen up.

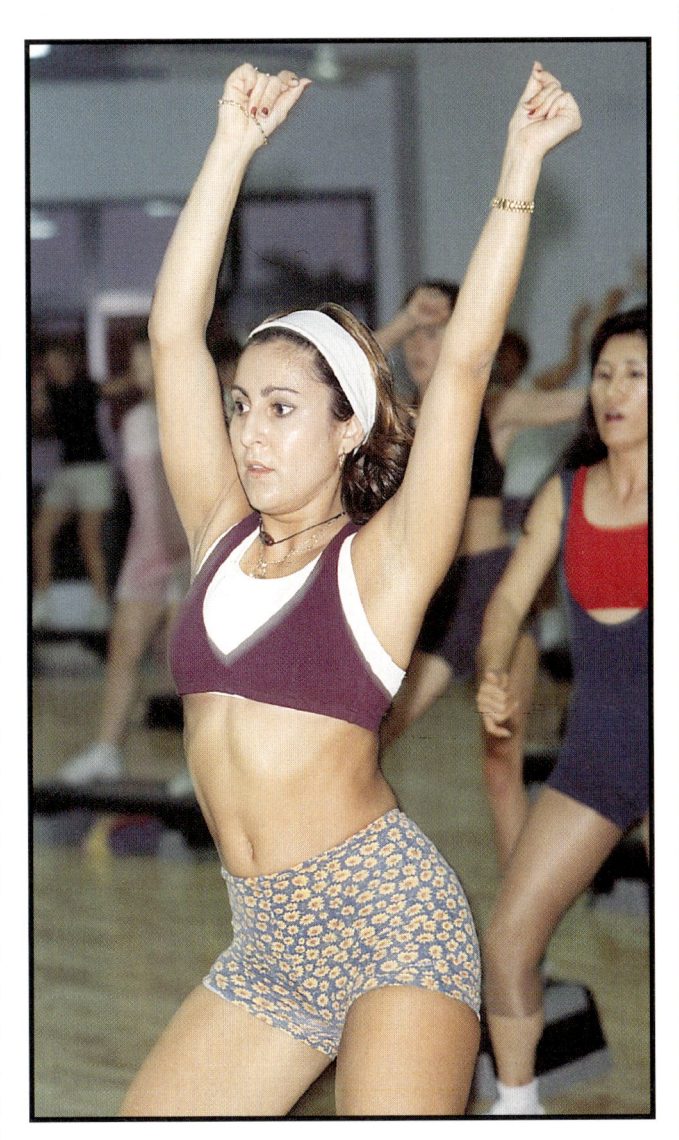

Aerobics classes are a great cardiovascular exercise. Breathing is all-important.

Get **UP**&**GO**!

How Your Body Works

Exercise and your cardio-respiratory systems

When you begin to think about exercise, your mind will start your body responding to your thoughts even before you take your first step. During this pre-exercise phase, you may have a sensation similar to nervousness or excitement (this is known as the 'fight or flight syndrome'). Your body is preparing itself by increasing the volume of blood pumped out by your heart each minute (which increases your heart rate) and increasing the number and depth of your breaths.

Once you start to exercise, your body will continue to respond and undergo changes. Your blood flow will increase until it meets the demands of your activity and more oxygen is transported around your body in your blood per minute. Your blood is redirected to areas where muscles are working and away from areas that are less in need of blood, such as the digestive system. Your blood pressure will increase steadily until your exercise intensity reaches a plateau, and your respiratory muscles will slightly increase your chest expansion.

When you finish exercising, your body will enter a recovery period during which the amount of blood being transported will decrease; your blood will be redistributed to all areas of your body and your blood pressure will return to normal. Also, your heart and respiratory rates will decrease. These changes increase and improve your body's ability to cope with everyday activities and stress.

The beneficial effects of exercise on the cardio-respiratory system include:

- Your heart rate is reduced at rest and at easy levels of exercise.
- Your heart increases in size and strength.
- Your respiratory rate is more efficient.
- Your blood pressure is reduced.

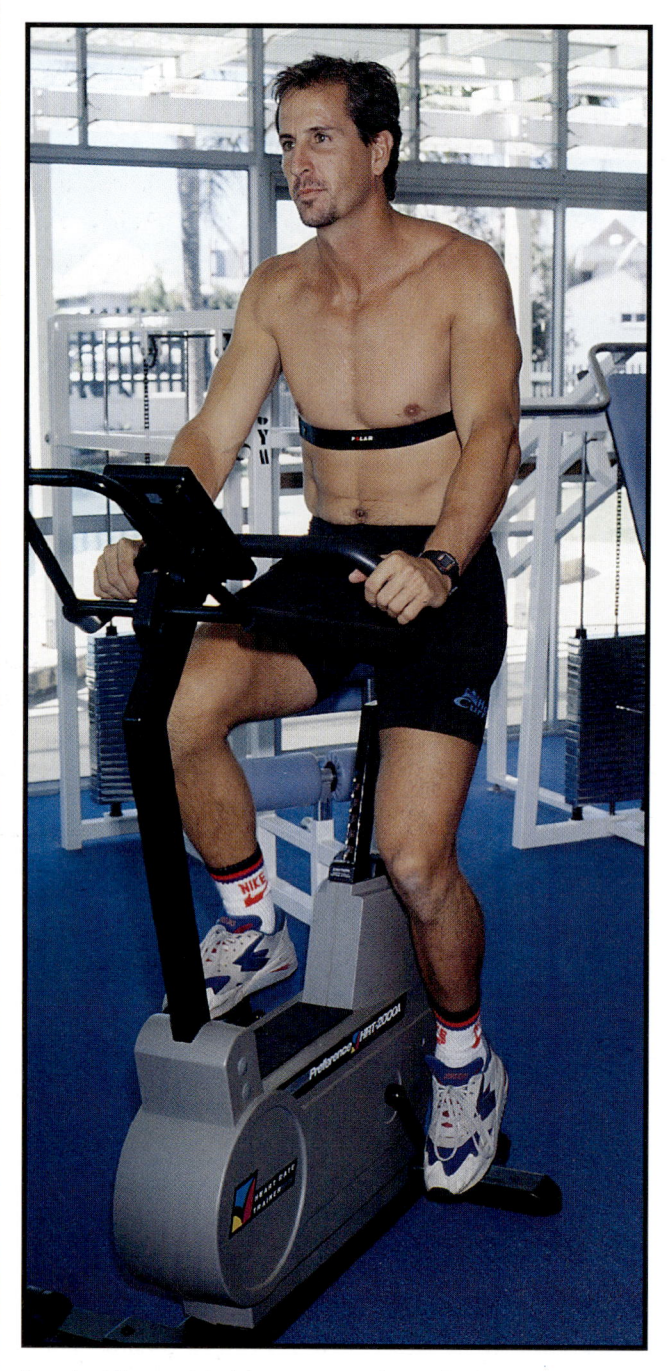

Exercise bikes are ideal for exercising the cardio-respiratory system.

Get UP&GO!

How Your Body Works

- You recover from exercise faster.
- You can engage in higher intensity activities more comfortably.
- Your ability to use different food fuels as an energy source increases.
- Your muscles absorb oxygen from blood more efficiently.
- Your stores of adenosine triphosphate (the main energy source used by your body) increase.

The digestive system

Your digestive system prepares food for absorption into your body. Long before you eat, the smell and sight of food starts the digestive process working. The salivary glands go into action, producing saliva which moistens the food, assists chewing and starts the digestion of starches.

Once swallowed, the food makes its way into your stomach where it is mixed with gastric juices and broken down into smaller particles. Acids and enzymes start digesting the protein but, contrary to what many people believe, none of the nutrients in foods are absorbed here. (However, it should be noted that alcohol is quickly absorbed here. This is because the body recognises alcohol as a toxin and wants to get rid of it quickly.)

From your stomach, food is released in small amounts into the small intestine where digestive enzymes breakdown the nutrients — the carbohydrates, proteins

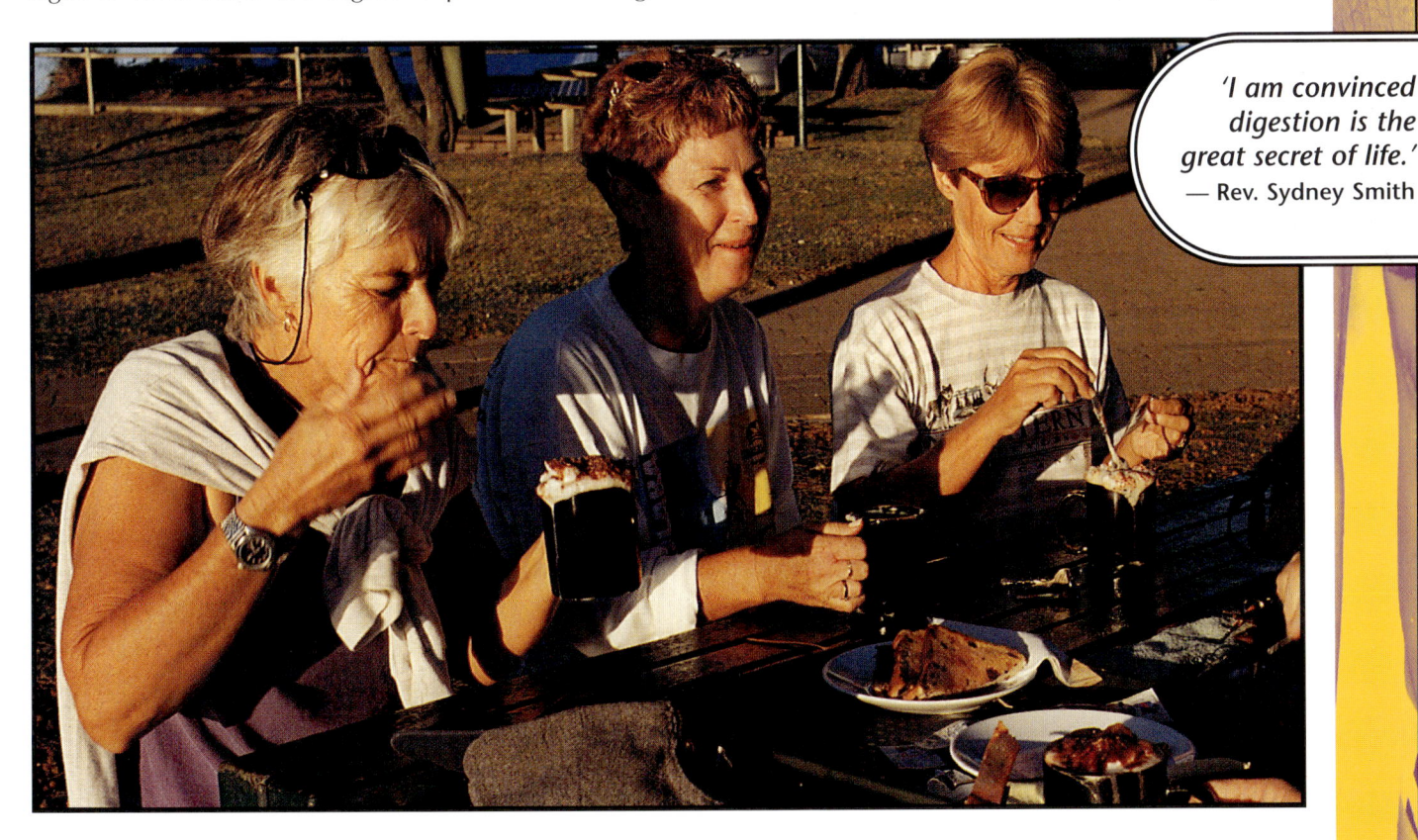

> *'I am convinced digestion is the great secret of life.'*
> — Rev. Sydney Smith

and fats — into smaller molecules: carbohydrates to glucose, proteins to amino acids, and fats to fatty acids. These smaller molecules can then be absorbed into the blood, along with some vitamins and minerals.

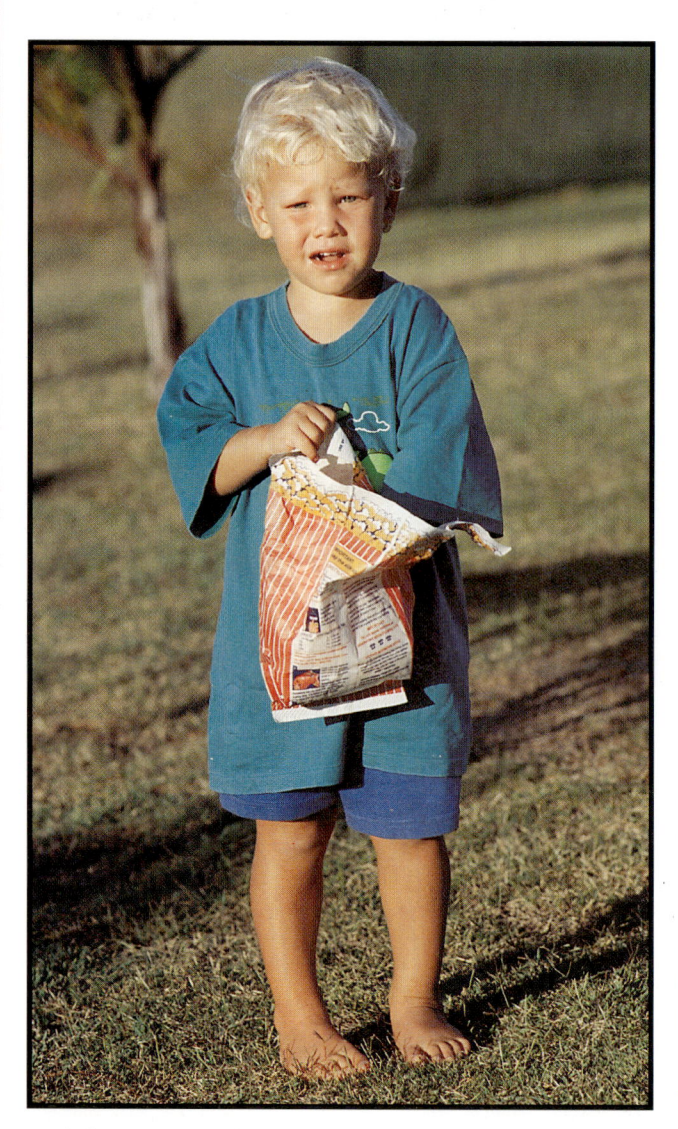

For kids, popcorn (without butter) is a great, low-fat, carbohydrate food.

The indigestible portion — fibre and resistant starch (a carbohydrate that's not digested in the small intestine) — moves on to your large bowel, where it is fermented by 'good' bugs to provide bulk. More water and vitamins are also absorbed here and the waste is excreted. Having adequate fluid in your diet is important to help move the bulk through your body and eliminate waste material efficiently.

Let's look at what happens to these nutrients. Carbohydrates are broken down into two main groups: sugars and starches. Through digestion, these are broken down into simple sugar units — glucose, fructose or galactose — which are absorbed from the small intestine into the bloodstream. The body uses glucose for energy, so once in the bloodstream fructose and galactose are converted to glucose. The glucose is now available for immediate use for energy, or it can be stored in the liver and muscles in the form of glycogen (long chains of glucose units.) As energy is required these glucose units are released. (Refer to 'The Energy Systems' on page 51 to see how energy is produced.) These glycogen stores are limited and can be depleted during exercise.

Fats are broken down into their simplest form — fatty acids and triglycerides — and these are absorbed into the bloodstream where they are used as energy or stored as body fat. The body has the capacity to store very large amounts of fat.

Protein is broken down into single units called amino acids, which are absorbed into the bloodstream and used as building blocks to repair body tissue, and to make enzymes and hormones.

No single food supplies all the nutrients you need, so a good balance of foods is absolutely essential. (Refer to 'Food for Health' on page 82 to help you work out a balanced diet.)

Listen to Your Gut

The bowel is a group of organs comprised of the stomach and the large and small intestines. Your bowel is your biggest friend. So big, in fact, that there is more weight of material in the bowel at any one time than the combined weight of all your organs put together! So big, that if you opened up your bowel and spread it out, the surface area would cover a double tennis court.

A slow bowel transit time (longer than 36 hours) indicates that your bowel is not propelling food through your gut very efficiently. This can lead to congestion and putrefaction.

The colour of your faeces will give you a good idea of how healthy you are on the inside:

- Light brown to brown is healthy.
- Yellow or green indicates diarrhoea (often this can be the result of a bowel sterilised by antibiotics).
- Black usually indicates that there has been bleeding from the stomach or upper digestive tract.
- Tan or grey suggests an insufficiency of pancreatic enzymes (necessary to breakdown proteins in food), a blockage of the flow of bile (necessary to breakdown fats in food), or too much fat in your diet (usually causing the faeces to float).
- Red may be due to bleeding from the lower digestive tract.

If you stop and listen to your gut, you may be aware of subtle messages such as: feeling full after eating or feeling as if you haven't fully evacuated your bowel after going to the toilet. You may be aware of 'grumbling' noises (due to gas bubbles generated by unfriendly bacteria in the bowel); dull or occasional sharp abdominal pains (caused by expanding gas in the bowel becoming trapped); a burning sensation in the stomach after eating (caused by too much acid in the stomach or an irritated stomach — gastritis) or after passing a bowel motion (acid generated in the bowel through irritation of the gut due to spicy foods or unfriendly bacteria); or constipation.

If you are experiencing any of the above, it really is time for you to improve your digestion. Be aware of what foods and drinks sit well in your stomach and those that seem to protest. If you constantly experience any of the above symptoms, you may have a specific food allergy and should seek some medical advice. Making healthy food choices is important, but you also need to prepare your digestive system. Remember to chew your food well. Imagine how hard it is for your body to digest chunks of unchewed food. Eat slowly. Chew food well. Enjoy the taste and savour the pleasure of a good meal. If you're in a hurry and really do need to snack on the run, try having a smoothie (a blended fruit and dairy drink), which doesn't require chewing.

Probiotics

Probiotics are living organisms which, when you eat enough of them, can help improve the action of bacteria which live in your gut. There are a large number of micro-organisms that live in your gut; some benefit your health and wellbeing, while some are harmful. The population of each is affected by illness, your diet and your age. Antibiotics can destroy the level of both bad and good bacteria in the gut. As you get older the level of bacteria in the gut decreases.

By adding helpful bugs through food — for example, lactic acid bacteria in fermented milk products — we can help maintain a healthy balance of bacteria in the gut. There are already a number of products on the market you can try — yoghurts with *lactobacillus acidophilus, bifidus, casei, GG* or *LC1* added, and fermented milk drinks such as Yakult and Shirota.

Exercise and your digestive system

Maintaining a good level of fitness allows the muscles and nerves of your digestive system to function more efficiently. It also improves your ability to absorb and process foods. There are long-term benefits to be gained for your digestive system if you exercise regularly: your metabolic rate will increase, helping you to burn more energy and maintain weight more effectively and your risk of constipation will decrease, because your bowel movements will become more regular.

The Musculoskeletal System

Your skeleton and muscles provide support and protection for your organs and allow your body to move.

Your skeleton

Your skeletal system — the structure of bones that make up your skeleton — serves several purposes. It provides:

- the basis for all movements developed by the muscles;
- the shape and form for all your body structures and features;
- protection for internal organs and softer underlying tissues;
- the site of formation of blood cells; and
- storage for minerals.

The skeleton begins to form during the first few weeks of life and continues to grow into adulthood. Certain factors, such as exercise and nutrition, influence the development and growth of bone. Vitamins D, C, and A are all essential to proper bone growth. (Refer to 'Vitamins for Vigour' on pages 72–73.)

Exercise and your skeleton

Regular exercise is the key to stronger bones. The main benefit of exercise is that it influences bone density by placing your bones under stress. This stress stimulates your bones, making them thicker and stronger. Weight training is one of the most effective activities in influencing bone density, especially among the elderly. A number of retirement homes now actively encourage their residents to exercise with weights.

How Your Body Works

Lack of exercise has the reverse effect: bones waste, becoming thinner and weaker. When elderly people slip or fall, they break bones very easily; including exercise in their daily routine may help to prevent their bones from becoming fragile.

Your muscular system

Your muscles are the final component of your body that creates movement. After your body has digested and processed food into nutrients and passed them around — along with oxygen via the cardio-respiratory system — and sent out messages from the brain via the neural network of nerves, the muscles have the energy to contract and a reason for doing so.

It is your muscular system that provides overall movement: movement of fluids, such as blood and urine; storage of minerals and fluids, such as glycogen; posture maintenance; and body heat.

If your body-fat levels are ideal, your muscular system accounts for nearly half your body weight. Your muscles are designed to convert energy obtained from the food you eat into energy for movement. If your muscles can convert the energy

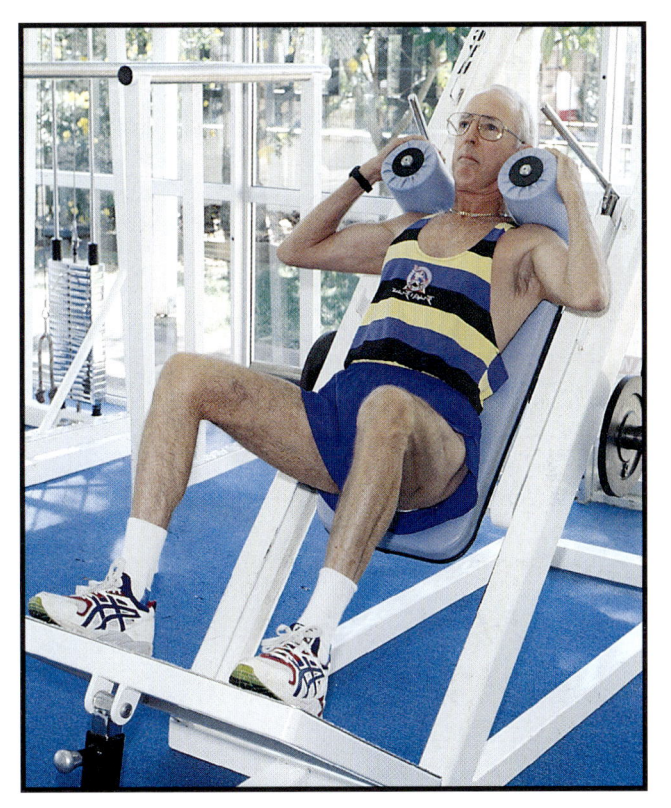

Resistance training is becoming very popular for older people. Try it for yourself, and don't be afraid to ask for assistance — gym staff are always ready to help.

ATP and PC — Important Chemicals

One of the most important chemicals necessary to make your muscles contract is ATP (adenosine triphosphate), the main energy used by your body for all types of actions. ATP is used by cells in their normal function; when muscles contract they use ATP to initiate movement. ATP is produced in the cells from the energy in food. A lack of carbohydrate in your diet can result in lower levels of ATP which will reduce your ability to perform physical activities. Another important chemical is phospho-creatine (PC), which is also a major source of energy for high-intensity activity.

How Your Body Works

available and you have trained your body to use this energy via movement, you will find it comfortable to exercise often.

Muscles contract after they have received a message from your brain. A number of minerals and chemicals are necessary to make this message activate the muscles.

Exercise and your muscular system

There are a range of benefits to be gained for your muscular system through regular exercise. Your muscular response to training depends on the type of training you do; however, you may find increases in:

- the volume and size of your muscle mass;
- your muscular endurance;
- your ability to extract nutrients and oxygen from your blood;
- your supplies of ATP-based energy stored in your muscles; and
- your strength of connective tissue and ligaments.

Your muscles can be trained for endurance and/or strength. People talk about having great muscle 'tone', mistakenly referring to their level of body fat and shape. The true meaning of tone is the tension of the muscle fibres in a muscle. If someone has great tone, you will only notice it if the person also has low body fat. You should aim for increased muscle definition and a low level of body fat.

The Nervous System

Your brain is your body's computer. It controls and regulates all your body's functions, sending out signals and instructions and receiving information. After receiving messages from its network of nerves, it processes them and sends back signals for a response.

Body tone is achieved through low levels of body fat and strong muscle definition.

'We can alter our lives by altering our attitudes.'
— William James

How Your Body Works

These signals are sent to various areas, including your digestive organs, your muscles and your eyes.

It is the signals sent to your muscles that create contractions. Your brain can be trained to signal the muscles to respond in different ways. It can increase its reaction time or increase its strength through specific types of training. For increasing strength, your brain learns to make more fibres in each muscle contract, therefore increasing the total number of contractions. For speed gains, your brain learns to make the muscle fibres contract more quickly.

Exercise and your nervous system

Your muscle-nerve coordination is improved by training and regular exercise. This enhances your balance, reaction time, coordination and agility. Generally, your nervous system responds more rapidly and efficiently with training.

Energy systems

Now that you have a grasp of how your body provides nutrients to working organs and muscles, you need to understand what actually happens to the nutrients and how they are used for energy.

There are three systems that provide energy for exercise:

1. ATP–PC system This system relies on ATP stores available in the muscles. (See the box on page 49.) It is used for explosive activities that require close to maximum effort. It can be restored very quickly and is available for use again after a short time.

The ATP stored in your muscles breaks down and releases energy. The energy given off from breaking up this chemical is used for exercise, tissue repair and daily functions. After you have used this energy, your body can replenish it through food to rebuild ATP. This is why

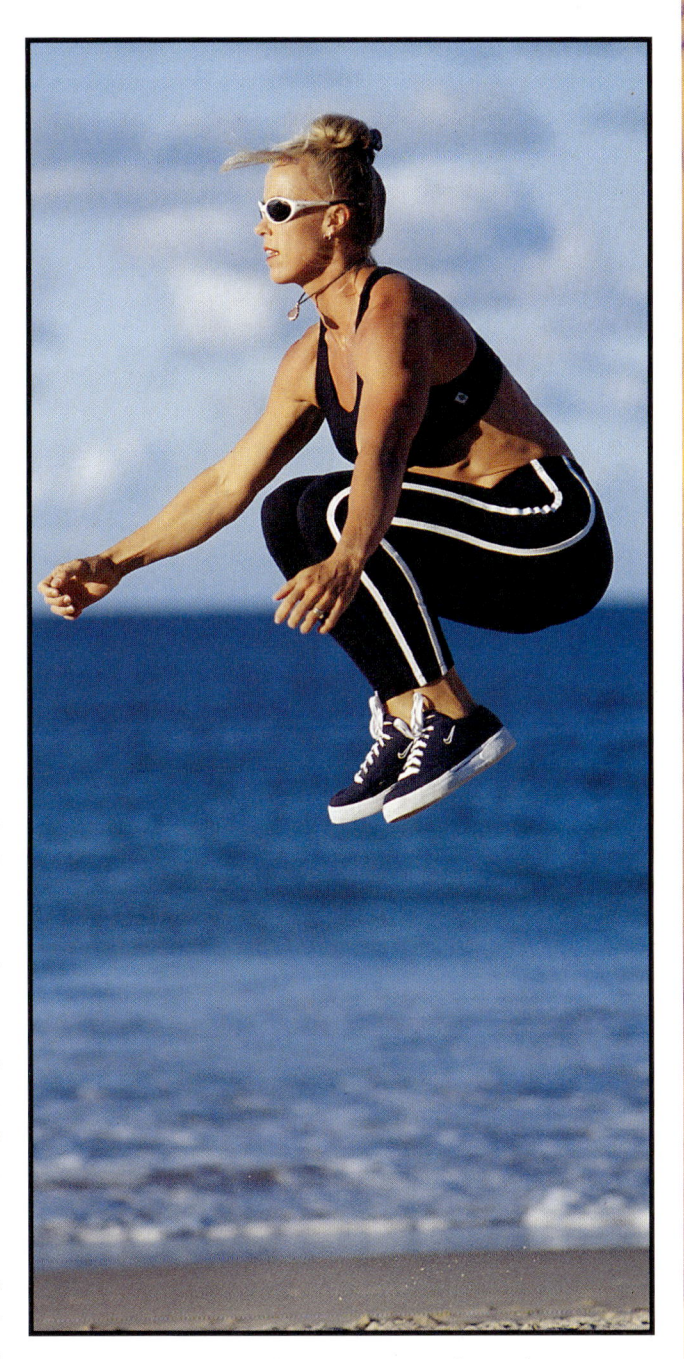

Explosive action such as plyometric training places a huge demand on the nervous system as well as muscle fibres.

Get UP&GO! 51

How Your Body Works

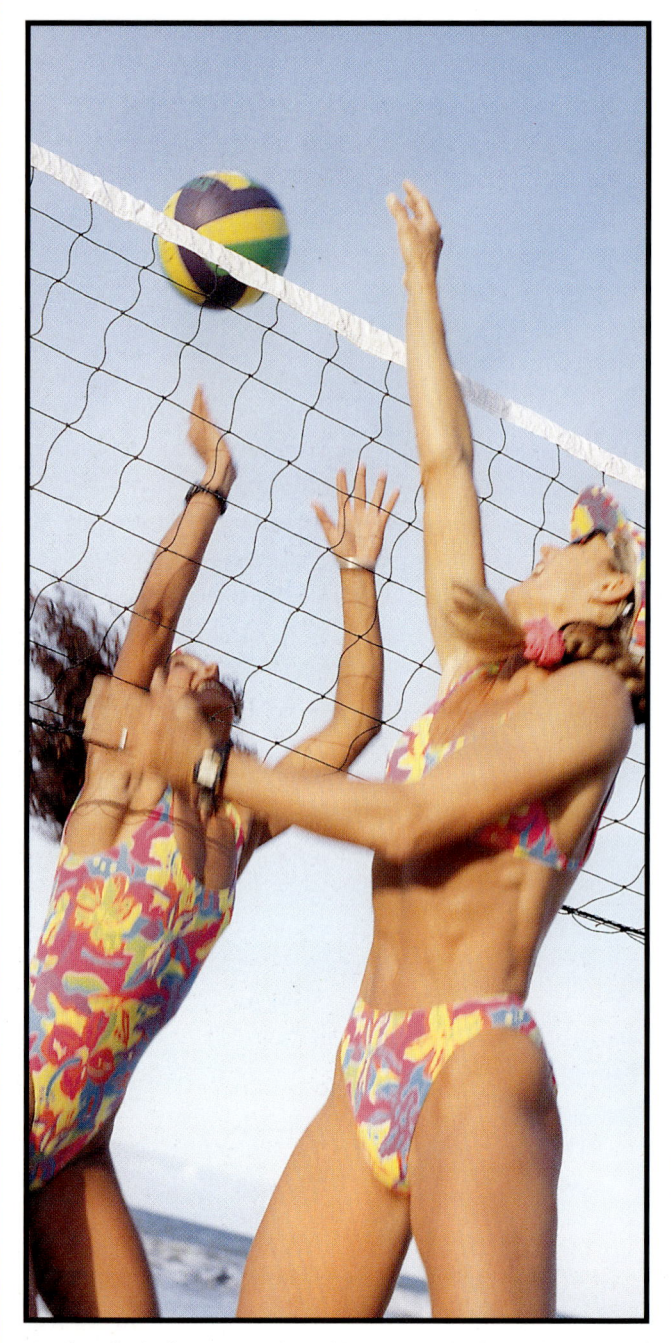

Beach volleyball is a great sport for anyone who loves the outdoors and doesn't mind having sand kicked in their face!

a proper diet is crucial for those who exercise regularly.

If the activity you are doing is very short, such as tennis or weights, and does not allow time for the oxygen levels to increase through a higher heart and respiration rate, then only ATP is available immediately for use. However, if increased oxygen is available, such as during an hour-long, brisk walk, then it is more likely to use fat stores as its main source of energy.

The ATP–PC system is important in sport for strength training, speed training, agility training, plyometric training — that is, any activity that makes a muscle contract very quickly, such as jumping and weaving in a volleyball game — and high-intensity interval training such as skill drills and sprint repeats. In everyday life, it's important for activities such as lifting heavy objects, sprinting to catch the bus, and chasing your kids around the house. It lasts for about ten seconds when used at a maximal level.

2. Anaerobic energy system This system relies on the by-product of ATP: lactic acid. Your body makes lactic acid from high-intensity exercise after ATP is used. Our body can recycle lactic acid and use it again to make more energy. It is this continual recycling of both ATP and lactic acid that we call the anaerobic energy system. It can last up to 35 seconds at maximal intensity, before the lactic acid level builds up so much that it prevents you from continuing. If you were to slow down and produce less lactic acid, your body would remove the excess and get you ready to go again. This energy is used for efforts of sustained intensity, such as sawing through a thick piece of timber or mixing a very heavy doughy bread mix. In sport it is used for team sports and events that require repeated high-intensity efforts with recovery periods between.

How Your Body Works

What Happens When You Exercise?

Different types of exercise use different fuels to provide the energy required — carbohydrate, fat and protein are all used as fuels for activity, although most exercise will use a combination of carbohydrate and fat. Carbohydrate is stored in the muscles as glycogen and released as glucose when energy is needed.

There are three main factors that affect which fuel the muscles use:
1. the intensity of the exercise (how hard you exercise);
2. the duration of the exercise (how long you exercise for); and
3. your level of fitness.

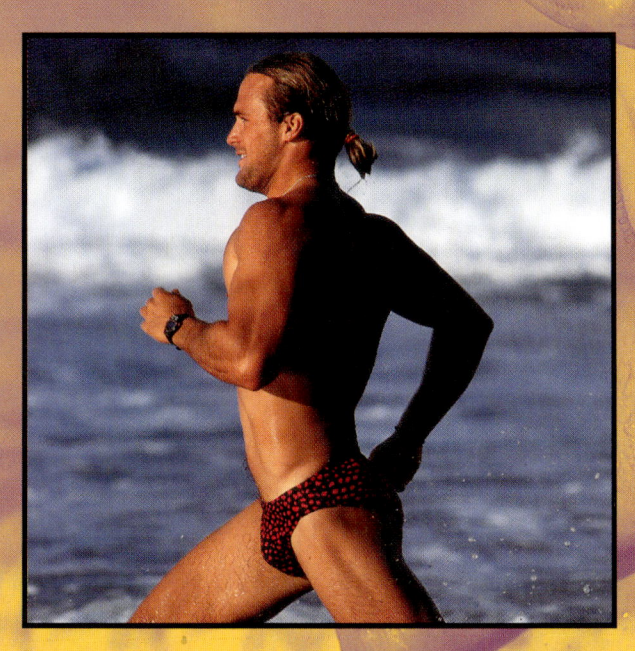

In general, the harder the effort required for the activity, the greater the energy needed and the more glycogen used. If your activity doesn't require much effort — for example, golf or washing the car — more fat than glycogen is used as the fuel source. However, these low-intensity activities don't use much fuel in total, so little fat is actually burned. However, there is a limit to how much glycogen can be stored in the body, and these stores are depleted during exercise. In contrast, body-fat stores — even on skinny people — never run out.

As the exertion level increases — for example, during jogging, swimming or brisk walking — the demand for energy (ATP) increases, and glycogen supplies most of this energy. If you keep this exercise up for 25 minutes or more, blood glucose and glycogen levels start to drop and fat starts to be burned as a fuel as well. The longer this kind of activity is maintained (if the pace is sustained), the more fat is used.

As your fitness level increases, your body becomes more efficient at preserving the glycogen stores and more fat is used as a fuel source during exercise. This means you are able to exercise for longer before becoming fatigued. When you first start to exercise you will probably find you will feel tired after 15–20 minutes, but after three weeks or so you will find you can exercise for longer before tiring. Remember, a well-hydrated body uses fuel much more efficiently.

Aim to increase your fitness level and to fuel up on energy-giving nutritious carbohydrates to improve your day.

How Your Body Works

3. Aerobic energy system This energy is derived mainly from the use of oxygen. When oxygen is available in your blood during lower intensity activity, the lactic acid levels aren't allowed to build up to a high level before they are recycled. This system is mainly used for activities that take longer to complete at a lower intensity. It uses fat stores more readily than any other energy system, but only if your fitness is at an average or higher level. The aerobic system can supply energy for a long period as long as you keep breathing and keep eating. It can supply energy for tasks such as walking the dog, mowing a large lawn, cleaning the house and gardening. In sport it is used in endurance running or activities that are lower in intensity and take longer than 15–20 minutes to perform.

How your energy systems fit together

When you are exercising, all your energy systems are required to supply energy. It would be almost impossible to find an activity that relied on only one energy system. For example, imagine you are cleaning the house. General housekeeping activities such as sweeping, mopping, moving around the house while tidying up and hanging out the washing all make use of the aerobic or oxygen system. There will be activities around the house that require very strong effort, such as lifting a laundry basket full of wet clothes, taking the rubbish out, moving a table to clean the floor, cleaning high windows, washing the dog and scrubbing a mark off the floor — all these will make use of the ATP–PC system. Occasionally, there will be a very stubborn stain or mark which requires an extra long or hard scrub to remove it. Sometimes, you might find you have to stop and recover before you continue rubbing. This is your lactic acid system working.

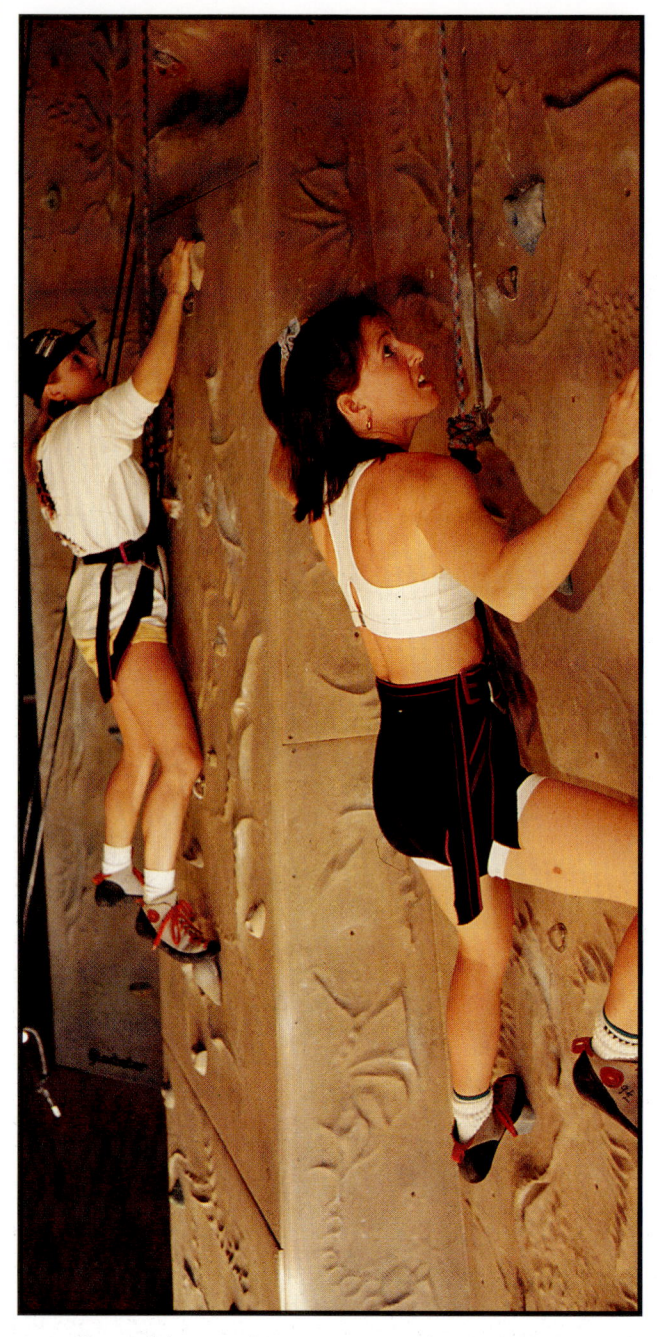

Great for confidence and concentration, indoor rock climbing is becoming extremely popular.

How Your Body Works

All systems work at the same time but to a different degree. Some activities will see an increase in energy from the ATP–PC system, while others will make use of the aerobic system. All three energy systems work in harmony and have specific abilities. Luckily, you don't have to change gears before you make use of a different energy source.

The Liver

Your liver is a large, complex organ that plays a role in virtually every process of metabolism. The liver is the body's equivalent of a bilge pump. Your body is constantly bombarded with toxic chemicals, from inside the body and from the environment. The liver converts and neutralises these toxic chemicals into water-soluble and safe by-products which can then be eliminated from your body.

There are two steps in this process of neutralising chemicals. First, when substances are initially presented to the liver, a group of enzymes convert them into compounds that are easier to handle. Second, the liver attaches molecules to these compounds to make them more water-soluble.

These two steps must be balanced for your liver to get rid of all the toxins effectively on a regular basis.

The liver also plays an important role in the metabolism of protein, fat and carbohydrate. When these nutrients are broken down into their smaller components — amino acids, fatty acids and simple sugars — they are absorbed into the bloodstream where they are either used or transported to the liver.

Some glucose (from carbohydrate breakdown) is stored in the liver in the form of glycogen. This glucose is released into the bloodstream to help maintain normal blood glucose levels essential to keep the brain functioning.

Because the liver glycogen stores are small, they can be depleted easily; this can have an effect on exercise performance, concentration and energy levels. (Refer to page 102 to see what you should be eating and drinking during exercise.)

Liver glycogen stores can be depleted overnight, so if you plan on taking early morning exercise make sure you have a meal with plenty of nutritious carbohydrates the night before and perhaps a nutritious bedtime snack. Athletes exercising strenuously for long periods (60–90 minutes) should aim to have cereal or fruit and yoghurt before they exercise to top up liver glycogen stores and take in carbohydrate during exercise to top up their blood glucose level (see 'Food for an Active Lifestyle' on pages 91–107).

A healthy liver is vital to a healthy body. By eating a well-balanced, healthy diet — including plenty of fresh fruit and vegetables — you can help keep your liver in top shape.

How Your Body Works

Your Metabolic Rate

Your metabolic rate (sometimes called resting metabolic rate) is the rate at which your body uses energy to keep you alive when your body is awake, but resting — including basic functions such as breathing, heart rate and body temperature. It is the speed at which your body 'idles'. It accounts for 60-70 per cent of your total daily energy expenditure. Metabolic rate varies with several factors having an influence:

Age

Your metabolic rate decreases with age partly due to loss of lean body tissue. Many people don't compensate for this in their eating habits. For example, at 50 years of age, you use approximately 6 per cent less energy at rest than you would have at 20 years of age; however, most people continue to eat just as much and often exercise less. Regular strength training can help prevent muscle loss.

> 'True enjoyment comes from activity of the mind and exercise of the body: the two are ever united.'
> — Baron Alexander von Humboldt

Dieting

If your energy intake is severly restricted your body will go into 'survival mode', and your metabolic rate will slow down. (Refer to 'Diets' Versus a Balanced Diet on page 89.)

Body fat

By reducing body fat and increasing muscle mass, you can increase your metabolic rate. The more lean tissue you have, the more energy your body uses. Muscles use energy even at rest; body fat uses no energy.

Sex/Gender

Women generally have a lower metabolic rate than men because they usually have less lean body tissue and lower body weight. This helps explain why men can usually eat more than women and not put on weight.

Research suggests that women are more energy-efficient at some exercises than men — for example, swimming and walking. This is just one of the many reasons why it's important to select a training program that suits your needs.

Your metabolic rate can be changed

Two main factors can affect your metabolic rate:
1. Regular physical activity will increase your metabolic rate, mainly by increasing your muscle mass. Also, after exercise, your metabolic rate stays up for several hours. The fitter you are, the longer your metabolic rate remains elevated. Even incidental activity, such as walking up stairs or vacuuming, will contribute to an increase in metabolic rate.
2. The process of eating and converting food into a form our bodies can use increases your metabolic rate.

Start the day with a healthy breakfast to kick-start your metabolism, and try eating smaller meals with a nutritious snack in between.

So, start increasing your level of activity and enjoy eating healthy meals regularly.

■ ■ ■

The health and wellbeing of each of our body's systems influences all others and, in turn, reflects our own health and wellbeing.

Listen to Your Body

When you are feeling unwell, do you head straight for the doctor? When I start to feel a sore throat coming on, or I can feel my glands becoming enlarged, I know I need to relax and get a bit more sleep, take a look at what I've been eating over the past couple of weeks, and make sure I've been drinking enough water. Usually, after a few days of extra sleep, better food and more water, the soreness in my throat disappears and my glands return to normal.

Of course, there *are* conditions and illnesses that do need a doctor's care, but by learning to recognise causes and symptoms of illness, you can learn to use preventative measures.

Kids can often get sick in their first week of school after a holiday period. They run themselves ragged during school holidays — with outings, late nights, parties, and treats that aren't everyday food — and once they slow down and get back into a routine, they feel tired and can't function at 100 per cent.

What about the New Year flu? Ever wondered if it was a result of an excess of alcohol, parties, late nights and eating out? If you are run down — or have been burning the candle at both ends — then if there is a bug or virus going around, the chances are you'll get it.

If you feel unwell, or are plagued by a recurring problem, look at what you can do to help yourself. I suffered from sinus pain for 20 years. One night, in desperation, I went to a doctor's surgery and asked for a prescription for my usual antibiotic. The doctor said he would give me the prescription, but I wouldn't need it if I tried something different.

He told me to stand on my head or hang over the end of my bed and let the sinuses drain for as long as I could stand it, then lie on my back on the floor. I went home and followed his advice, and have not taken an antibiotic since.

This simple self-help remedy made me wonder what else I could cure myself of and led me to read and learn all I could about natural remedies and prevention. I haven't taken an antibiotic in three years and am able to treat myself through stress reduction, food, water, sleep, and fresh air and sunshine.

When you're feeling off-colour, listen to your body and ask yourself the right questions:

- Why do I feel like this?
- Have I been drinking enough water?
- Have I skipped meals?
- Have I been getting to sleep at a reasonable hour?
- Have I been getting any exercise?
- What can I do to help myself?

Also be aware that you can make a vast difference to the quality of your life by standing guard over your mouth. This means keeping a check on what goes into it (eating and drinking habits) and what comes out of it (attitude, self-talk). You don't need a doctor to make these decisions for you.

Health is your most precious commodity. No matter what material success you have, if your body or mind is racked with pain or disease, the pleasures of the world are meaningless. Prioritise your health needs into each day and take control of your own health.

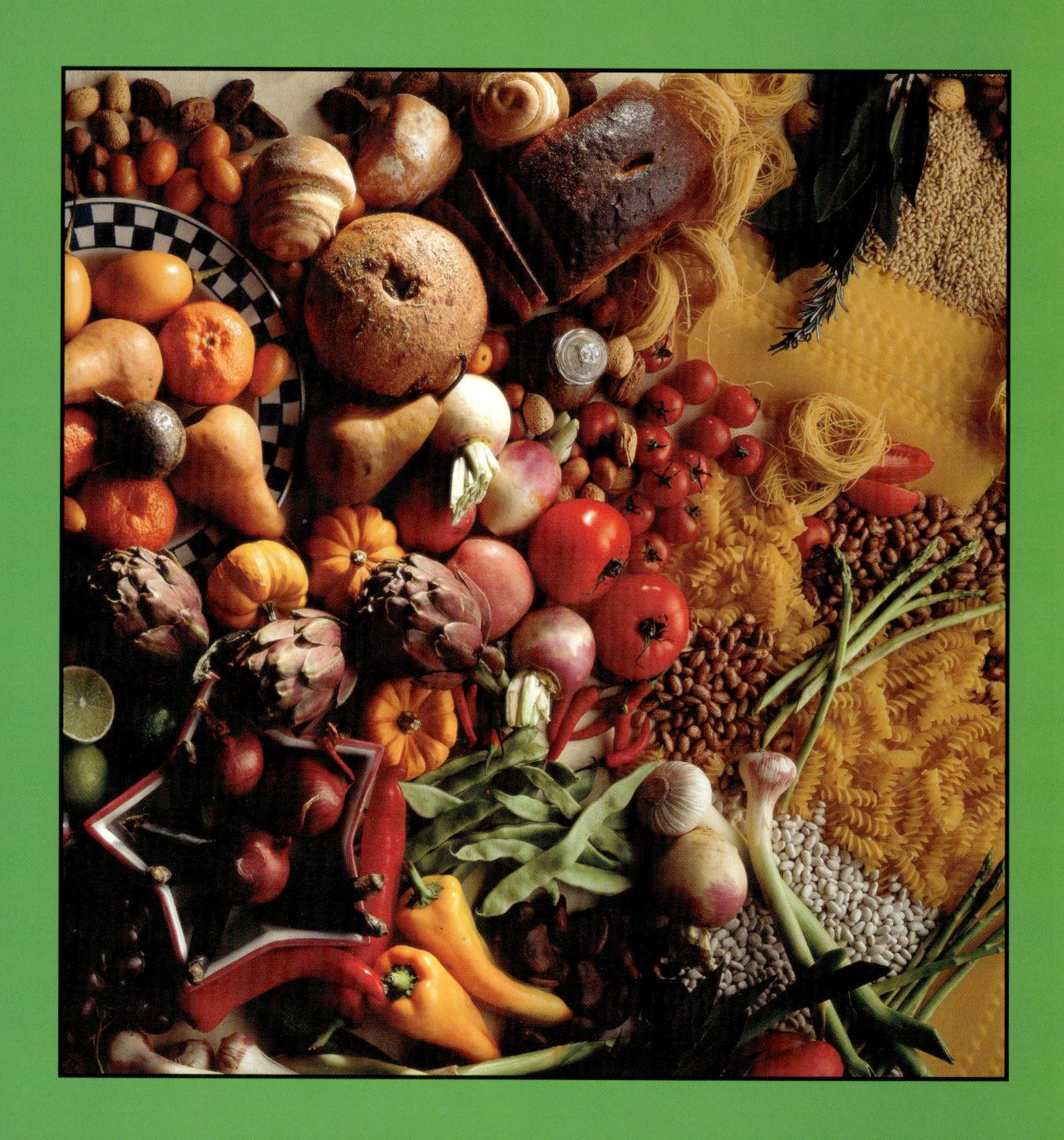

Food & Nutrition

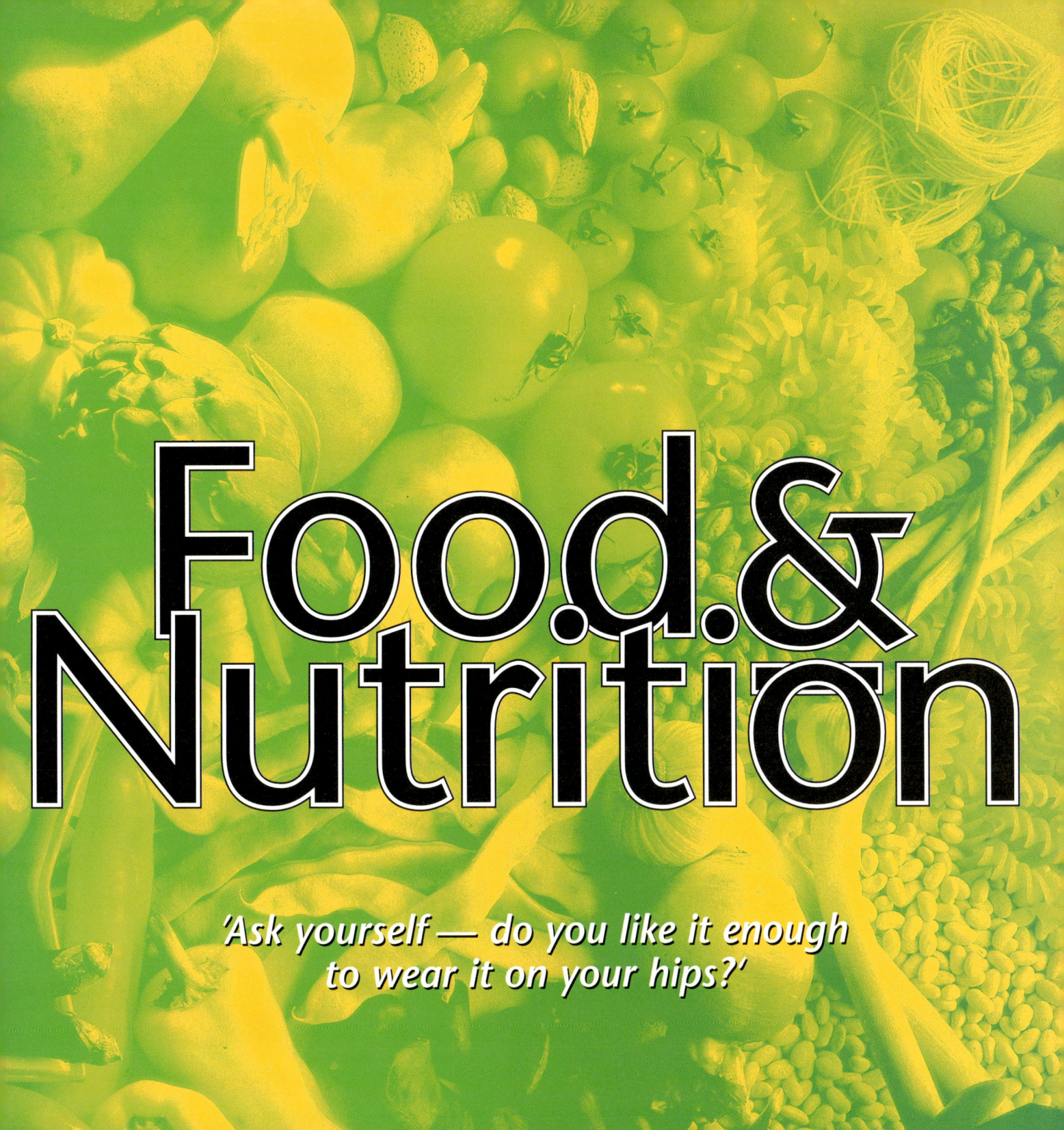

'Ask yourself — do you like it enough to wear it on your hips?'

Food for Life

'Eat well to live well.' If only it was as easy as it sounds! When your days are busy, good nutrition can suffer. Eating well needs to become a habit. You can improve the way you feel just by making healthy eating habits a priority in your life, but first you have to understand what eating well means. In this chapter you'll learn what nutrients are contained in the food you eat, how they function in your body, and in what proportions you should be including them in your diet to ensure that you are eating well.

Eating Well

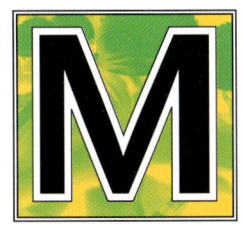

Many people think good nutrition means eating lots of brown rice and bean sprouts, and never eating chips or chocolate — they're wrong! There are no 'good' or 'bad' foods per se. Eating well means enjoying a well-balanced diet from a wide variety of foods — choosing more of some foods and less of the rest — all in moderation.

Eating well also means being aware that everything you put in your mouth has a direct effect on your body. When you change your eating habits you will feel a difference. When you are eating well, you won't feel as tired in the afternoons or as mentally drained. You'll have more energy and clearer thoughts; you and your body will function better.

What's In The Food You Eat?

Food is the fuel for your body — it satisfies hunger and gives you the energy to 'get up and go'.

Food contains nutrients that are all vital to good health: protein, fat and carbohydrates — essential for energy and growth; and vitamins and minerals — which we need in smaller amounts to help release the energy from food and keep the body functioning

Food for Life

normally. Food also contains fibre and water, both of which are necessary for a healthy body.

Your body needs the right mix of nutrients to function well. When food is digested in the body, energy is released; the amount of energy from each food is measured in kilojoules or calories. The various nutrients in food provide different amounts of energy:

Nutrient	Energy provided per gram
Protein	4 calories/17 kilojoules
Fat	9 calories/38 kilojoules
Carbohydrate	4 calories/17 kilojoules
Alcohol	7 calories/29 kilojoules

Everyone needs energy, but how much energy you need depends on a number of things, including your activity level, body size, sex and age. If you maintain a healthy weight for your height you're probably including enough kilojoules in your diet to fuel your body's needs. (This does *not* necessarily mean you are eating a well-balanced diet, though!)

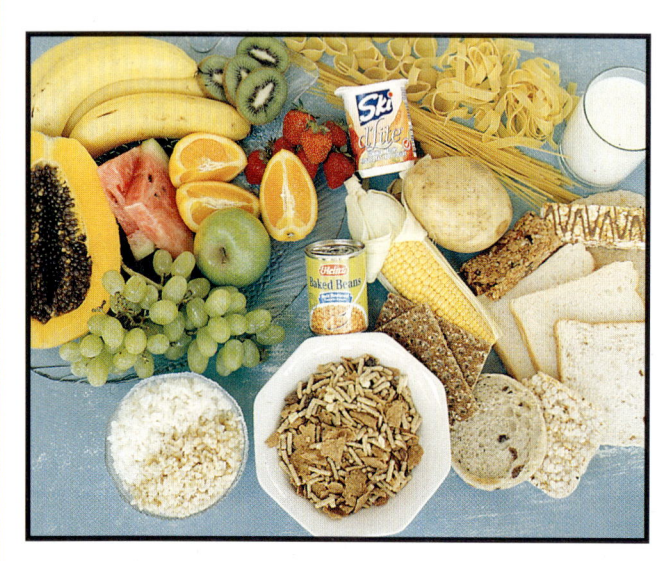

A sample of nutritious carbohydrates. Include these often in your diet.

Let's look at how our bodies use the various nutrients:

Carbohydrates

Carbohydrates are the most readily available form of energy in the body. Through digestion, carbohydrates are broken down into simpler forms which, when absorbed into the bloodstream, are available as glucose for energy. If your body doesn't need the energy immediately, glucose is stored in your liver and muscles with water, as glycogen.

Carbohydrates are generally divided into two groups:

1. Simple carbohydrates (sugars): those which are sweet tasting such as sugar, soft drinks, fruit and milk products.

2. Complex carbohydrates (starches): starchy vegetables such as potatoes, corn and grain products (breads, rice, pasta, etc).

However, I prefer to think of them in terms of the health value my body gets from them:

1. Nutritious carbohydrates: breads, grains, cereals, legumes, fruits and vegetables, and milk products (these foods should supply over half of your daily energy needs).

2. Sugar-based carbohydrates: foods containing sugars, such as soft drinks, honey and jam.

3. Non-useful carbohydrates: those foods that contain carbohydrate but are also high in fat — for example, pies, chips, croissants, chocolate and most processed foods.

Food for Life

Nutritious Carbohydrates

Breads and cereals

Breads and cereals are an important source of energy, fibre and B group vitamins. Wholegrain varieties are more nutritious — choose them whenever you can. Include a variety of breads and cereals — bagels, pita breads, rice, polenta, couscous, cracked wheat.

Fruit

Fruit is carbohydrate-rich, packed with vitamins — especially A and C — and fibre. It has also been shown to be a great source of antioxidants (which help to boost your immune system) and phytochemicals (natural chemicals that help to protect your health by fighting disease). (See page 80.)

Vegetables

Mum was right — Eat your vegies! Vegetables are naturally full of vitamins and minerals, and starchy vegetables (such as potato, sweet potato and corn) are rich in carbohydrates. Vegetables are also proving to be the most valuable source of phytochemicals. The more colourful the vegetable, the richer it is in phytochemicals. Try to include fresh and raw vegetables in your diet as often as you can. Frozen vegetables have a similar nutrient value (though possibly not as great a phytochemical value); make sure you don't allow them to thaw before you cook them.

Fruits and vegetables are often neglected by busy people. They'll eat fruit if it is sliced or in fruit salad, but often won't take the trouble to just pick up a piece and eat it. If this sounds like you, start including fruit with your breakfast. Try a banana or pawpaw on your cereal, or drink some fruit or vegetable juice. Several studies have shown that people who eat plenty of fruit and vegetables have a lower incidence of heart disease and some cancers.

Pine–Orange Blast

This refreshing drink is an easy way to get a dose of vitamins and carbohydrates for energy. It will also provide a third of your daily fibre needs.

1 slice of pineapple, chopped
1 orange, peeled and chopped
Blend until smooth.
Pulp of 2 passionfruit
Dilute with water if necessary. Stir and drink.

(Leaving the orange unpeeled will increase the fibre content and make the drink more 'chunky'.)

Nutritional summary
- Protein 4 grams ■ Fat 0 grams ■ Carbohydrate 22 grams
- Kilojoules 475 ■ Calories 113
- Fibre 11 grams (14 grams if orange peel is included)

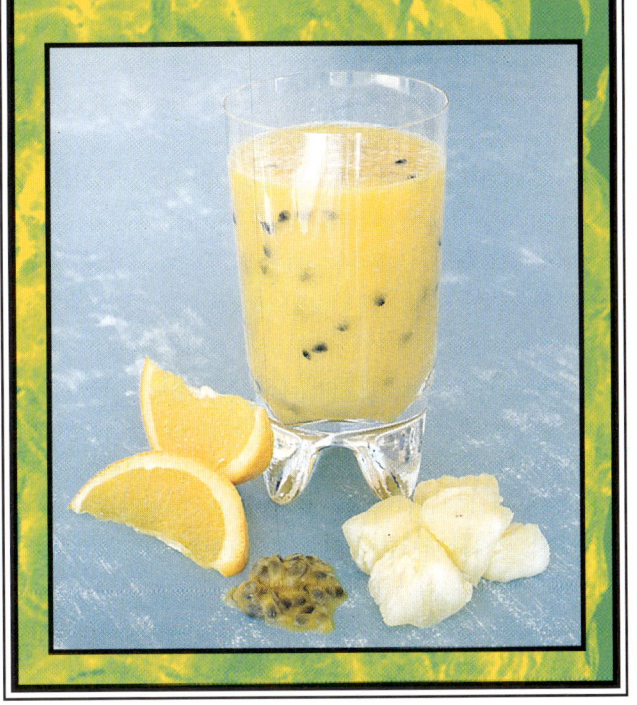

Food & Nutrition

Get UP&GO!

Food for Life

Banana Soy Smoothie

This is a good source of fibre, as well as being low in fat. It's a meal in a glass — rich in carbohydrate for energy, as well as being filling.

- 1 chopped banana (small)
- 1 teaspoon honey
- 180ml cold low-fat soy milk
- 2 tablespoons low-fat natural yoghurt
- 1/4 cup bran cereal

Blend until smooth.

Nutritional summary
- Protein 14.3 grams ■ Fat 0.5 grams
- Carbohydrate 48.5 grams
- Kilojoules 1357 ■ Calories 284
- Fibre 5.5 grams

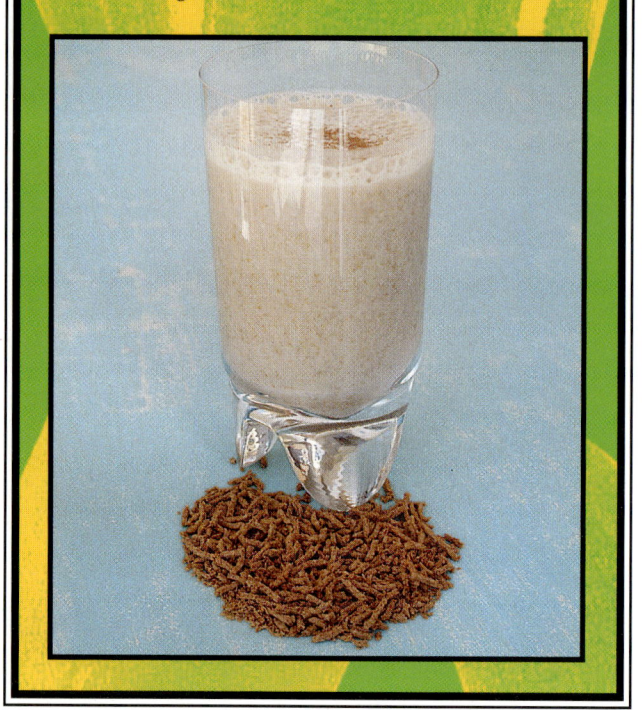

Legumes

Dried beans (such as baked beans, soy beans, kidney beans), dried peas and lentils are a valuable source of both carbohydrate and protein, as well as fibre and phytochemicals. Include them often.

Low-fat milk products

Low-fat dairy and soy milk, and low-fat yoghurt, are all useful sources of carbohydrates and protein — readily available and easy to consume. These products are also a rich source of calcium. (You should note that soy products are not naturally high in calcium. Check that your choice of low-fat soy milk has been calcium-enriched to a similar level as cow's milk.)

Sugar-based Carbohydrates

Sugars, honey, syrups, jams, soft drinks, sport drinks, lollies and iceblocks are all full of energy, but they provide you with very few vitamins or minerals. If you are an active person, you may need to include a small amount of these foods or drinks to help you meet your daily energy requirements, but make sure this doesn't mean you neglect your nutritious carbohydrates.

Non-useful Carbohydrates

When you choose carbohydrate foods it's important that you don't make them high-fat choices. Non-useful carbohydrates should only be used occasionally. These are the ones prepared with lots of fat — processed foods such as pies, chips, biscuits, cakes, quiches, lasagne and chocolates. Try an alternative snack such as a fresh wholemeal scone, a fruit bun, a piece of fruit or a tub of low-fat yoghurt, all of which contain less than 2 grams of fat.

Food for Life

Carbohydrates: Questions and Answers

Q: Are potatos and bread fattening?
A: No. Carbohydrate foods such as potatos, bread, grains, fruit and vegetables are naturally low in fat. The big problem is the way we often choose to prepare them — for example butter on bread and vegetables, creamy sauce on pasta, cream on fruit. It is true that all foods will make you fat if eaten to excess, but carbohydrates are natural appetite suppressants, more so than any other foods. They are filling, not fattening.

Q: 'Snakes'-type sweets and meringues don't contain any fat, so can I eat as much as I like?
A: No. While these foods don't contain any fat, if you overindulge in them you'll choose less of the more nutritious foods and miss out on vitamins, minerals and fibre. It's also easy to consume more energy than your body uses, and this excess energy is then stored as fat.

Q: Why do I often feel tired towards the end of the afternoon?
A: There are several things you need to consider: Have you eaten enough nutritious carbohydrates earlier in the day? Did you have lunch? Have you been drinking enough water?

If you answered 'yes' to all these questions and you still feel tired, you may function better on smaller, more regular intakes of carbohydrates throughout the day. This will help keep your blood glucose level, as well as your energy level, steadier. Try small meals or snacks of nutritious carbohydrates every three hours or so. (But don't make this an excuse for overeating.)

Q: I don't feel hungry in the morning. Besides, if I miss breakfast, won't it help me lose weight?
A: No. How often, in the morning rush to get to work and the kids off to school, is breakfast missed or substituted by a coffee or a juice? When trying to lose weight, many people forget that their body still needs carbohydrate as an energy source. A low-fat, nutritious carbohydrate breakfast will actually stimulate your metabolism. Research shows that breakfast-eaters generally have a lower daily fat intake and lower body-fat levels. Those who skip breakfast often have a high-fat snack midmorning to compensate for missing breakfast. Many of the foods we have at breakfast time are a vital source of fibre, minerals and vitamins that are difficult to make up for during the day (milk on your cereal, for example). People who miss breakfast often find their energy levels drop later in the day. If you *really* can't manage breakfast first thing in the morning, try a fruit smoothie, a milk drink, or a breakfast bar and juice, and then follow up with a nutritious midmorning snack.

If you have children, ensure that they start the day with a healthy breakfast. Children who miss breakfast often:

- perform worse at school than those who eat breakfast;
- have poor concentration, and are more irritable.
- are more likely to suffer from iron, calcium and vitamin deficiencies;
- have a greater chance of becoming obese later in life — like adults, they will often choose a high-fat snack midmorning to make up for missing breakfast.

Breakfast really is the most important meal of the day.

Food & Nutrition

Get **UP&GO!**

Protein

Protein is made up of amino acids — your body's building blocks — which are used for growth, building and repairing tissue, and making red blood cells, hormones and antibodies. There are 22 amino acids which we need for good health. Our body is able to make some of the acids, but eight of them (nine in children) — known as essential amino acids — must come from the food we eat.

All animal foods — meats, poultry, fish, eggs and dairy foods — are rich in protein and contain all the essential amino acids. These foods are also often high in fat, so choose low-fat dairy products, lean meats, skinless poultry and watch your serving size.

Plant-based foods — breads, breakfast cereals, grains, lentils, dried beans and peas, soy products, nuts and seeds — are a valuable source of protein. However, plant-based foods are missing at least one of the essential amino acids. By including a wide variety of plant-based foods in a balanced diet, you get all the essential amino acids your body needs.

Vegetarian Diets

Australians have traditionally eaten more meats and animal products than grains, fruits and vegetables. Today, with the emphasis on healthy living, people are being encouraged to swing the balance in favour of plant-based foods.

The potential benefits of vegetarian-style eating are many, including a lower risk of heart disease, high blood pressure, some cancers and diabetes. It's becoming more common for people to eat little or no meat, but a healthy vegetarian diet needs to be well-planned to ensure it's well-balanced. It's not healthy to omit meats and fill up on fruit and

What are Legumes?

Legumes are dried peas (chickpeas, split peas, etc), beans (kidney, soy, lima beans, etc), lentils and bean sprouts. They are low in fat and full of fibre, protein and iron, and rich in phytochemicals.

Some people avoid legumes because they are embarrassed by the flatulence they can cause.

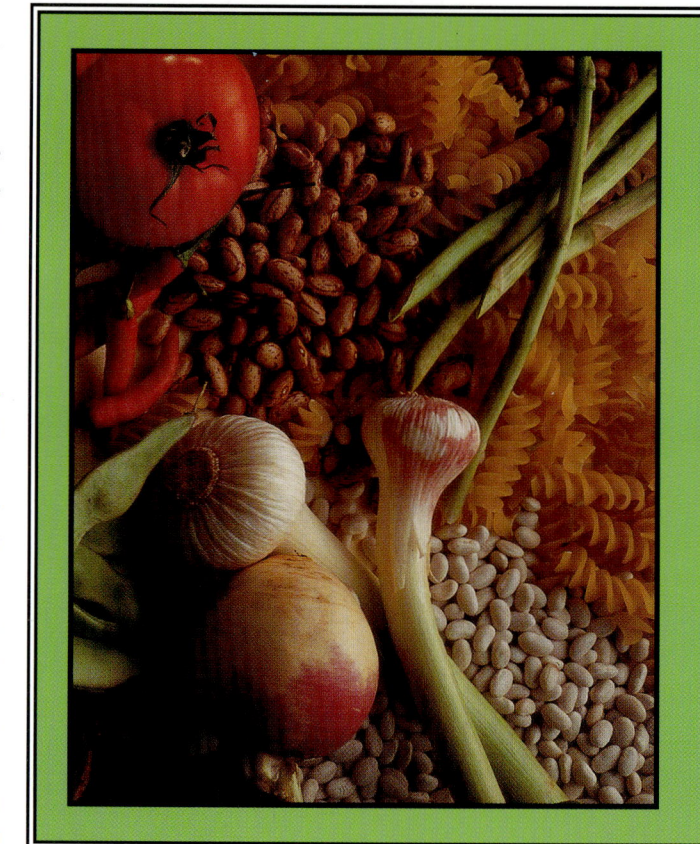

This occurs when some of the starch in legumes isn't fully digested and ferments in the lower bowel, producing gases. You can reduce this problem by changing the water in which you soak the legumes, and by cooking them well. You can also buy them pre-cooked in cans and vacuum-packed bags, ready to heat and add to your favourite recipe.

Tips for a Healthy Vegetarian Diet

- Regularly consume wholegrain foods from a wide variety of grains such as wheat, corn, barley, rice, oats and millet.
- Regularly consume a wide variety of fruits and vegetables — eat them raw and often.
- Regularly consume nuts and seeds — try them in salads, stir-fries, on cereal or in spreads.
- Regularly consume legumes and lentils, including tofu, baked beans, kidney beans, soy beans and chickpeas.
- Use low-fat milk or milk products — cow's, goat's, fortified soy or rice milk.
- Choose iron-fortified breads and cereals.
- Monitor the fat content of your diet.

If you are in doubt about your diet, get some advice from a dietitian or nutritionist.

vegetables. If you choose not to eat meat, you need to substitute lentils, beans, peas, nuts, tofu and tempeh, and use a variety of grains.

There are three main types of vegetarian diets:

1. Ovo-lacto vegetarians: those who eat eggs and dairy products but no meats, poultry or seafood.

2. Lacto vegetarians: those who will include dairy products but no meats, poultry, seafood or eggs.

3. Vegans: those who eat nothing of animal origin whatsoever.

Those choosing a vegan diet need to pay particular attention to good food choices. Animal foods are a vital source of vitamins B12 and B2, iron, zinc, calcium and iodine, and some essential fatty acids. In a vegan diet these must be found in plant-based foods. By choosing fortified soy milks, and fortified breakfast cereals and breads, and ensuring you include a wide variety of foods in your diet, this can be achieved — with the exception of vitamin B12, which may need to be supplemented. However, it's almost impossible for pregnant women and growing children to meet their nutritional requirements on a vegan diet. The high carbohydrate content of the diet may make it filling before all their nutrient needs have been met. Others who may be at risk of vitamin or mineral deficiencies include teenage girls and women on fad diets, athletes and pregnant women.

Some vegetarians choose dairy foods as a protein source with little thought to the fat content. A healthy vegetarian diet should be low in fat, especially saturated fat — you should choose fat-reduced dairy products and wholesome snacks.

Fats

Fats are a source of stored energy that have several important functions:

- as a carrier for the fat-soluble vitamins A, D, E and K;
- as a source of essential fatty acids — essential because they can't be made in the body; we can only get them from our food and they are essential to good health;
- they contribute to the pleasurable taste, texture and smell of food; and
- they provide essential protection for your internal organs.

To look good and stay energetic, a healthy body does need a certain amount of fat. In the first few years of life, dietary fat is an important source of energy. The problem is that people tend to eat too much fat, too often, leading to a poorly balanced diet and long-term health problems.

Have you heard the saying, 'eat too much fat and get fat'? Fat supplies twice as much energy as protein and carbohydrate foods and more than alcohol. However, the body isn't able to use this energy efficiently (your body prefers carbohydrates as an energy source) and it's readily stored as body fat if your total energy intake is greater than your body's requirement.

All Fats Aren't Equal in Health

High blood cholesterol appears to be one of the major risk factors in heart disease. Cholesterol is carried in the blood by 'lipoproteins'. Low-density lipoprotein (LDL) is the 'bad' cholesterol which blocks the arteries. High-density lipoprotein (HDL) is the 'good' cholesterol which has a protective effect against heart disease.

When you have your cholesterol checked, it's good to know these individual levels as well as your total cholesterol level to help you assess your risk of heart disease.

While all fats have some saturated, polyunsaturated and mono-unsaturated fat in them, they are classified according to which type is dominant. The type of fat you choose is important as these different fats have varying effects on your blood cholesterol.

Saturated Fats

These are usually found in animal foods — fatty meats, poultry skin, full-fat dairy products (milk, yoghurt, cheese, cream, butter) — and coconut and palm oil. It's the saturated fat hidden in processed foods — such as biscuits, crisps, cakes, quiche, pies and chocolate — that contributes a very large percentage of the fat in our diet. Saturated fats really are the bad guys; they raise the total blood cholesterol level, as well as the 'bad' cholesterol fraction that clogs up blood vessels and is associated with some cancers. Saturated fats should be severely restricted in your diet.

Unsaturated Fats

These can be broken down into polyunsaturated and mono-unsaturated fats.

Polyunsaturated fats

Are found in most vegetable oils and oily fish. They contain the following essential fatty acids:

1. Omega 6 fatty acids (from linoleic acid)

These are widely distributed in plant foods — safflower, sunflower, linseed (flaxseed), sesame seeds and soy beans; the seeds, oils and margarines containing these; legumes and raw nuts.

2. Omega 3 fatty acids (from linolenic acid).

These are found in abundance in cold-water fish — salmon, tuna, sardines, trout and mackerel — and in small amounts in linseed, canola and soy beans.

A balance between the Omega 3 and 6 fatty acids is important for good health. The Omega 3 fatty acids have many nutritional benefits for a healthy cardiovascular and immune system. The Australian diet tends to be higher in Omega 6 fatty acids through the consumption of margarines and vegetable oils. To correct this balance we should be eating more fish, seafood, linseed and soy products, and choosing olive and canola oils.

Try some of the wonderful new soy and linseed breads, or one of the many varieties of low-fat soy milks and yoghurts. Also try adding some marinated tofu to your stir-fry dishes. Look for the various flavoured tinned tunas and salmons to add to a pasta or spread on a bread roll. Include fish two to three times a week if possible.

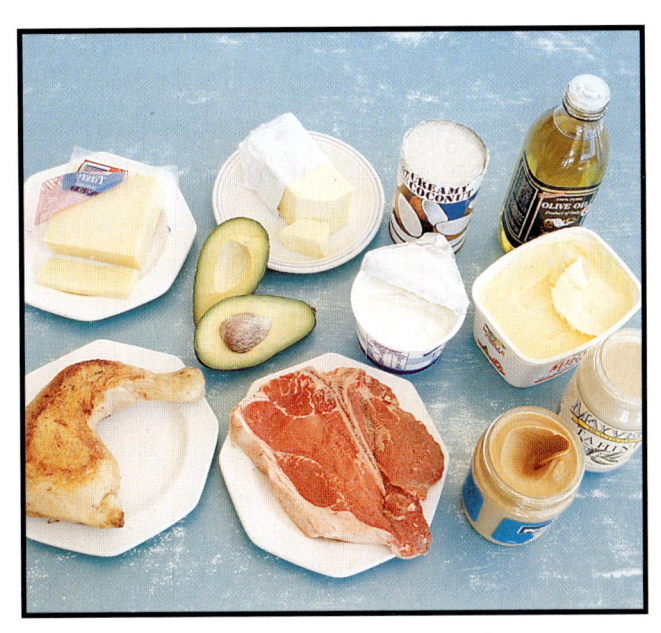

Can you spot the fats that are better for your health?

Mono-unsaturated fats

The main sources of mono-unsaturated fats are olive and canola oil, olives, avocados and most nuts. Both mono-unsaturated and polyunsaturated fats help to lower the total cholesterol level, lowering the 'bad' cholesterol without lowering the 'good' cholesterol.

Trans fats

There is also another type of fat — trans fatty acids. These are found naturally in meat, full-fat dairy products, and processed foods, and are also formed during the processing of vegetable oils. Trans fatty acids increase the 'bad' cholesterol and decrease the 'good' cholesterol. This is another reason to stay away from processed foods and to choose lean meats and low-fat dairy products.

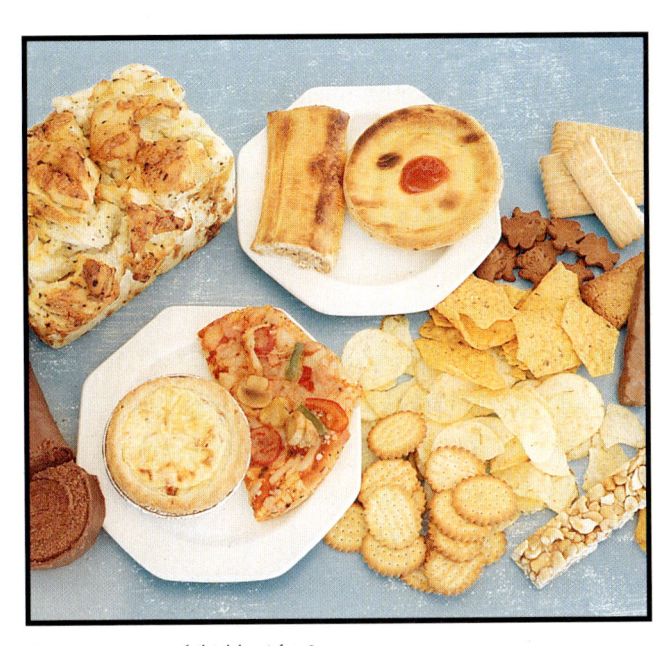

Are you aware of 'hidden' fats?

Fatty Hints

Here are some tips to help you reduce your fat intake:

- Try marinating meat before grilling or barbecuing; this is a much healthier alternative to adding a creamy sauce to cooked meat. When marinating, instead of reaching for the oil try using different herbs and spices — garlic and ginger are good choices. If you're stir-frying, cut the marinated meat into thin strips and cook quickly over a high heat to seal in the juices.
- Watch your serving sizes. As a rough guide, the portion of meat you eat should be no larger than the size of your palm.
- Choose fish, legumes or lentil dishes in place of red meat or poultry on a regular basis.
- Choose reduced-fat or low-fat milk products.
- Avoid foods containing coconut or palm oil, and vegetable oils of unknown origin.
- If you're a takeaway food freak or you eat out regularly, think about your choices. Stay away from the deep-fried, battered and mornay-type foods. Ask for interesting breads instead of chips, and have the dressings and sauces served separately so that you decide how much goes on.
- Learn to read food labels. Compare different brands of similar products for fat content. Aim for less than 7g fat per 100g.
- Be aware of advertising claims, such as the word 'lite'. Does it refer to the fat content? It could refer to the colour or taste (in olive oil), to the salt (in crisps), or to the sugar (in cakes).

> 'Most people end up digging their grave with their teeth.'
> — Anthony Robbins

Try some of these low-fat alternatives:

- **Milk, yoghurt** — use skim or reduced-fat varieties, and reduced-fat fortified soy milks.
- **Cream** — use evaporated skim milk, or ricotta cheese mixed with fat-reduced milk.
- **Sour cream** — use low-fat natural yoghurt, or buttermilk.
- **Cream cheese** — use baker's/continental cheese.
- **Cheese** — Save for adding taste to meals. Try a little Parmesan or Romano, which are strong in taste. On sandwiches, try cottage, ricotta or baker's cheese.
- **Oil** — use olive or canola oil. A non-stick pan is a good investment, as you won't need to use as much oil. Use a spray pack — this will stop you from 'splashing' in too much oil. Stir-fry in stock or wine as an alternative.
- **Dressings** — use 'oil-free' dressings. Try balsamic vinegar or lemon juice as a substitute. Make creamy dressings using low-fat yoghurt as a base.
- **Dips** — try low-fat natural yoghurt mixed with ricotta as a base, adding herbs and flavours as desired.
- **Pastry** — try filo pastry, brushing with water or low-fat milk every couple of layers.
- **Biscuits and cakes** — try using a lot less fat than a recipe requires. Fruit cakes, scones, pikelets and fruit-based muffins use much less fat than most cakes and biscuits.
- **Crisps/snacks** — try pretzels, home-made pita crisps or unbuttered popcorn.

Fats: Questions and Answers

Q: What kind of fat should I use?
A: You should cut down on all trans and saturated fats. For optimum health, mono-unsaturated fats are the best choice. Do without butter on your bread — use Gold N' Canola margarine, avocado, hommos, tahini or a nut butter instead. Choose either a cold-pressed virgin olive oil (also rich in phytochemicals) or canola oil on your salad or for cooking. Choose lean meats, use fat-reduced dairy foods, cut down on processed and snack foods, and avoid fatty takeaway foods. Remember, fats are fat and oils are fat. Whatever you choose, they all have the same high energy value and should be consumed in limited amounts.

Q: What's cholesterol?
A: Cholesterol is a white waxy substance (a natural steroid alcohol) that is found in our blood, tissues, bile and fat. Cholesterol in the blood can be produced by the liver or derived from animal foods that are high in fat, especially saturated fat.

Eggs, prawns, calamari and offal are high in cholesterol but don't have any real effect on blood cholesterol. Use in moderation.

By cutting down on saturated and trans fats you can reduce your cholesterol intake. Be aware that food labelled 'cholesterol free' doesn't necessarily mean it is free of saturated fat (for example, coconut milk) or 'fat free' (for example, margarine).

Q: How much fat should I have?
A: Going to the extreme of trying to eliminate fats and oils means your body will miss out on essential fatty acids, fat-soluble vitamins (especially vitamin E) and some minerals, especially iron and zinc.

Most women and children require between 35 and 60 grams of fat per day, while most men need between 50 and 70 grams. For a moderately active female who does aerobics three to five times a week and walks twice a week, fat consumption should be 50–60 grams of fat per day. A similarly active male should consume 60–70 grams of fat per day.

If you're trying to lose body fat, then around 30 grams (no less) of fat per day for women and 40 grams per day for men is recommended. Obviously, the more active you are, the higher your energy requirements are and the more fat you may need, but remember to choose the fats that are best for your health. Invest in a fat and fibre counter to keep track of how much fat you are consuming.

Q: Should I restrict fat in my children's diet?
A: It's important that you don't restrict the fat in the diets of children up to the age of five. Their growth demands are so high that it becomes difficult for them to get enough energy if fats are restricted. They also need the essential fatty acids for normal growth. Children up to the age of five should have full-fat milk products included in their diets.

Vitamins

Vitamins are essential to good health. Our bodies can not manufacture them so we need to get them from our food. Vitamins assist chemical reactions in the body; they help to release energy from food and act as disease-fighting antioxidants to make your blood and immune system healthy. Below is a guide to just some of the vitamins you should be including in your diet.

Vitamins for Vigour

Vitamin	Main functions	Good sources
A	■ Keeps your skin, eyesight and mucous membranes healthy. ■ Aids your immune system. ■ Acts as an antioxidant.	Liver, oily fish, butter, cheese, egg yolk, carrots, pumpkin, rockmelon, mango, paw-paw, broccoli, spinach.
B1 (thiamine)	■ Helps release energy from food. ■ Essential for carbohydrate food metabolism. ■ Used in normal function of heart and nervous system. ■ Maintains muscle tone.	Fortified breakfast cereals, some breads, liver, kidney, lean pork, nuts, dried peas, yeast, yeast extract.
B2 (riboflavin)	■ Helps release energy from food. ■ Helps keep your eyes and nervous system healthy.	Milk, yoghurt, cheese, egg whites, offal, green vegetables, fortified cereals, yeast extract.
B3 (niacin)	■ Essential for metabolism of carbohydrate, protein and fat. ■ Assists healthy growth. ■ Keeps your skin healthy.	Lean meat, fish, pulses, peanuts, fortified breakfast cereals, breads, eggs, milk.
B6 (pyridoxine)	■ Aids in metabolism of protein. ■ Helps your immune system. ■ Assists in the formation of red blood cells.	Lean meat, poultry, fish, liver, eggs, wholegrain breads, cereals, soy beans, nuts, yeast extract.
B12 (cyanocobalamin)	■ Assists in the formation of red blood cells (a lack of which can lead to anaemia). ■ Helps keep your nervous system healthy. ■ Aids in metabolism of folate.	Foods of animal origin: lean meats, poultry, fish, eggs, milk. Vegetarians need fortified soy milks to supply B12.

Vitamin	Main functions	Good sources
C (ascorbic acid)	■ Assists healthy growth, especially bones, teeth and gums. ■ Helps immune system. ■ Aids the absorption of iron.	Fruits and vegetables, especially citrus fruits, berries, kiwi fruit, pawpaw, broccoli, spinach, capsicum.
D (calciferous)	■ Needed for absorption of calcium and phosphorus for healthy bones and teeth.	Oily fish, fish liver oils, butter, cheese, fortified margarines, sunlight on your skin.
E (tocopherols)	■ Helps keep cell membranes and body tissue healthy. ■ Acts as an antioxidant.	Vegetable oils, unsaturated margarines, wheat germ, nuts and seeds.
K	■ Essential for normal blood clotting.	Green leafy vegetables: broccoli, brussels sprouts, cabbage; eggs, cheese.
Folic acid	■ Vital in the production of DNA. ■ Important in the formation of red blood cells (prevents anaemia). ■ Important before and during pregnancy to prevent the risk of neural tube defects.	Dark-green, leafy vegetables, liver, pulses, yeast wholegrain cereals. (Note: Folate is destroyed by cooking, so include some fresh green vegetables in your salads.)

How to Protect the 'Vitamin Value' in Food

The fresher the fruits and vegetables, the higher their vitamin content. There is some loss of nutrients in the freezing, canning and drying of foods, but the way in which fresh produce is stored and prepared will also affect their vitamin value. Don't cut up fruits or vegetables only to let them stand for a long time before cooking or consuming raw. Exposure to air destroys some vitamins. Try to avoid buying produce that has been pre-cut. Squeeze juice just before you drink it; don't squeeze a whole container of juice and leave it in the fridge — the vitamins will disappear. Lightly steam, stir-fry or microwave your vegies to reduce vitamin losses in cooking. Leave the skins on fruit and vegetables whenever possible, this is where the vitamins are richest.

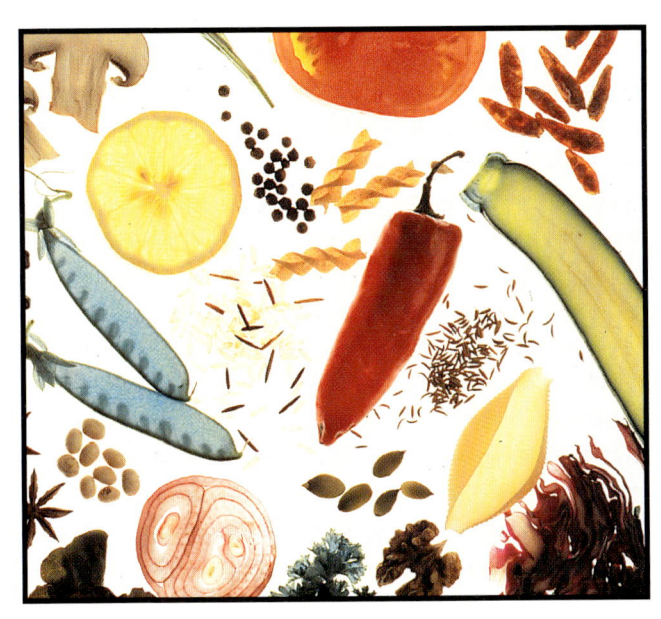

Natural foods are packed with essential vitamins.

Minerals

Minerals play an important role in healthy blood and bones, and in the proper functioning of your nerves and muscles. They also help enzymes in the production of energy.

There are at least 20 different minerals and trace elements needed for a healthy body. Minerals are important for healthy blood, strong bones, proper functioning of nerves and muscles, and in various chemical reactions. By choosing the right foods, you'll provide your body with enough of the minerals it needs. Below is a guide to just some of the minerals you should be including in your diet.

Minerals for Maintenance

Mineral	Main functions	Good sources
Calcium	■ Essential in the formation and maintenance of strong bones and teeth. ■ Important in nerve function. ■ Necessary for contraction and relaxation of muscles. Note: Excess protein, caffeine and salt in your diet will deplete calcium stores.	Milk and dairy products (such as yoghurt, cheese and milk), salmon, almonds, oranges, baked beans, broccoli. (Dairy foods are the best source of calcium. If you don't use dairy foods, try soy milk with added calcium.)
Copper	■ Is part of many enzymes. ■ Necessary for a healthy nervous system. ■ Helps iron in the formation of red blood cells. ■ Important for bone growth.	Shellfish (oysters, crab), liver, kidney, wholegrains, nuts, cocoa.
Fluorine	■ Helps build healthy bones and teeth. ■ Helps fight against tooth decay.	Toothpaste, fluoridated drinking water, tea.
Iodine	■ Necessary for normal function of thyroid gland.	Seafood, seaweed (sushi), iodised table salt.
Iron Note: Women and athletes especially need to watch their intake.	■ Necessary to carry oxygen in the blood from your lungs to all parts of the body. ■ Helps make oxygen available to your muscles for physical activity. ■ Triggers chemical reactions that release energy from food. ■ Essential for keeping your immune system in tip-top shape.	There are two types of iron in our food: 1. haem iron, which is found in flesh foods such as red meat, fish and poultry; and 2. non-haem iron, which is found in plant-based foods such as breads, cereals, green leafy vegetables, legumes and eggs. Non-haem iron is not as well absorbed by your body as haem iron.

Mineral	Main functions	Good sources
Magnesium	■ Helps build healthy bones and teeth. ■ Aids energy metabolism. ■ Important for muscle contraction. ■ Helps keep your nervous system healthy.	Present in a wide variety of foods, including green leafy vegetables, pulses, wholegrains, nuts, dried fruits.
Phosphorus	■ Works with calcium to build bones and teeth and keep them healthy. ■ Helps B group vitamins release energy from cells. ■ Helps absorption of other nutrients.	Lean meat and poultry, fish, milk, cheese, wholegrains, nuts, seeds.
Potassium	■ Helps sodium maintain fluid balance. ■ Helps normal heart function and blood pressure. ■ Essential for a healthy nervous system.	Fresh fruit, especially bananas, citrus fruits and avocados; nuts, dried fruits, raw vegetables.
Selenium	■ Associated with vitamin E as an antioxidant.	Lean meats, fish, milk, avocados, vegetables (although, depends on selenium content of soil)
Sodium	■ Helps potassium maintain fluid balance. ■ Essential for a healthy nervous system. ■ Important for muscle function.	Table and cooking salt, processed meats, yeast extract.
Zinc	■ Essential for normal growth, reproduction and overall good health. ■ Aids the immune system. ■ Vital to our sense of taste. ■ Part of many enzymes and insulin. ■ Helps the body make protein and use carbohydrates efficiently.	Fish, oysters, lean meats, poultry, milk, wholegrain cereals and breads, nuts. As with iron, zinc is better absorbed from animal sources.

As you can see, there are many minerals that are essential for maintaining good health, but some deserve special mention.

Calcium

Osteoporosis is a condition where bones lose calcium, and become brittle and break more easily. It's a bigger concern for women than men, but both men and women lose calcium from their bones as they age. Those that need to pay particular attention to their calcium intake include pregnant and breastfeeding mums, children and adolescents, post-menopausal women, vegetarians and young females — especially those who do regular strenuous exercise and carry little body fat, and those who follow strict diets.

'There is only one success — to be able to spend your life in your own way.'
— Christopher Morley

Check out the good sources of calcium in the Minerals for Maintenance chart. If you fall into any of the above groups, include at least three serves from the milk product choices outlined in Steps to Healthy Eating on page 84.

Iron

Iron is needed in the blood to get oxygen to your working muscles. If your iron levels are low, you'll feel very tired and your exercise performance will suffer. Iron deficiency is common in women, particularly those who exercise a lot and may restrict their food choices. Meat is the best dietary source of iron because it contains haem iron which is the most readily absorbed form of iron. Check out other good sources of iron in the Minerals for Maintenance chart. Choosing a vitamin-C rich food with your iron source will significantly enhance the absorption of iron.

Do You Need a Vitamin or Mineral Supplement?

If you eat a healthy, well-balanced diet, you should get all the vitamins you need from your food. However, there are times when our vitamin needs are higher — during illness, stress and lifestyle changes — and certain groups of people for whom a supplement may be useful. For example, women are usually advised to take a folate supplement if planning a pregnancy and an iron and folate supplement to meet increased needs during pregnancy. Others at risk of developing a vitamin deficiency include heavy drinkers and smokers, the elderly, children and teenagers on fad or crash diets, and vegans. There is some evidence to suggest a vitamin E supplement may protect against certain cancers and heart disease.

No amount of vitamin or mineral supplements will compensate for a poor diet. In their natural form, vitamins and minerals act with other nutrients to increase their efficiency. This chemical balance can be upset by larger doses of one or more vitamins or minerals, decreasing the absorption of others or causing toxic levels in the body.

So, before you rush out to buy a supplement, look carefully at your diet. If you think you are at risk, seek advice from a nutritionist.

Antioxidants

Antioxidants occur naturally in plant foods, especially in the skin and juice of fruits and vegetables. We also find them in wine and tea. Antioxidants help boost the immune system and mop up 'free radicals' which can damage body cells. (Free radicals are produced in the body, but levels are also increased by exposure to pollution, smoking and sunlight.)

There are many known antioxidants, including vitamins A, C and E, zinc and selenium. We don't really know exactly how these antioxidants work in the body but we do know that the interaction between all of them is important in preventing disease.

By including plenty of fruits and vegetables, wholegrains, nuts and seeds in a varied diet, you'll get a good balance of antioxidants for better health.

Food for Life

Water

Water constitutes approximately 62 per cent of the body (69 per cent for children); it's one of the body's most essential nutrients. After oxygen, water is the nutrient we need most to keep us alive. You could last several weeks without food, but your body could only go a few days without water.

Water is involved in the digestive process and the elimination of waste products. Water transports nutrients to the cells and tissues, lubricating joints and eyes, and helping to regulate body temperature. It also plays an essential role in keeping your bodily functions at their peak.

Dehydration

When your body tissues don't have enough water to function efficiently, you enter a state of dehydration. This can lead to headaches, fatigue, poor concentration, constipation, irritability and bad breath.

Do I hear you say: 'But I always drink when I'm thirsty'? Thirst is a poor indicator of your fluid needs. By the time you begin to feel thirsty you've already started to become dehydrated. Don't wait until you're thirsty — drink regularly throughout the day.

Children are much more susceptible to dehydration than adults. They sweat less efficiently than adults and are therefore at greater risk of overheating during exercise or in hot weather. Often they are preoccupied and too busy to think of drinking until they are thirsty. Encourage them to drink regularly, especially before, during and after exercise.

Water is the cheapest and most readily available fluid source. Acceptable alternatives are a sports drink, fruit juice or diluted cordial. Steer away from soft drinks as a fluid source, as they are high in sugar and not good fuel replacers.

Tips to Keep You Hydrated

Get into the habit of having a glass of water on waking and half an hour before each meal.

- Try drinking a glass of water while the jug is boiling for a cup of tea or coffee.
- If you're enjoying some wine, beer or spirits, remember to drink plenty of water. Have a glass of water in between drinks.
- Remember to drink plenty of water in winter too, as internal heating at home or in your workplace will dehydrate you.
- Freeze a bottle of water and put it in your car to have while you're on the run during the day.
- Keep a bottle of water on your desk at work or in class to sip regularly. Try setting yourself a routine — for example, drink on the hour.
- Always keep a jug of water in the fridge. Try adding lemon or mint for flavour.

Strong tea, coffee, cola drinks and alcohol are diuretics — that is, they increase the flow of urine, causing the body to lose fluid. Enjoy them for flavour and pleasure, but remember to replenish your body's fluids with liquids that hydrate. Aim to consume at least 1.5 litres of caffeine-free fluids each day — more if you exercise or if it's hot.

Alcohol

Alcohol is a concentrated source of energy that can contribute significantly to your total energy intake. When alcohol is consumed, it's readily absorbed in preference to other nutrients, which means less dietary fat is used for energy. So, if you're fit and healthy and happy with your body, enjoy a glass of wine with your meal if you wish, but if you are trying to lose body fat you'll need to be more conscientious. The more kilojoules you consume in alcohol, the more fat kilojoules there are available to be stored as body fat.

Drink	Cals	Kj
Beer 375ml can/stubbie		
Regular (4–5% alcohol)	134	563
Reduced alcohol (3.3% alcohol)	94	394
Lite (0.9% alcohol)	39	161
Wine		
250ml (standard glass)	85	355
Champagne		
250ml (standard glass)	77	324
Spirits		
whisky, rum, gin		
1 nip (30ml)	60	252
Port		
(60ml)	89	374

Which water should I drink?

In recent years the marketplace has been flooded with bottled water, water coolers and water filters. It's great to see so many businesses with water coolers for staff and customers/clients — sometimes the sight of one reminds you that you're thirsty or need a drink. With all these water products available, many people are wondering if they should still drink tap-water.

In Australia, town water is checked regularly by the local authorities for contamination, so it's safe to drink. You may not like the taste, or you may be concerned about chemicals in tap-water and prefer to use bottled or filtered water. The point is, you have a choice.

If you're more likely to drink water when it's bottled or filtered, then make that choice. If you drink filtered water, clean your filter on a regular basis and replace it when necessary. If you're travelling in countries where the water may be contaminated, it's sensible to use bottled water for both drinking and cleaning your teeth to reduce the risk of illness.

Fibre

Dietary fibre is that part of plant foods that isn't digested by the enzymes in your gut. It's found in cereals, breads, grains, legumes, fruit and vegetables, seeds and nuts. Fibre aids digestion; keeps your gut happy, healthy and regular; helps lower blood cholesterol; and helps reduce the risk of some cancers. A diet high in fibre is important to help control weight — high-fibre foods are filling and satisfying, so choosing these will help prevent overeating.

There are two types of dietary fibre: soluble and insoluble.

1. Soluble fibre dissolves in water and forms a gel, adding to faecal bulk and keeping it soft. Soluble fibre can help lower cholesterol, regulate blood sugar levels and aid in the prevention of bowel cancer. It is found in oats and oat bran, barley, legumes, breads, most fruits — especially apples and citrus fruits — vegetables and linseeds.

2. Insoluble fibre helps keep your gut regular and healthy. It helps prevent constipation and speeds up the transit time of our stools — this is important as it minimises the time any bad chemicals may stay inside your body. It is found in wholegrain breads and cereals, bran, nuts, seeds, some fruits (especially in their skins) and vegetables.

To keep you healthy on the inside, it's important to include a range of high-fibre foods in your diet to ensure you get enough of both soluble and insoluble fibre. You need at least 30 grams (in total) per day. If you need to bolster your fibre intake:

- choose wholegrain or bran-based cereal, or sprinkle bran on top of your regular cereal;
- substitute beans and lentils for meat on a regular basis;
- choose raw fruit (eat their skins, if edible); instead of juice, try dried fruit; and
- include fresh vegetables in your diet frequently, especially corn, peas, cabbage, broccoli and cauliflower.

If you need to increase the fibre in your diet, do so gradually or you may find your gut won't react kindly. It's always important to consume plenty of fluids and this is especially important if your diet is high in fibre.

Check out the fibre content on the labels of your favourite breakfast cereals and breads. Use the chart below to choose fibre-rich foods to help you reach your 30+ grams fibre target per day:

Suggested food	Fibre content (in grams)	Suggested food	Fibre content (in grams)
1 cup of white rice (cooked)	1.8	1 cup regular pasta (cooked)	2.8
1 cup brown rice (cooked)	3.0	1 cup wholemeal pasta (cooked)	8.5
1 small potato (peeled)	1.0	1/2 cup of corn	2.0
1 small potato (skin on)	1.5	1 medium carrot	4.0
1 kiwi fruit	3.0	1 medium apple	3.0
3/4 cup baked beans	10.5	an average serve of broccoli	4.0
lentil burger patty	7.0	50 grams of nuts	3.5

Great Foods to Eat Regularly

Bananas: Great for the active, busy person. Readily packaged, they're full of carbohydrate and potassium and rich in magnesium, which helps you deal with stress.

Lean beef: A good source of iron-rich protein. Avoiding red meats may lead to iron deficiency and fatigue.

Broccoli: Along with cabbage, cauliflower, brussels sprouts, capsicum and turnips, broccoli contains some powerful anti-cancer properties. Full of vitamins A, C, folate and riboflavin.

Carrots: The best source of vitamin A, an immunity enhancer. Carrot juice has an excellent balance of vitamins and minerals.

Chilli: Capsaicin in chilli gives it the 'fire'. It stimulates your metabolic rate and endorphins, the 'feel good' hormones, and is a great source of vitamin C. Red chilli is a good source of beta-carotene (used to make vitamin A).

Citrus fruits: Oranges, grapefruits and mandarins are great sources of vitamin C, folate and thiamine. It's best to eat the fruits themselves, rather than their juices, because the membranes contain fibre and antioxidants.

Fish: A valuable source of Omega-3 fatty acids which are important in fighting heart disease, and for relief from rheumatoid arthritis and possibly asthma. Fresh, canned or smoked, you should eat fish at least three times a week. Herring, mullet, trout, salmon, tuna, mackerel and sardines are richest in Omega-3. Fish is also a good source of zinc and iron.

Phytochemicals

Phytochemicals are naturally occurring chemicals found in plant foods, which play a significant part in maintaining good health. They are found in fruits and vegetables, nuts and seeds, whole cereals, oats, legumes, herbs, olive oil, wine and tea. Choose well-coloured fruits and vegetables. These are richer in phytochemicals.

Phytoestrogens are a type of phytochemical, found in soy products and linseeds. We don't yet know the full effects of phytoestrogens on our

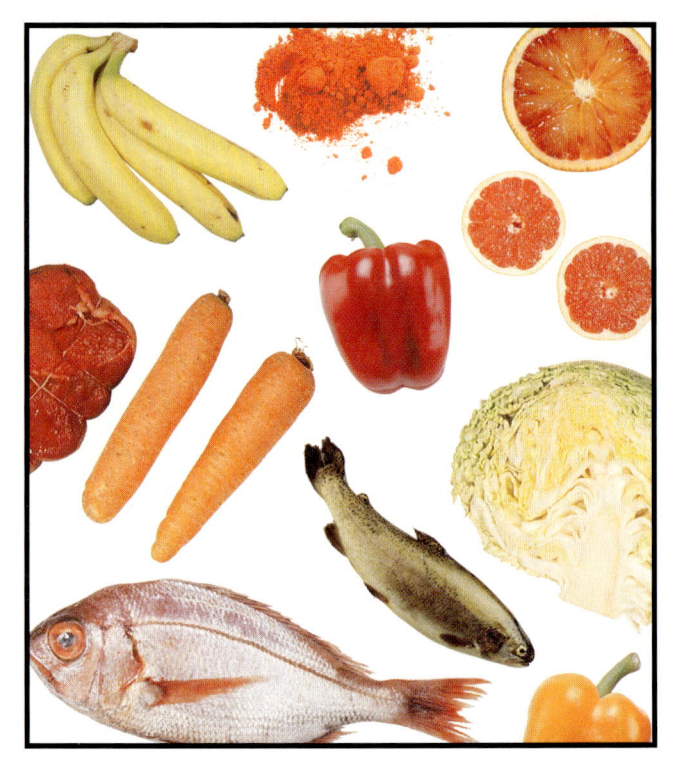

Food for Life

bodies, but studies have shown they may help with the symptoms of menopause, help protect against some cancers, help reduce cholesterol and protect against osteoporosis.

By regularly including soy products — fat-reduced soy milk and yoghurt, tofu, tempeh, soy beans, miso and the soy and linseed breads and cereals that are now available — along with legumes, fruits and vegetables, and plenty of herbs and spices, you will boost your phytochemical intake, a step towards optimum health. There is no one 'miracle food' — you should enjoy a wide variety of foods in moderation.

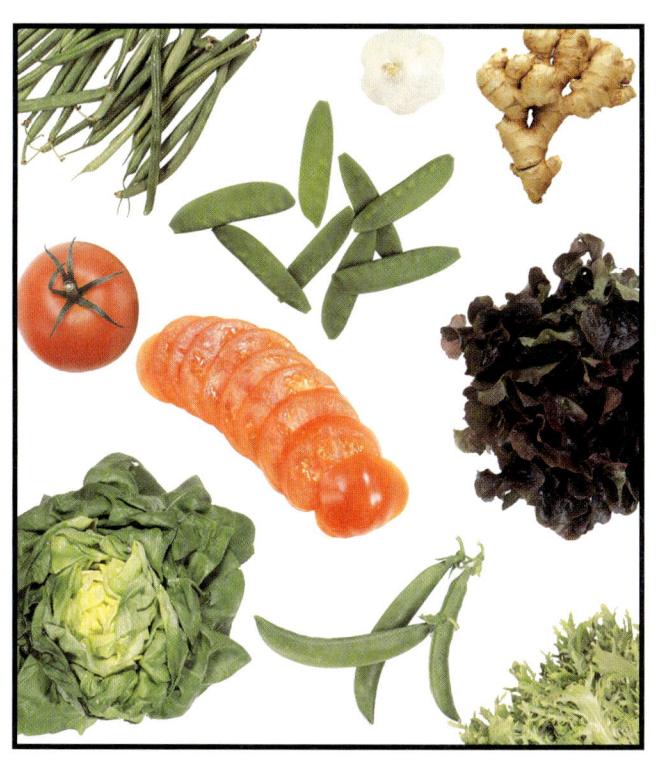

Garlic and ginger: Garlic has long been used to treat colds and flu and ginger is known to help digestion. Both have powerful antioxidant properties and should be used regularly for both taste and health.

Green leafy vegetables: Spinach, Chinese greens, snow peas, rocket, endive, etc. are all packed with nutrients like vitamins B and C, beta-carotene, folate, magnesium, and lots of minerals and fibre.

Oats: Full of carbohydrate for energy. Rich in soluble fibre for a healthy gut, lowering cholesterol and keeping blood sugar levels stable.

Soy beans: A vital source of protein and iron for vegetarians. Full of fibre, B group vitamins and magnesium. Soy contains natural oestrogen and when eaten regularly as beans, tofu, miso or soy milk, it may help with the symptoms of menopause.

Tomato: Besides being rich in vitamin C, tomatoes contain the antioxidant lycopene (related to vitamin A), carotene, salicylic acid — a natural aspirin — and folate.

Yoghurt: A good source of calcium and protein, and healthy bacteria that helps to keep your gut happy and healthy. Choose reduced-fat varieties with added *lactobacillus* bacteria. Some people who are lactose intolerant may be able to tolerate yoghurt.

■ ■ ■

Now that you have a better understanding of what's in the food you are eating, make a conscious effort to be aware of what you are putting in your mouth. In the next chapter, you will look closely at your own diet and see what changes you need to make to ensure that you are eating well.

Food for Health

You will often hear people telling you to make sure you eat a balanced diet. But what does this actually mean? This chapter will give you a comprehensive overview of what a balanced diet is — focusing on the main food groups and the three keys to a healthy diet: balance, variety and moderation. We will then take a close look at your own eating habits and discover what food groups you may be neglecting. We will also discuss the difference between 'diets' and a balanced diet.

A Balanced Diet

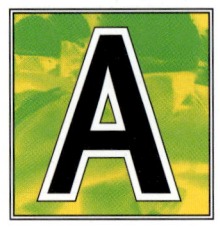

A balanced diet is one that provides your body with all the nutrients — carbohydrates, protein, fats, vitamins and minerals — as well as adequate water and fibre. It should also supply you with a sufficient amount of energy (kilojoules) to fuel your body.

Balance, Variety and Moderation

The keys to a healthy diet are balance, variety and moderation.

Balance

If you consider what you eat in a day, you'll probably find that over half of your food choices come from meat and meat alternatives, milk products and fats, with breads, grains and cereals, and fruit and vegetables running a poor second. This is not a well-balanced diet. For better health, the balance needs to swing in favour of the plant-based foods — which are low in fat, full of energy-giving carbohydrate, high in fibre and rich in phytochemicals. On a well-balanced plate, lean meat (or a meat alternative) should constitute about 25 per cent of your meal, with the remainder being made up of vegetables, grain foods (pasta, rice, bread, etc) or fruit.

Variety

Aside from breastmilk, there is no one food that provides our bodies with all its needs. Many people think that if they eat fruit and vegetables, breads and cereals, meat, fish and milk products they are giving themselves a variety of foods. However, often their choices within these groups are quite limited.

All foods contain different amounts of nutrients — for example, citrus fruits are rich in vitamin C but not in vitamin E; plant-based foods vary in the phytochemicals they contain; and different forms of fibre affect your body in different ways. For best health and protection against disease, you need to include a variety of foods to ensure you get the healthy balance your body needs.

Look at the variety of foods in your diet. Include a variety of grains — wheat, oats, barley and rye — and try some of the interesting grain breads that are available. Look at your protein choices. Do you include fish regularly, or lentils? Do you eat a wide variety of vegetables? There are around 50 different types available at any one time in the fresh food section of most supermarkets. Eating a variety of foods from the various food groups will ensure that you get a good mixture of all the nutrients you need.

Moderation

A healthy, well-balanced diet means you are eating enough nutritious food to give your body the energy and nutrients it needs. If you are maintaining a healthy weight for your body, then you are probably eating the right amount of food (although this doesn't mean you are necessarily eating a well-balanced diet).

Eating should be a pleasurable and sociable part of life. Unfortunately, too many people eat too much too often. Many people eat beyond hunger through boredom, loneliness, unhappiness, etc.

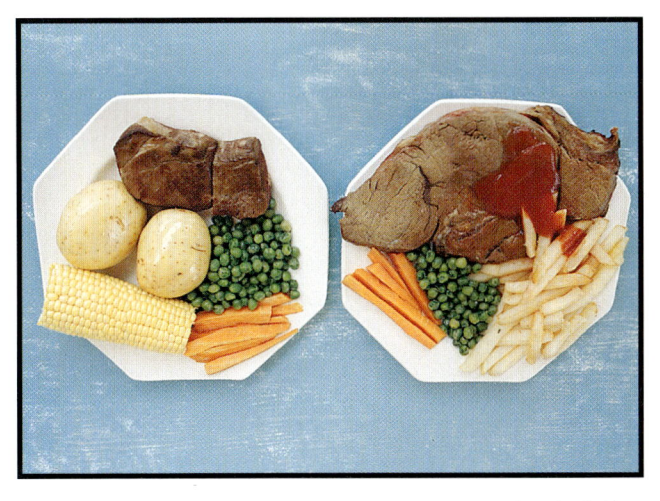

Check the balance of the meals you eat. Does your plate look like the well-balanced plate on the left?

Enjoy the less healthy foods occasionally, but don't binge. Many people claim they have a sweet tooth and can't live without their 'sugar fix'. Try cutting down on the sugar you add to tea and coffee, and halve the amount of cakes and biscuits you consume each week. After a few weeks you'll surprise yourself: you'll probably find some of your favourite foods too sweet, or that you can only manage a tiny piece of cake.

Learn to enjoy the natural sweetness of fruit and vegetables (try fresh carrots, pumpkin, peas and corn). Save the chocolates for special times and then choose the very best. Go for quality, not quantity.

You may have a 'fat tooth' — in other words, you're always reaching for the chips, pies, cheese, nuts, cream buns and the like. Try cutting down your choices of these by half each week. If you use full-cream dairy products, try fat-reduced products instead. Also try to limit your salt intake — try herbs and spices to add flavour.

These are all *learned* tastes. So, learn to use much less and enjoy the real flavour of healthy food.

Food for Health

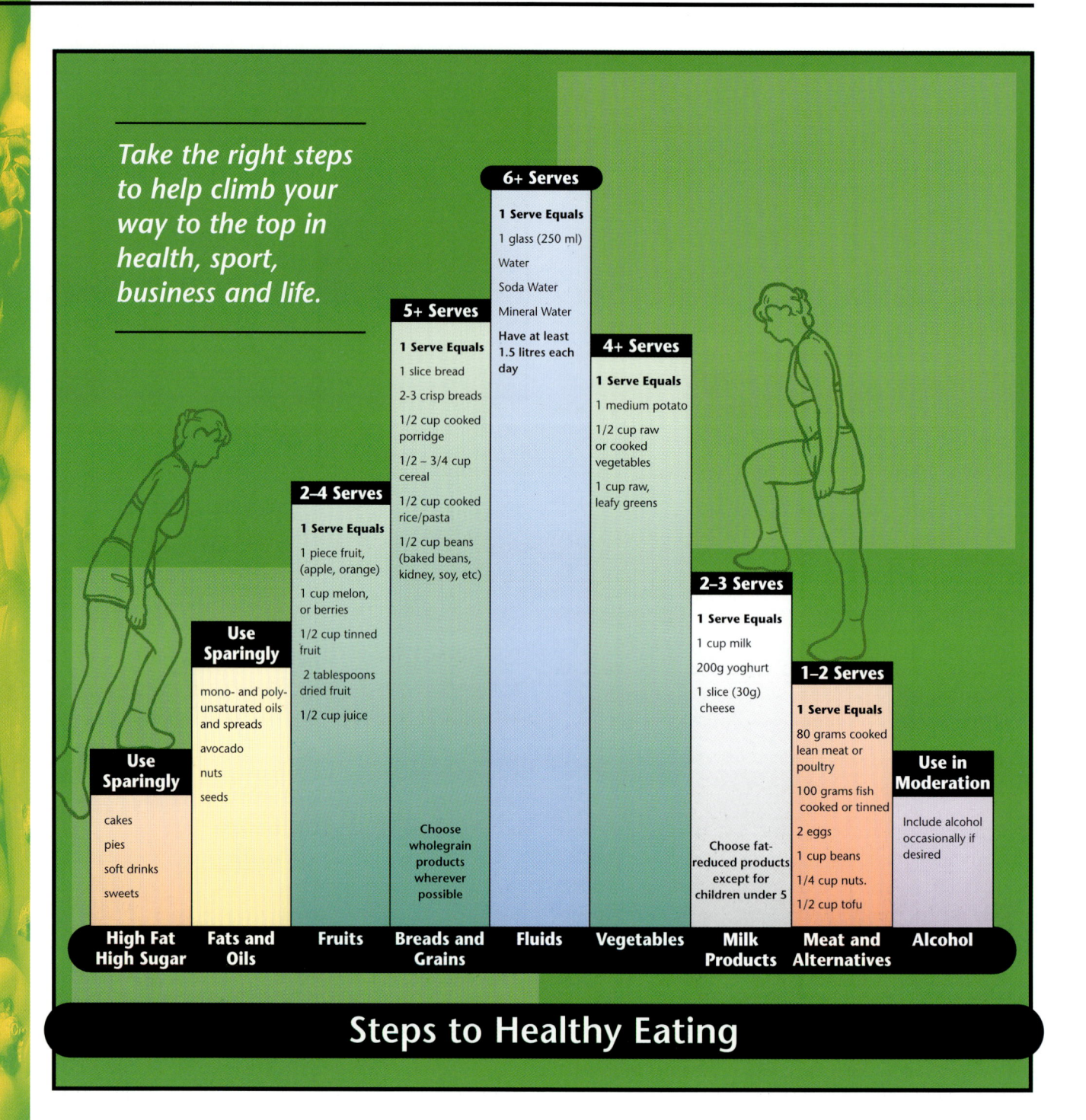

Take the right steps to help climb your way to the top in health, sport, business and life.

Steps to Healthy Eating

High Fat / High Sugar — Use Sparingly
- cakes
- pies
- soft drinks
- sweets

Fats and Oils — Use Sparingly
- mono- and poly-unsaturated oils and spreads
- avocado
- nuts
- seeds

Fruits — 2–4 Serves
1 Serve Equals
- 1 piece fruit, (apple, orange)
- 1 cup melon, or berries
- 1/2 cup tinned fruit
- 2 tablespoons dried fruit
- 1/2 cup juice

Breads and Grains — 5+ Serves
1 Serve Equals
- 1 slice bread
- 2-3 crisp breads
- 1/2 cup cooked porridge
- 1/2 – 3/4 cup cereal
- 1/2 cup cooked rice/pasta
- 1/2 cup beans (baked beans, kidney, soy, etc)

Choose wholegrain products wherever possible

Fluids — 6+ Serves
1 Serve Equals
- 1 glass (250 ml)
- Water
- Soda Water
- Mineral Water

Have at least 1.5 litres each day

Vegetables — 4+ Serves
1 Serve Equals
- 1 medium potato
- 1/2 cup raw or cooked vegetables
- 1 cup raw, leafy greens

Milk Products — 2–3 Serves
1 Serve Equals
- 1 cup milk
- 200g yoghurt
- 1 slice (30g) cheese

Choose fat-reduced products except for children under 5

Meat and Alternatives — 1–2 Serves
1 Serve Equals
- 80 grams cooked lean meat or poultry
- 100 grams fish cooked or tinned
- 2 eggs
- 1 cup beans
- 1/4 cup nuts.
- 1/2 cup tofu

Alcohol — Use in Moderation
Include alcohol occasionally if desired

Get UP&GO!

Your Diet

Now that you have a good understanding of what nutrients are contained in the foods you eat and what a balanced diet should include, it's time to examine your current diet. Keeping a food and fluid diary will allow you to take a close look at your eating patterns and establish whether or not your diet is well-balanced. You should try to keep your diary for at least a week so that you can see a pattern in your eating habits.

Write down *everything* that goes into your mouth at *the time* it goes in. Also keep a record of the *amounts* of food and drink that you consume, and how it's *prepared* eg fried, barbecued.

Keeping the diary requires you to understand what type of food you are eating. If you're not sure what food group something falls into, refer to Steps to Healthy Eating on page 84. Some foods will fit into more than one group — for example, a creamy carbonara sauce contains cream (fat), cheese, and some meat (bacon) and is served with pasta.

Let's look at a couple of examples to get you started.

Consider this Sample of a Day's Food and Fluid Intake:

Breakfast:
1 bowl of wholegrain cereal with low-fat milk, and banana sliced on top.
1 cup of weak black tea.

Morning tea:
2 pikelets with jam, no butter.
1 cup of white coffee.

Lunch:
1 small wholemeal pocket bread spread with avocado and filled with salad vegies, bean sprouts and low-fat cheese.
1 apple.

Afternoon tea:
1 tub low-fat fruit yoghurt.

Dinner:
Bowl of stir-fried Hokkien noodles with sliced lean beef, snow peas, broccoli, capsicum, mushrooms, water chestnuts, a few cashews, garlic and ginger (stir-fried with a little olive oil and balsamic vinegar).
1 glass of wine. 1 cup of herb tea.

Other snacks:
5 glasses water, 1 can mineral water, 3 rice crackers, handful of dried fruit.

This diet has provided:

- 7 servings of breads/cereals/grains;
- 5 servings of vegetables;
- 3 servings of fruit;
- 3 servings of milk products;
- 2 servings of meat;
- 2 servings of fats and oils;
- 1 serving of sugary carbohydrate; and
- adequate fluid and fibre.

This is a healthy and balanced daily intake.

These meals and snacks could be broken down into the following categories and recorded in your diary as follows on page 86:

Food for Health

Food and Fluid Diary

| | Fluids | Nutritious carbohydrates ||| Milk and milk products | Meat and meat alternatives | Fats and oils | Sugar | High-fat carbohydrates | Other (including alcohol) | Fibre |
		Breads, cereals and grains	Vegetables	Fruits							
Breakfast											
wholegrain cereal		1									x
low-fat milk	150 ml				½						
banana				1							x
weak black tea	180 ml									x	
Morning tea											
2 pikelets		1									
jam								1			
white coffee	—				½					x	
Lunch											
pocket bread		2									x
low-fat cheese					1						
avocado			½				1				
bean sprouts			½			½					x
salad			1								x
apple				1							x
Afternoon tea											
low-fat fruit yoghurt					1						
Dinner											
noodles		2									
lean beef						1					
vegetables (lots)			3								x
oil and vinegar							1				
nuts						½	1				x
wine	—									x	
herb tea	150 ml										
Other snacks											
water/mineral water	1.6 ltrs										
rice crackers		1									
dried fruit				1							x
Total	2.1 ltrs	7	5	3	3	2	3	1	—	3	9

Example of a balanced day's eating. Draw up your own food and fluid diary (copy blank chart on page 88) and fill in for 7–10 days.

Get UP&GO!

Here is Another Example:

The following example is not a well-balanced diet. Too many high-fat carbohydrate foods are chosen, and more fresh fruit should be included. The fluid intake may appear adequate but the choices are poor. For example, coffee, strong tea, cola drinks and alcohol help dehydrate your body. For every alcoholic or caffeine-based drink you need to drink an extra glass of water.

Breakfast:
1 bowl of wholegrain cereal with full-cream milk, tinned peaches.
1 slice white toast, buttered, with honey.
1 coffee with milk.

Morning tea:
1 black tea.

Lunch:
Hamburger on buttered wholemeal roll with onions and salad.
1 vanilla slice.
1 Coke.

Afternoon tea:
1 coffee with milk.
2 sweet biscuits.

Dinner:
Large steak, chips, and salad with a creamy dressing. Large bowl of ice-cream.
1 glass wine.

Other snacks:
1 beer.
1 black tea.
2 chocolate biscuits.
2 glasses water.

So, let's break this day down, too.
This diet has provided:
- 4 servings of breads/cereals/grains;
- 5 servings of vegetables;
- 1 serving of fruit;
- 3 servings of milk products;
- 4 servings of meat;
- 4 servings of fats and oils;
- 7 servings of high-fat carbohydrates; and inadequate fluid and fibre.

Your Food and Fluid Diary

Copy the chart on page 88 to create your own food and fluid diary so you can take a close look at your diet. For this exercise to be worthwhile, ensure that you eat normally — don't change your diet just because it's on record!

You can take this exercise as far as you like. If you have a thorough understanding of food and its nutrients, you might like to keep a diary that includes the main categories of nutrients to see if you are including enough carbohydrate, protein, etc. Or you might like to look at adding special categories that relate to special needs. For example, girls, women, athletes and pregnant women, in particular, might like to monitor their iron consumption to see if they are gaining an adequate supply from their current diet. Adolescents and pregnant women might like to check that they are including enough calcium and protein in their diets. If you know your body has special needs, include an extra column or columns in your diary to monitor these needs.

Food for Health

Your Food and Fluid Diary – Date:

	Fluids	Nutritious carbohydrates				Meat and meat alternatives	Fats and oils	Sugar	High-fat carbohydrates	Other (including alcohol)	Fibre
		Breads, cereals and grains	Vegetables	Fruits	Milk and milk products						
Breakfast											
Morning tea											
Lunch											
Afternoon tea											
Dinner											
Other snacks											
Total											

Food & Nutrition

Get **UP&GO!**

Food for Health

'Diets' Versus a Balanced Diet

The word 'diet' is derived from the Greek word 'diata', which means 'way of life'. Unfortunately, most people think of a diet as something they 'go on' to lose weight, which implies restricting the variety and amount of food you eat, limiting social eating pleasures and testing your willpower — not something you can make a way of life.

Most diets work on the principle of weight loss rather than fat loss. When food intake is severely restricted, your body reacts by losing weight. Weight lost quickly consists of roughly half muscle and water, and half fat. This results in a slower metabolic rate, so once you start eating normally again, your body actually uses less energy and the excess is stored as fat.

There's no magic formula for successfully losing body fat. If you've been on the diet merry-go-round for years, you'll probably know this already. Losing body fat and keeping it off isn't about dieting. It's about adopting healthy, long-term eating habits — a diet that's based on balance, variety and moderation — and becoming a more active person. The first steps you can take are reducing the amount of fat you eat and becoming more active. Fat loss is much slower than weight loss (around 0.5–1 kilogram per month) and the loss may not even show on the scales if you are exercising and developing muscle. A changing body shape is often the best guide to successful body-fat loss.

In a nutshell, you need to look at making long-term changes to the way you think about food, fitness and life:

- Improve your day-to-day eating habits and reduce the fat in your diet.
- Become an active person — increase the amount of time you spend on general activity in a day.
- Be committed to change. Habits can't be changed in a week — after all, you've probably been doing things in a certain way for years. To change habits, you need to change your attitude.
- Include regular exercise that you enjoy.
- Always set yourself realistic goals.
- Be patient. By reducing the fat in your diet and eating more carbohydrates you'll achieve a slower but more permanent decrease in body fat. A weight loss of around 1.0 kilogram per month is realistic and sustainable. Even a total loss of 6 to 8 kilograms over a year can improve your metabolism and reduce the risk of health problems.

The key to looking trim, taut and terrific is to set yourself realistic goals for better food choices. Make changes to your lifestyle that will help you to eat a healthy balanced diet and allow you the time to commit to regular exercise while enjoying these changes along the way.

Is Your Diet Balanced?

When you have written in your food and fluid diary for a week, sit down and examine your eating habits. Was your diet well-balanced over the week? Did you have the required number of serves each day? Did you neglect a particular food group?

> 'For overweight people, food is a major event. For healthy, trim people, food is something they eat when they're hungry.'
> — Dr. John Tickell

Also consider the time of day you are consuming most of your food. Are you having a good breakfast and lunch and a light dinner, or are you concentrating your food intake late in the day, or straight after an exercise session?

Did your week become 'bad' halfway through, or at the weekend? Who are you with when you eat — family, friends, alone? Does this affect the type of food you eat or the amount? Also consider the amount of time you allow yourself to eat. Do you eat on the run? Do you grab high-fat, high-sugar snacks? How stressed were you throughout the week? Did stress have an impact on your diet?

Are you considering balance, variety and moderation in your diet?

Remember, an indulgent meal out on a Saturday night accounts for less than five per cent of your weekly food intake. It's what you do *most* of the time that determines how well you eat. So, when asking yourself the above questions, look at your eating pattern over a week or a longer period of time, not just for one day. With your increased knowledge, you can now make changes to ensure your diet is well-balanced.

Once you've studied your diary to see where changes need to be made, continue to keep a record of your food intake for a while, and then relate it to your energy levels and exercise performance.

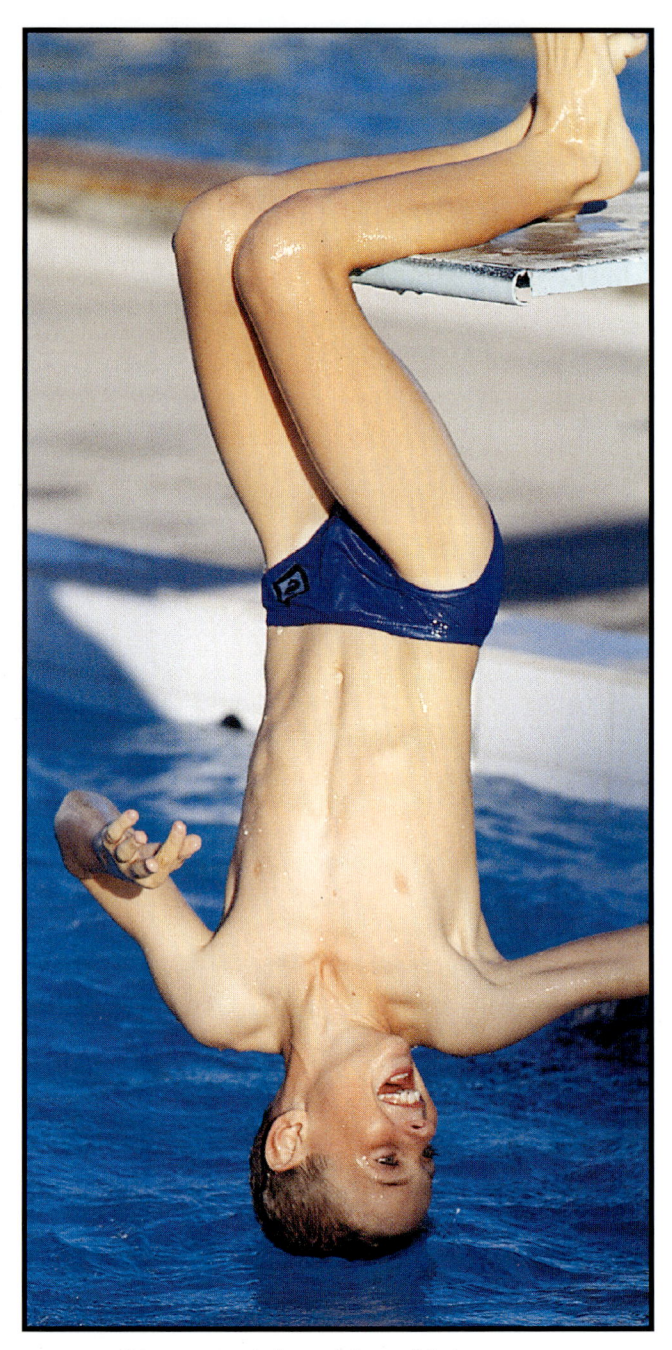

However old you are, a balanced diet will help you enjoy an active lifestyle.

Food for an Active Lifestyle

Whether you exercise to keep fit or you compete at an amateur or professional level, the basic principles of eating well need to be followed if you are to get the most out of your training. This chapter will look at refining these basic principles to suit the individual athlete's needs. By choosing the correct foods and fluids at the right time, you'll improve your training and give your body the chance to perform at its best.

Fuelling Your Muscles

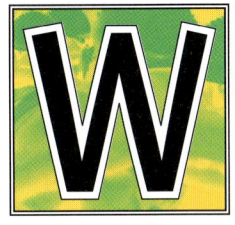

When we eat carbohydrate foods — starches and sugars — they are broken down in the body to glucose. This glucose maintains blood glucose levels and is used as energy or, if it's not needed immediately, it's stored in your muscles and liver in the form of glycogen. During exercise, glycogen is used as fuel and, just as a car can run out of petrol, your body can run out of glycogen. Glycogen stores are limited, only supplying fuel for up to 90 minutes of continuous intense exercise. These stores need to be continually topped up by carbohydrate in your diet.

If you want to exercise or train efficiently, you must ensure that you've got enough glycogen in your muscles before you start. This means eating plenty of nutritious carbohydrates to fuel your muscles, which will help you to train at your best for longer and to recover more quickly between sessions.

How Much Carbohydrate Do You Need?

The more you exercise, the more carbohydrate you should include in your diet. The amount you need relates to your activity levels and your body weight. Use the following chart as a guide to how much carbohydrate you need.

Food for an Active Lifestyle

Carbohydrates will be supplying over half your daily energy needs. As a rough guide, a recreational athlete (with a moderate activity level) would need between 300 and 400 grams of carbohydrate per day, while an endurance or professional athlete (that is, one with a heavy activity level) would need between 500 and 700 grams per day.

When you fill up on carbohydrates, choose nutritious carbohydrates that will maximise your vitamin and mineral intake. You may need to supplement your diet with some sugar carbohydrates to help you reach your carbohydrate goal, but make nutritious carbohydrates your first choice.

Use the Carbohydrate Calculator on page 93 to help you work out what you should be including in your diet to reach your daily carbohydrate requirements.

How to Calculate Your Carbohydrate Needs:

For example: A 90-kilogram footballer who exercises for 1–2 hours per day would need 6–7 grams of carbohydrate per kilogram he weighs (ie, 90 X 6–7 = 540–630 grams carbohydrate per day).

To translate this into food servings turn to the Carbohydrate Calculator. Each serving equals 15 grams of carbohydrate. From the example above: 540–630 ÷ 15 = 36–42 serves per day.

Carbohydrate Requirements

Activity level (Refers to how hard and how long you are actually exercising)	Grams per kilogram of body weight per day
Light — less than 1 hour per day (walking or aerobic sessions 3–5 times a week)	4–5
Light to moderate — 1 hour per day (participate in team sports)	5–6
Moderate — 1–2 hours per day (medium-to-high-intensity exercise, serious amateur)	6–7
Moderate to heavy — 3 hours per day (intense training — for example, triathlete)	7–8
Heavy — 4 hours or more per day (continuous, intense exercise — for example ultra-endurance athlete)	9–10

Source: Adapted from L. Bourke, *Complete Guide to Food for Sports Performance* (Allen & Unwin, Sydney, 1995).

Food for an Active Lifestyle

Carbohydrate Calculator

Each serve contains 15 grams of carbohydrate.

Breads, cereals and grains — aim to include at least 6 serves from this group every day.

- 1 slice bread
- 1/2 bread roll or fruit bun
- 1/2 English muffin or crumpet
- 1/2 small pocket bread
- 1/4 large Lebanese bread
- 1 small scone or pikelet
- 1/2 breakfast bar
- 2/3 fruit muesli bar
- 25 grams pretzels
- 2 thick rice cakes
- 3 thin rice cakes
- 2 Ryvita crispbreads
- 4–6 cracker biscuits
- 1 1/2 VitaBrits
- 1/2 cup Sports Plus
- 1/2 cup cooked rolled oats
- 3/4 cup Corn Flakes or Weeties
- 2 tablespoons untoasted muesli
- 3 cups unbuttered popcorn
- 1/2 cup cooked pasta
- 1/3 cup cooked rice, noodles
  (Not the instant variety.)

Vegetables — include these every day.

- 1/2 cup corn, sweet potato, parsnip
- 1 small–medium potato
- 1 1/2 cups cooked vegetables
- 1/2 cup lentils, baked beans, etc

Fruit — include at least 3 serves every day.

- 1 medium piece — apple, orange, pear
- 1 small banana
- 1 cup berries, melon or pawpaw
- 2/3 cup canned fruit
- 2 small plums, nectarines or mandarins
- 1 small mango
- 1/2 cup fresh fruit salad
- 15 grapes (small handful)
- 1 medium slice pineapple
- 1/2 cup (125 ml) fruit juice
- 1/4 cup dried fruit

Dairy foods — include at least 2 serves every day.

- 300 ml full-cream milk or soy milk
- 200 gram tub low-fat plain yoghurt
- 250 ml reduced-fat milk or soy milk
- 100 gram tub low-fat flavoured yoghurt
- 250 ml calcium-enriched, reduced-fat milk
- 100 gram tub Fruche
- 2 scoops Vitari
- 3 tablespoons skim milk powder

Drinks and sugar-based foods — use this group to top up your carbohydrate quota or in recovery.

- 250 ml sports drink
- 150 ml soft drink
- 200 ml cordial (diluted 1:4)
- 3 tablespoons Milo, Ovaltine or Sustagen Sport
- 125 ml Sustagen drink
- 1 tablespoon glucodin or sugar
- 1 tablespoon jam, honey, syrup
- 4 jelly beans or snakes
- 1/3 cup jelly
- 2 tablespoons low-fat ice-cream

Get UP&GO!

Achieving Your Carbohydrate Target Intake

If you can't quite meet your carbohydrate target, don't panic — everyone's body is different. If you are within 50 grams of your target you are doing okay. At first it may seem like you're constantly eating to achieve your target. Don't give up! Try drinking some of your carbohydrates in the form of fruit smoothies or sports drinks, or try adding skim milk powder to your milk drinks, soups or mashed potatoes.

You may need to look at cutting back on your fibre. Wholegrain foods, fruits and vegetables are full of fibre and quite filling, which can make it difficult for you to fit in a lot of food. Try using white breads and pasta, and choose juice occasionally. If you still feel uncomfortable, then reduce your carbohydrate target a little and see how you feel and perform.

As an athlete, a guide to whether or not you're getting enough fuel for your exercise needs is your weight. If you're losing weight unintentionally, you'll need to increase your energy intake, include more carbohydrate and check that you're getting enough protein. If you're gaining body fat, first check that your fat and protein intakes aren't too high; then cut back a little on carbohydrate, if necessary.

The GI Index

Not all carbohydrates are the same. Previously, we believed that sugary foods, such as jam, were absorbed quickly — causing a sharp rise in blood glucose levels — while the starchy foods, such as bread and potatoes, were absorbed much more slowly. Recent research has shown that things aren't that simple.

Case Study

Jane is a 32-year-old mum who likes to keep fit and enjoys playing netball on Saturday afternoons. She trains with her team for two hours every Thursday evening and does three aerobic classes and two strength/cardiovascular sessions each week. On Sundays she often enjoys a walk or a bike ride with her family.

Although Jane thought she was eating well, she was complaining of feeling tired — especially towards the end of the week. She kept a detailed food and fluid diary for a week and made an appointment to see a dietitian.

Assessment of Jane's diet showed that carbohydrate was only providing around 40 per cent of her daily energy intake — not enough to keep her muscles fuelled for her exercise. In the past couple of years Jane had cut down on her red meat intake and a blood test revealed that her iron levels were low, adding to her lethargy.

Jane maintained her weight at around 60 kilograms and was carrying only a little excess body fat. The dietitian pointed out that Jane needed 5–6 grams of carbohydrate per kilogram of her body weight — that is, $60 \times 5\text{–}6 = 300\text{–}350$ grams of carbohydrate — per day to ensure her glycogen stores were fuelled. To boost her iron levels she needed to include red meat at least four times a week and to choose an iron-fortified cereal. She was encouraged to include vitamin-C rich food with vegetarian meals to help improve iron absorption from plant foods. Tea and coffee can impair iron absorption so she should drink them between meals.

Food for an Active Lifestyle

Following is a sample of how Jane is now eating. Most days Jane would also have a 500 ml sports drink (30 grams) or include another piece of fruit (15 grams). She drinks 1.5–2 litres of water each day.

	Grams of carbohydrate	Serves
Breakfast		
1 cup wholegrain cereal	30	2
with 1/2 cup low-fat milk	7	1/2
Sliced banana or strawberries	15	1
1 tablespoon of chopped nuts sprinkled on top of cereal	15	1
1 slice wholegrain toast with honey	15	1
Cup of herb tea and a glass of water	–	
Morning tea		
Scone with jam	30	2
Cup of coffee	–	
Lunch		
Wholegrain roll spread with avocado	30	2
30 grams lean roast beef	–	
Lots of salad	–	
250 ml orange juice	30	2
Afternoon tea		
Breakfast bar, or a tub of low-fat fruit yoghurt	30	2
5 rice crackers or a handful of pretzels	15	1
Dinner		
Serving of lean meat, chicken, fish or tofu	–	
1 1/2 cups of rice or pasta, *or* a jacket potato and 1/2 cob of corn, with lots of vegies	45	3
An occasional glass of wine	–	
After Dinner		
Piece of fruit or a Milo drink	15–30	1–2

A total of 295–325 gms or 19 1/2 – 21 1/2 serves.

At first, Jane had trouble eating all the food she needed, but as she started eating more regular meals and choosing nutritious carbohydrate snacks, she found she had more energy for both her sport and her family. The dietitian also advised Jane on the importance of good recovery nutrition and Jane found this helped to improve her training sessions.

Check your serving sizes — how much cereal do you really put in your bowl? How much milk do you really pour on top?
Be aware of what you really do eat and drink, so you can record amounts correctly in your diary.

Food for an Active Lifestyle

> *'Nothing comes from doing nothing.'*
> — William Shakespeare

We now know that the rate and extent of the rise in the blood glucose level is influenced by a number of factors, including the type of starch or sugar consumed, the amount of fat and fibre in the food, and the refining and processing the food has undergone.

The Glycaemic Index (GI) ranks foods containing carbohydrate according to the speed at which they are digested and enter the bloodstream as usable energy. Glucose is absorbed the fastest and is ranked GI=100. Foods with a high GI raise blood glucose levels quickly — for example, jelly beans. However, this energy burst doesn't last long compared to foods with a low GI, such as a low-fat yoghurt, which gives a slower, but longer-lasting source of energy.

How can we use the GI to our advantage?

For athletes, choosing foods according to their GI can help enhance performance. Choosing a meal rich in low GI foods at least 2 hours before exercise may help endurance athletes (or anyone who exercises continuously for more than two hours a day) by helping to delay fatigue. Remember to allow adequate time for digestion before exercising. During exercise, high GI foods are a good choice; they help top up your blood glucose level. Choosing high GI foods (or drinks) immediately after exercise (ie, within 20–30 minutes) is an ideal start to the important refuelling and rehydrating processes.

Foods with a low GI promote a greater feeling of fullness than high GI foods. So, by including more low-fat, carbohydrate-rich foods with a low GI, you'll find you need to eat less food (energy) to feel full. This is a bonus for those who are having a problem with weight control.

Many people experience a drop in energy late in the morning or afternoon, usually around three to five hours after eating. Have you ever felt like you need a nap at 3 or 4 p.m.? Signs of low blood glucose are varied, but include irritability, poor concentration, headache and a loss of energy. By choosing more foods with a low GI, it's possible to prevent large swings in blood glucose and energy levels.

Look in the box opposite for some low and high GI food suggestions — use them to your advantage.

Low GI	High GI
Uncle Toby's Rolled Oats	Corn Flakes
Uncle Toby's Natural Muesli	VitaBrits
All Bran/Sultana Bran	Puffed Rice
Apples	Bananas
Pears	Watermelon
Oranges	Potatoes
Apple juice	Breakfast bars
Beans, lentils	White and wholemeal bread
Basmati rice	Rice cakes
Wholegrain breads	Calrose rice
Pasta	Sport drinks
Flavoured milk	Glucose
Fruit yoghurt	Sucrose (table sugar) and honey

Adapted from Foster-Powell and Brand Miller, *The GI Factor*, Hodder and Stoughton, Sydney, 1996.

Food for an Active Lifestyle

Is Protein the Answer to Bigger Muscles?

There is a common misconception that muscles are made of protein, and that eating lots of protein will produce bigger muscles. This myth has created an industry worth millions of dollars.

The correct weight-training program, combined with good nutrition, will increase the size of your muscles. Exercise does increase your protein needs above that of an inactive person, but the fact that you'll need more food to meet your energy requirements will provide you with this extra protein.

How Much Protein Do You Need?

Check the chart below if you're just starting out on a strength-training program. If your training sessions are long and strenuous, aim for the higher end of the scale. For example, a 95-kilogram weightlifter in a muscle-gain phase would need 171 grams of protein per day (95 x 1.8 grams). Pregnant and breastfeeding athletes will need to make sure they get at least 10 grams of protein more than their daily requirement every day. A 63–kilogram pregnant female doing four swimming sessions a week would need 73 kilograms (63 x 1.0 = 63 + 10 = 73). You can see from the Protein Calculator on page 98 that it's not too difficult to reach your target by eating a reasonable amount of a variety of foods.

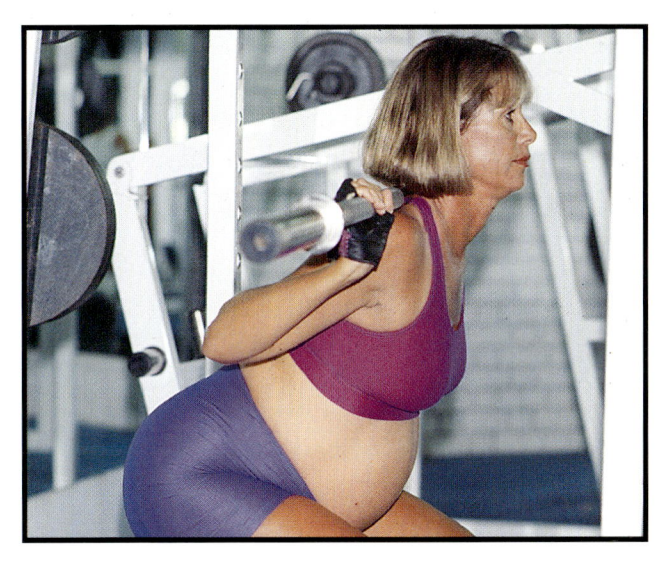

Use common sense when pregnant — you can continue to train right up to birth if you feel like it, however consult your doctor beforehand.

Protein Requirements

Activity level	Grams per kilogram of body weight per day
Sedentary person	0.75
Light exercise	1.0
Strength/speed training	1.2–1.8
Endurance athlete	1.2–1.8
Adolescent and growing athletes	2.0

Source: P.W.R. Lemon, *Do Athletes Need more Dietary Protein and Amino Acids?*, International Journal of Sports Nutrition, vol 5, 1995, supplement: s39—61.

Food for an Active Lifestyle

Protein Calculator

Each serve contains 5 grams of protein.

- 25 grams lean meat, poultry, cooked (for example, a slice of ham on a sandwich)
- 25 grams fish (cooked)
- 1 medium egg
- 30 grams nuts
- 2 thick slices bread
- 1 1/2 cups breakfast cereal
- 1 cup pasta or rice (cooked)
- 1/2 cup baked beans
- 1/3 cup lentils/beans (cooked)
- 75 grams tofu
- 150 ml skim milk
- 1 heaped tablespoon skim milk powder
- 20 grams Sustagen
- 100 ml reduced-fat, high-calcium milk
- 1/2 tub (100 grams) low-fat yoghurt
- 1 slice reduced-fat cheese
- 200 ml soy milk

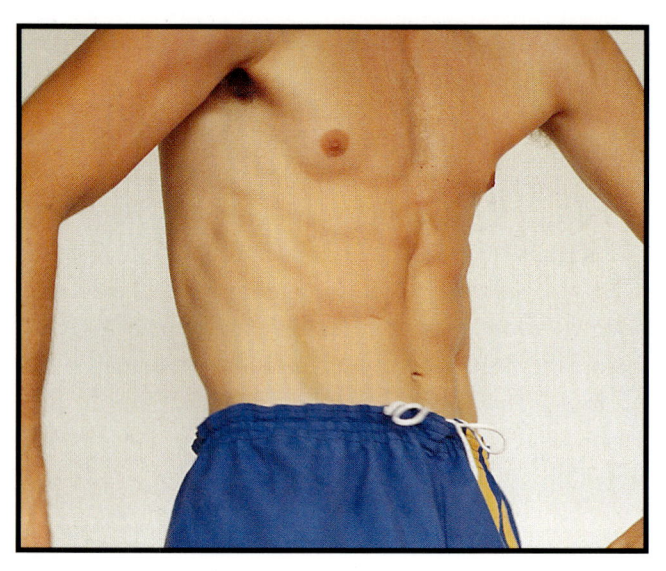

Do the best with what you have. By eating and training smart you can change your shape.

Shaping Up

When people think of improving their shape, the two main areas of concern are building muscle (building up) and losing body fat.

Building up

Whether you wish to increase your muscle mass to improve your strength for sport or to improve your shape, there are several factors that need to be considered:

Your genetics: Check out what your relatives looked like at your age — it will give you an idea of your potential for building yourself up. Males: if your male relatives were solid, then you have more of a chance of building up than if they were slight. Work with what you've got and be happy with your body type.

Your training program: A properly designed weight-training program is essential for building bigger muscles. Muscles won't get bigger or stronger unless they are worked.

Your eating habits: Are you feeding your body adequately?

You need:

- an adequate amount of protein to build muscle;
- enough carbohydrate to fuel your muscles so they can work efficiently at your training sessions; and
- enough energy to keep your body going.

Food for an Active Lifestyle

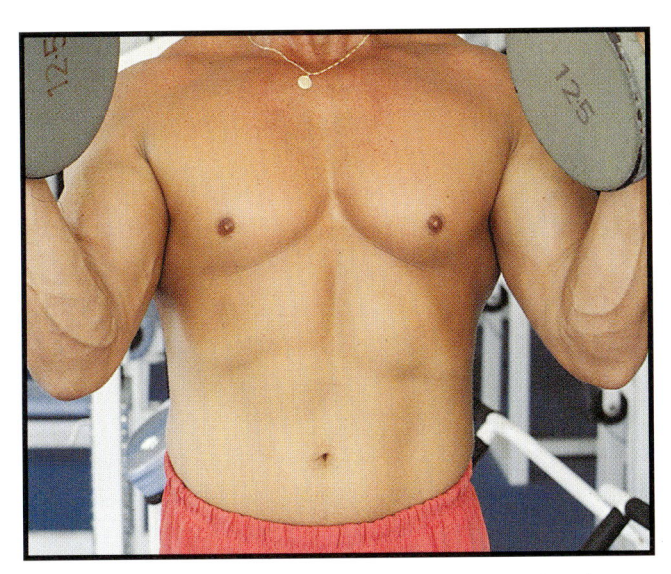

Weight gain of 0.5kg per week is realistic for building muscle. Rapid weight gain usually means an increase in body fat as well.

Given that your training and genetics are working for you, your diet might be your limiting factor. Consider the reasons why you might not be fuelling your body with enough energy:

- You're too busy with training, work, etc to buy and prepare food or to eat enough food to train and grow, let alone gain weight.
- Young males already have high energy demands for growth; when you add training needs, it may mean trying to eat more than you feel like.
- You prefer not to train with food in your stomach and you don't feel like eating for several hours after training.
- You neglect carbohydrates in favour of protein-based foods.

A weight gain of 0.5 kg per week is realistic. Rapid weight gain usually means an increase in body fat as well. Check this with girth and skinfold measurements. (See pages 138–141.)

Have patience — increasing muscle mass takes time.

Tips to Help You Build Up

- Eat regular meals — don't skip meals or rely on your appetite. Use your watch and schedule your snacks and meals every three hours to fit in with your daily routine.
- Try to eat six or more times per day.
- If you're on the run, you may prefer liquid snacks to food because they're easier to digest quickly. Make nutritious, low-fat fruit smoothies, or use milk-based drinks such as Sustagen Sport, Endura Opti, Ensure Plus, or milk with skim milk powder added.
- Try snacking on sports bars and drinking sports drinks during exercise.
- Plan ahead with meals and snacks. Pre-prepare pasta and rice dishes so you have something ready for dinner when you arrive home tired.
- Keep breakfast bars in your car, and other snacks at work.
- Replace tea and coffee with high-energy drinks — sports drinks and enriched milk-based drinks.
- Try reduced-fat milk and yoghurt, and legumes — they're a good source of protein and carbohydrate.
- Control your fat intake — remember, excess fat is stored as body fat, not muscle.
- Include a protein food at mealtime, but don't overdo the serving size.
- Feeling full? Cut down on your fibre. Choose more white breads and pasta. Have fruit juice instead of fruit

Food for an Active Lifestyle

Lisa's Health Drink

A good source of energy (carbohydrate) that's low in fat and gives you lots of the important antioxidants. This is a great breakfast drink if you don't feel like eating.

- 1 orange (juiced)
- 1 small banana
- ½ cup chopped pawpaw
- 1 egg
- 1 teaspoon honey

Blend all the ingredients together until smooth.

Nutritional summary
- Protein 9 grams ■ Fat 5 grams
- Carbohydrate 44 grams
- Kilojoules 1075 ■ Calories 257
- Fibre 5 grams

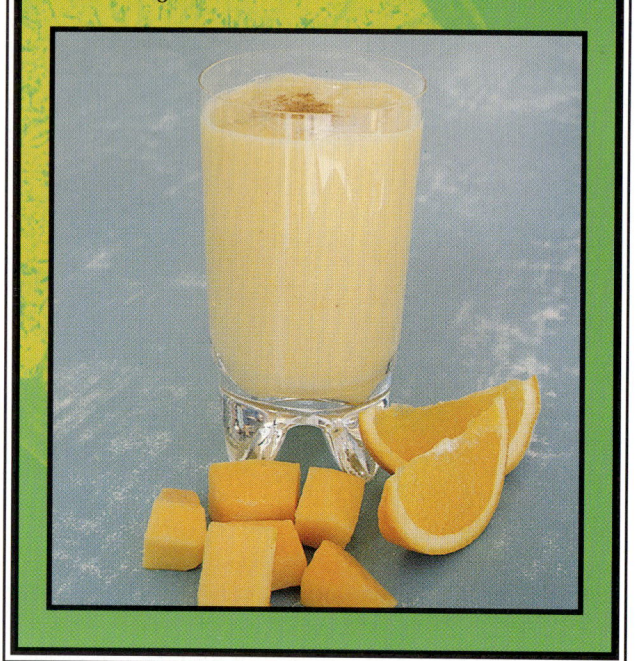

Losing body fat through healthy eating

From the recreational exerciser to the elite athlete, the amount and distribution of body fat is a common area of concern.

We all need a certain amount of body fat to maintain good health — women require more than men to maintain a healthy reproductive system. In the section entitled 'Understanding Your Body', we discussed the different types of bodies, so you have probably worked out which type best matches your body. Remember that this is your genetic shape and there is nothing you can do to change your bone structure. You should be aiming to be fit and healthy at a weight and body-fat level that is comfortable for you and that you can maintain without a constant struggle.

Body-fat levels are determined by the balance between the amount of energy (kilojoules/calories) consumed in food and drink and the energy used for metabolism and activity. This balance is also influenced by our individual adaptation to changes in eating and exercise. Fat loss is a result of using more energy than you take in. To lose body fat you need to change your eating habits. When overweight people cut down on dietary fat, weight (and body fat) will be lost because fewer kilojoules will have been eaten. If you become more active at the same time, the benefits will be even greater.

In their quest to lose body fat, already lean people often cut dietary fat to unhealthy levels and base their diet on fat-free carbohydrates. Although the body has a preference for carbohydrate as a fuel source, an excess of kilojoules/calories from any source will be stored as fat.

Excess body fat is a risk factor for many common diseases and, for athletes, can impair performance. Bathroom scales are not the best guide to an athlete's body-fat levels. More appropriate ways to measure body fat are discussed in 'Test Your Fitness' (in the

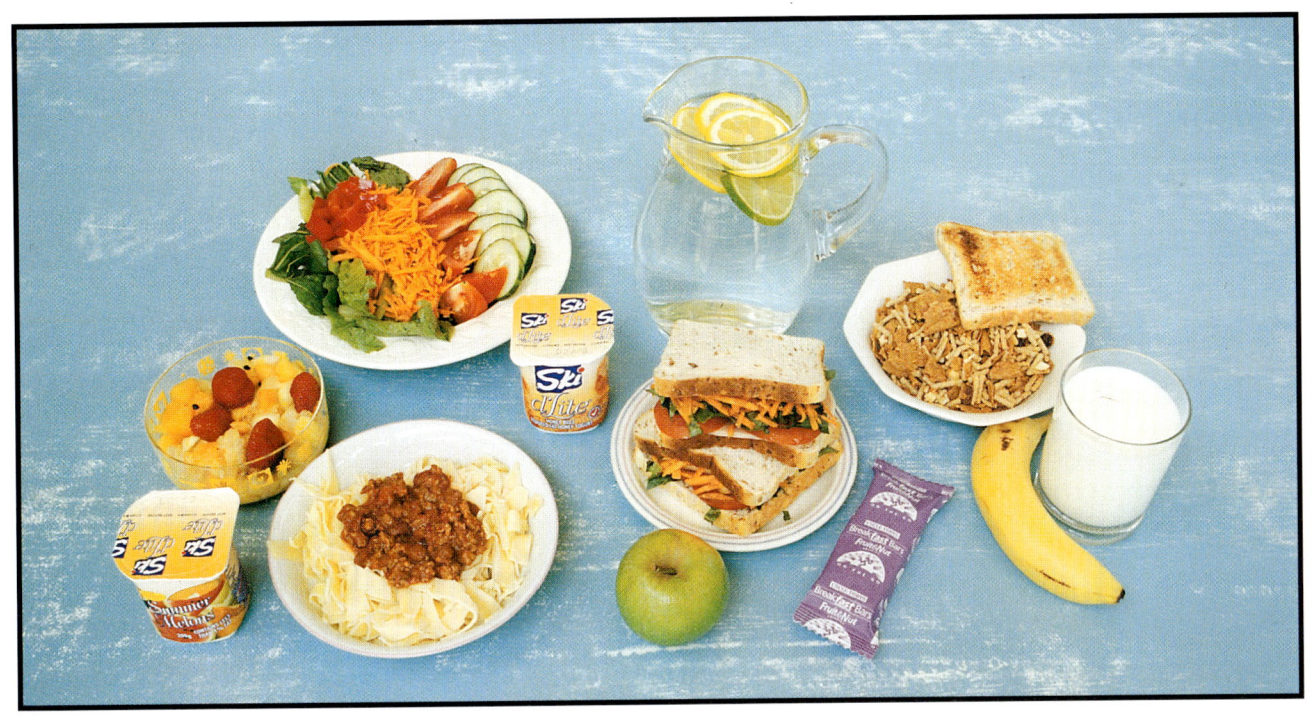

Eat well — reap the benefits. What do you eat in a day? Does it give you the energy you need?

section Training and Fitness). Before starting on a fat-loss program, try to have your body fat measured to determine how much fat you need to lose and to give you a realistic goal. (Many 'solid' people are surprised to find that they have quite low body-fat levels. A solid appearance can be due to muscle.) If this isn't possible, at least keep a record of your girth measurements along with your weight. A great guide to fat loss is when your clothes start to feel loose.

Healthy eating is essential if you are to lose body fat and still have enough energy to exercise efficiently.

- Keep up your carbohydrate intake — choose nutritious carbohydrates and watch how much of the sugar and non-useful carbohydrates you choose.
- Police your fat intake — cut down but not out, and avoid saturated fats and processed foods.
- Make sure you're getting enough protein, vitamins and minerals and that you include a variety of foods in your diet.
- Choose foods that are satisfying and filling, those lower in GI and higher in fibre.
- Eat regularly throughout the day so that you don't binge eat.
- Keep up your fluids, at least 1.5 litres of water a day.
- Continue to enjoy your food — it's what you eat *most* of the time that counts. Include high-fat carbohydrates and alcohol occasionally if you wish.
- Check skinfold or girth measurements along with weight to monitor change (every 4–6 weeks).
- Be patient and realistic — fat loss is a slow process.
- Aim to loose fat over a period of months not weeks.

Food for an Active Lifestyle

Eating to Compete

If you're going to compete in your chosen sport, following some basic nutritional principles can help give you the edge and keep you competitive. What you eat before, during and after you compete can make a huge difference to how well you perform. Whatever you do, it's important that you put these principles into practice during training so that you can assess yourself and then fine-tune things before the big day. There is no magic food. Each person has their own preference. Be aware of how different foods act in your body and what gives you the energy to exercise.

Carbohydrate Loading

Carbohydrate loading is simply increasing the body's store of glycogen to its maximum level to maintain a fuel supply for *endurance* exercise. Early methods of carbohydrate loading prior to competition were quite stressful on the athlete. Today, the plan is to have a high carbohydrate diet every day and gradually reduce your training in the days before competing.

If you are competing in a marathon, your pre-race strategies are a little different to someone having a weekly game of football or netball. Let's look at the tactics.

For endurance athletes:

■ To get maximum glycogen stored in your muscles and liver — taper your training load in the week leading up to your event and eat a high carbohydrate diet (around 9–10 grams of carbohydrate per kilogram of body weight) for two to three days before competing.

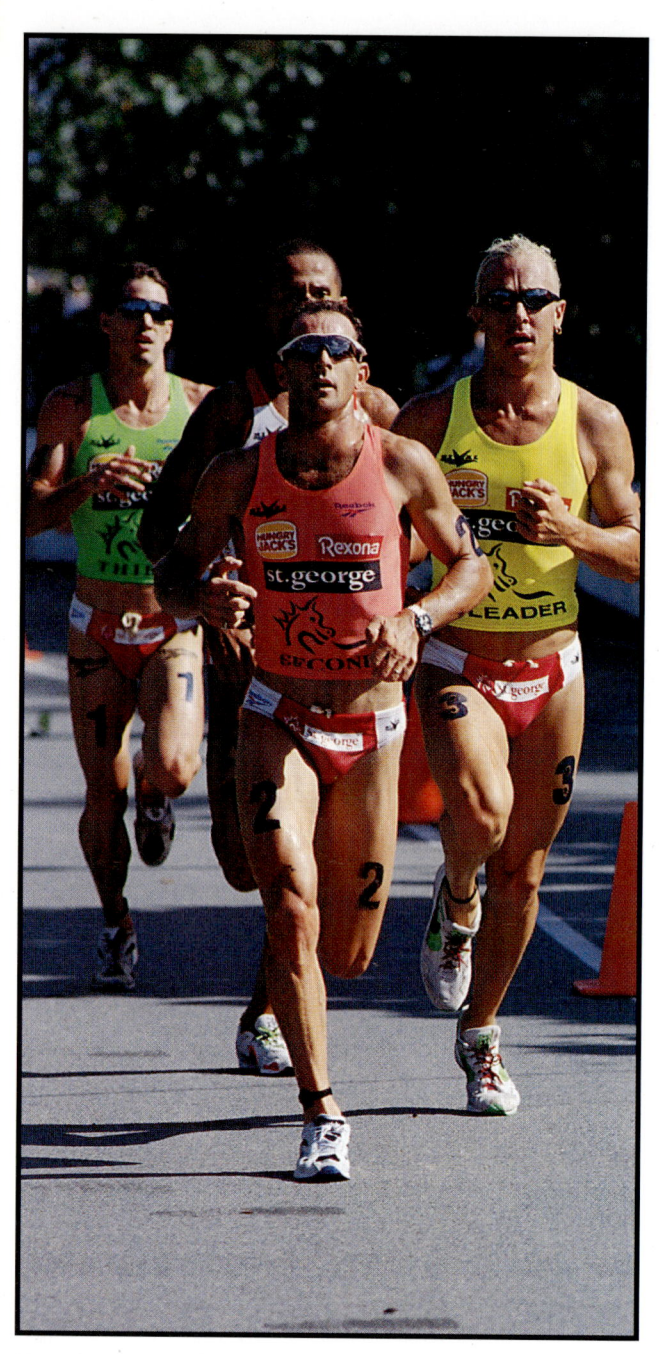

Keep your head and your heart in the right direction and you'll never have to worry about your feet.

- Drink extra fluids to ensure good hydration. Limit alcohol and caffeine-based drinks.
- Make sure you get enough protein in your diet and try trading some fat for extra carbohydrate.

If you compete each week, you should:

Maintain your usual high carbohydrate diet throughout the week, and the day before competing:

- Be especially conscious of consuming enough high carbohydrate foods.
- Consume extra fluids to keep you well-hydrated. (Clear urine indicates a well-hydrated body.)
- Eliminate unnecessary extras. Avoid high-fat snacks, takeaways and salty foods.
- Limit caffeine-based drinks.

The pre-event meal

This is your final chance to top up glycogen and fluid stores before competing. Experiment during training to establish what suits you best, but never try anything you aren't familiar with before an important event.

Your last meal should be two to four hours before you compete to allow for complete digestion and absorption. Eat enough to feel comfortable, and eat foods you enjoy.

This meal should:

- be high in carbohydrates — to maximise fuel stores;
- be low in fat — high-fat meals take longer to leave the stomach;
- include fluids — to assist hydration;
- exclude coffee, tea, cola and alcohol — they promote fluid loss; and
- not be too high in fibre — to avoid gastric upset during exercise.

Try some of these pre-event meal suggestions:

- cereal with reduced-fat milk and fruit
- low-fat fruit smoothie
- toast with spaghetti (or baked beans if tolerated)
- pancakes with syrup
- muffins or crumpets with honey
- pasta with a tomato sauce
- fruit salad with yoghurt
- banana sandwich
- low-fat rice pudding

If you need to eat something closer to the event, up to one or two hours before, choose snacks of fruit, bread, juice or a sports drink. If you're nervous and don't feel like eating, try a liquid meal, such as a fruit smoothie, or a liquid meal replacement such as Ensure, Sustagen or Endura Opti. Make an effort to eat well the day before your competition — remember to have a good snack before you go to bed the night before.

You should apply these principles to eating before you train as well. Make sure you have an afternoon snack — for example, a tub of yoghurt or some fruit — if you are exercising after work. Don't rely on lunch at noon or 1 p.m. to get you through a training session at 6 p.m. Sometimes it's not practical or comfortable to eat several hours before competing or training, especially if you train very early in the morning. Make sure your meal the night before is high in carbohydrate and you have a carbohydrate snack before bedtime. During training, try to have some diluted fruit juice, a sports drink or fruit. If you train hard for longer than an hour, try to have some carbohydrate, such as diluted juice or toast and jam (something that feels OK in your stomach), before you train and use a carbohydrate drink during training. Eat the rest of your breakfast when you finish training. Regardless of how long you train for, make sure you remember your fluids.

Food for an Active Lifestyle

> 'The mind is the limit. As long as the mind can envision the fact that you can do something, you can do it.'
> — Arnold Schwarzenegger

Some suggestions for meals and snacks the night before:

- pasta with a tomato-based sauce and a little meat
- stir-fried chicken, meat or fish with plenty of noodles or rice, and vegetables
- Large jacket potato filled with baked beans and a salad
- fruit with yoghurt or pancakes

And, of course, drink plenty of fluids.

What to eat during the event

What you eat and drink during a training session or competition depends somewhat on what you are doing.

For the recreational exerciser — someone who is doing sessions lasting 45–60 minutes — if your everyday diet includes plenty of nutritious carbohydrates and fluids, you should concentrate on replacing your fluid losses during exercise. There is some evidence that a carbohydrate drink may improve performance of high-intensity exercise of around an hour. Try a sports drink to see if this works for you.

Activities or training sessions lasting 60–90 minutes (the average football/netball game) won't fully deplete the body's carbohydrate stores, so take every opportunity to replace fluids and leave food for your recovery.

For endurance athletes (those exercising continuously for more than 90 minutes), fluid replacement isn't enough; carbohydrates need to be replaced to provide energy and help maintain blood glucose levels. You'll need to replace carbohydrates at around 30–50 grams per hour to delay fatigue. That's a 500–1000 ml sports drink or a large banana. Check out the Carbohydrate Calculator on page 93. It's important that fluid and fuel replacement is started early in your activity or training, in the first 20–30 minutes — don't wait until you're tired or thirsty.

What if you have several events in one day?

Your aim between events is to refuel and rehydrate. How you do this depends on the time you have and how your stomach handles food during competitions.

If your break between events is less than an hour, stick to fluids — either water, a sports drink or a juice. For longer breaks, again try fluids or a light snack such as a smoothie, fruit or yoghurt.

If you have at least two to three hours, try a rice or pasta meal, a honey or banana sandwich, rice cakes with jam, low-fat yoghurt or a bowl of cereal.

Replacing Fluids

Regardless of what sport you play or what type of exercise you choose, fluids are essential — you should drink as often as possible. Dehydration and overheating are major issues for people who exercise for long periods, especially when it's hot. Sweating can lead to dehydration — you can lose more than a litre of fluid in an hour when exercising in warm weather. You may not notice sweat losses if you're paddling a canoe, swimming, or cycling, so it's important for you to know how much fluid your body needs and that you make the effort to replenish it. You only need to be slightly dehydrated to see a drop in your performance, so get into the habit of drinking regularly.

How much do you need to drink when you exercise?

This depends on a number of factors, including how hard and long you train and how hot it is when you're exercising.

Food for an Active Lifestyle

You should aim to drink enough fluid to replace your sweat losses. This is easier in cool conditions or during low-intensity exercise. A simple way to tell if you're drinking enough is by checking the colour and quantity of your urine. If it's dark in colour and scant, you need to drink more. Be aware that B-group vitamin tablets can make your urine dark, so you should also check the volume.

For the serious athlete, the accurate way is to weigh yourself immediately before and directly after training (in the same clothes and before towelling off any sweat). Take into consideration any fluid or food consumed during the session and any toilet stops. A 1 kilogram drop in body weight equals 1 litre of sweat lost.

You should be aiming to match your fluid intake with your sweat losses as closely as you can *during* your exercise. If this isn't an option, then you must replenish your fluids after your exercise. Monitoring your weight changes regularly enables you to check how well you replace fluid losses and to adjust your intake according to training and climatic variations.

What should you drink?

Which drink you choose will depend on your particular exercise, taste preference, budget and, most of all, what works best for you. Maintaining good hydration is the important thing. You will be inclined to drink more of something that tastes good.

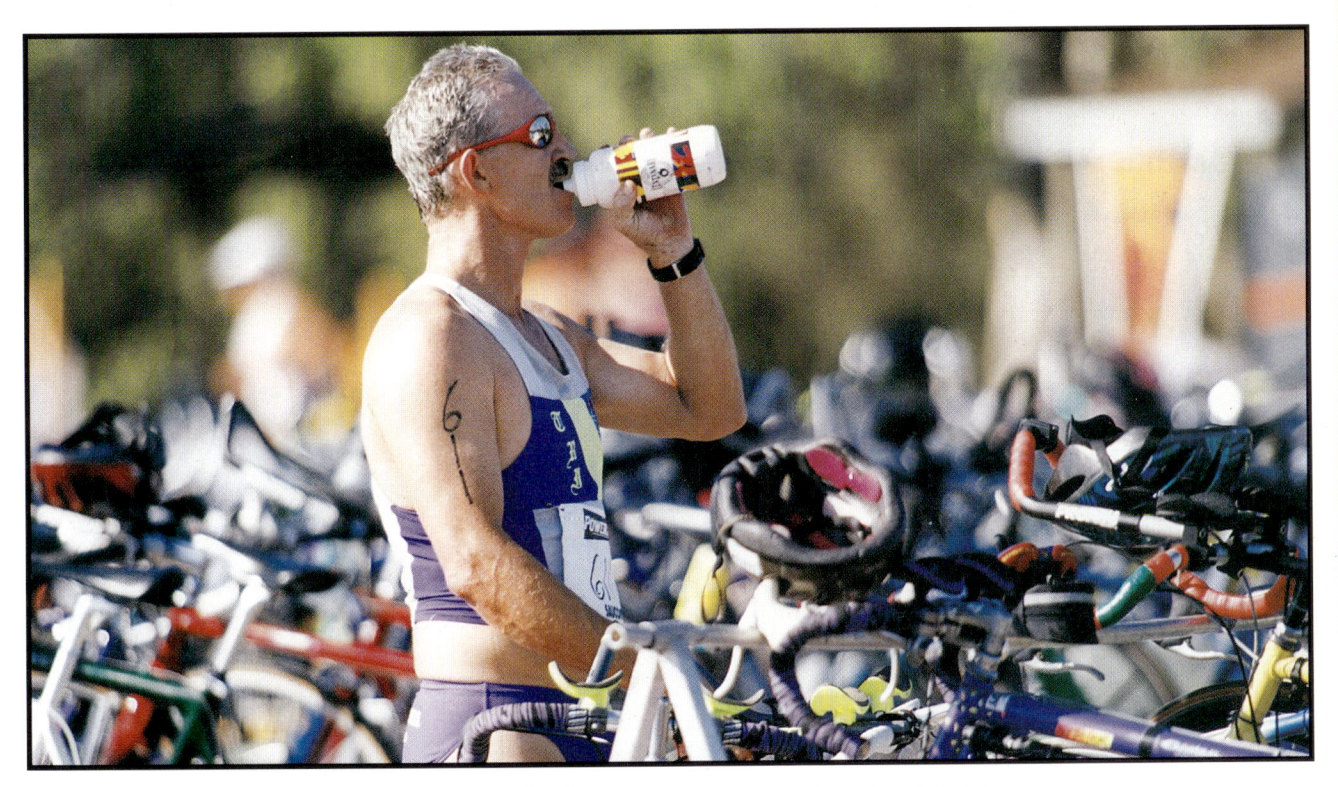

Dehydration and sweat loss is a major issue for people who exercise for long periods, such as triathletes. Replenishing your body fluids regularly is a must.

Tap-water is readily available, and cheap, and a perfectly suitable choice as a fluid replacement.

Juices, soft drinks, flavoured mineral waters and cordials all offer a source of both carbohydrate and fluid replacement. However, these highly concentrated sweet drinks are not absorbed quickly and should be diluted (half and half with water; cordial 1:10) if used during exercise.

Sports drinks are designed to provide a convenient way of replacing both fluid and carbohydrate during and after exercise. Because these drinks taste good, they may encourage you to consume more fluids. Taken during exercise, the carbohydrate will help delay fatigue by topping up blood glucose levels and conserving muscle fuel stores. This is especially important if you do strenuous exercise for longer than 60–90 minutes. The electrolytes, sodium and potassium found in some sports drinks improve their taste and help to promote retention of the fluid absorbed. Look for a sports drink containing 4–8 grams of carbohydrate per 100 ml and some sodium. When used correctly sports drinks can help exercisers at all levels, but they won't make up for a poorly balanced diet.

Alcohol, like caffeine and cola-based drinks, has a diuretic effect. Alcohol taken after exercise can slow down repair of damaged soft tissue. So, make sure you rehydrate before you indulge.

Fluid Facts

- **Drink to prevent thirst.**
- **Drink before you exercise. Drink more than your thirst indicates — it will be uncomfortable at first, but try to get used to starting exercise with a comfortably full stomach.**
- **You should drink 500–1000 millilitres in the two hours before you exercise. Sip gradually, even if you aren't thirsty. This is especially important if you sweat a lot or your group of activities offers little opportunity to consume fluids.**
- **Drink early and often during your exercise. Top up every 15 minutes with 150–250 millilitres. If it's hot, or you sweat a lot, you may need more.**
- **Drink after you exercise. Replace your losses beyond the point of satisfying your thirst.**
- **Aim to drink at least 600–800 millilitres of fluid for each hour of exercise. Take every opportunity during your activity to rehydrate — half-time, breaks of play, at change of ends.**
- **Make sure your drinks are cool, but not icy cold. Really cold drinks are harder to drink quickly in large amounts, often in a short period of time.**
- **Be aware that dehydration increases your risk of cramps.**
- **A well-hydrated athlete performs better and recovers more quickly.**
- **Alcohol and cola drinks are not rehydrating fluids.**

Food for an Active Lifestyle

Recovery

One of the secrets of success in sport and training is refuelling and rehydrating your body well after you have finished exercising or competing. The number-one goal after a hard exercise session should be to replace fluid losses and ensure that muscle glycogen stores are replenished. The hour after you finish exercising is vital to good recovery. Your muscles are looking to refuel and, in fact, in this time your muscles replenish their glycogen stores much faster than normal. Your muscles need to be refuelled before your next session if you expect to perform well.

Try to consume 50–100 grams of carbohydrate (see the Carbohydrate Calculator on page 93) within the first thirty minutes after exercising and continue refuelling regularly until your next session. This is particularly important if you train more than once a day. Consider choosing foods that have a high GI rating (see page 96) to help refuel your muscles quickly.

Often the last thing on your mind after training or competing is food. If this is the case, try choosing a carbohydrate drink — such as a sports/electrolyte replacement drink — which will help replace glycogen stores and fluid losses.

Fluid losses need to be replaced completely — beyond the point of your thirst. You should be passing pale and copious amounts of urine. It's also important to replace sodium that may have been lost in sweat, as this will aid in restoring the body fluid balance. Choosing a sports drink and including foods such as yoghurt, bread or cereal will boost your sodium intake.

Remember, better recovery means a better training session next time.

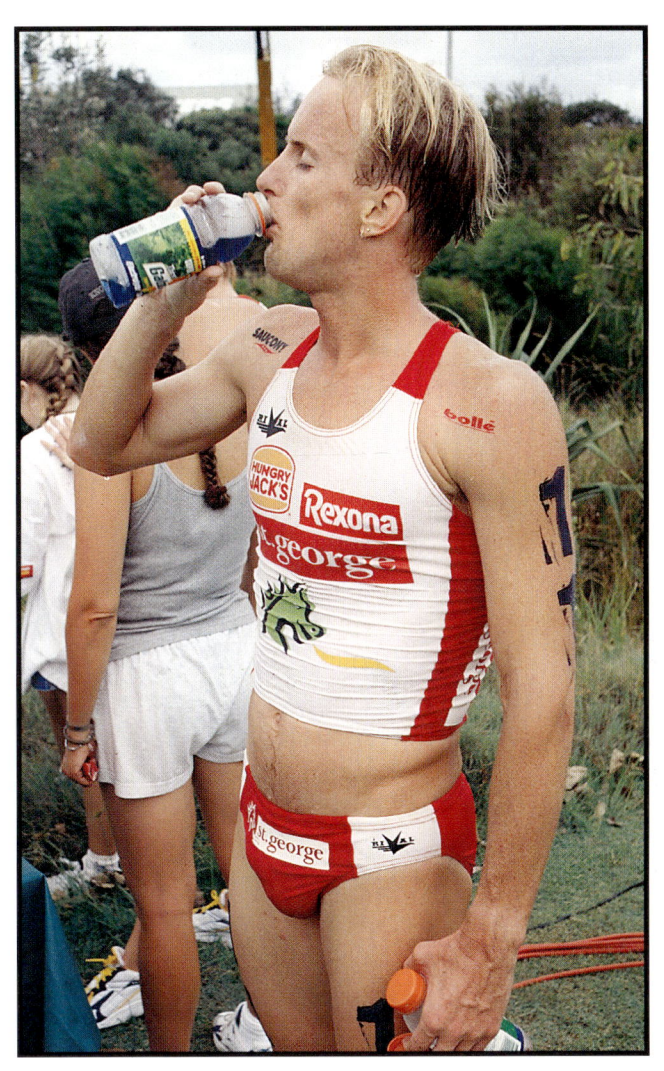

Refuelling and rehydrating your body after exercise or competition is vital to good recovery.

■ ■ ■

Whether you exercise for pleasure, fitness or to compete, I hope the nutritional strategies in this chapter will help you improve the way you exercise and give you an edge over your opposition. *Go for it!*

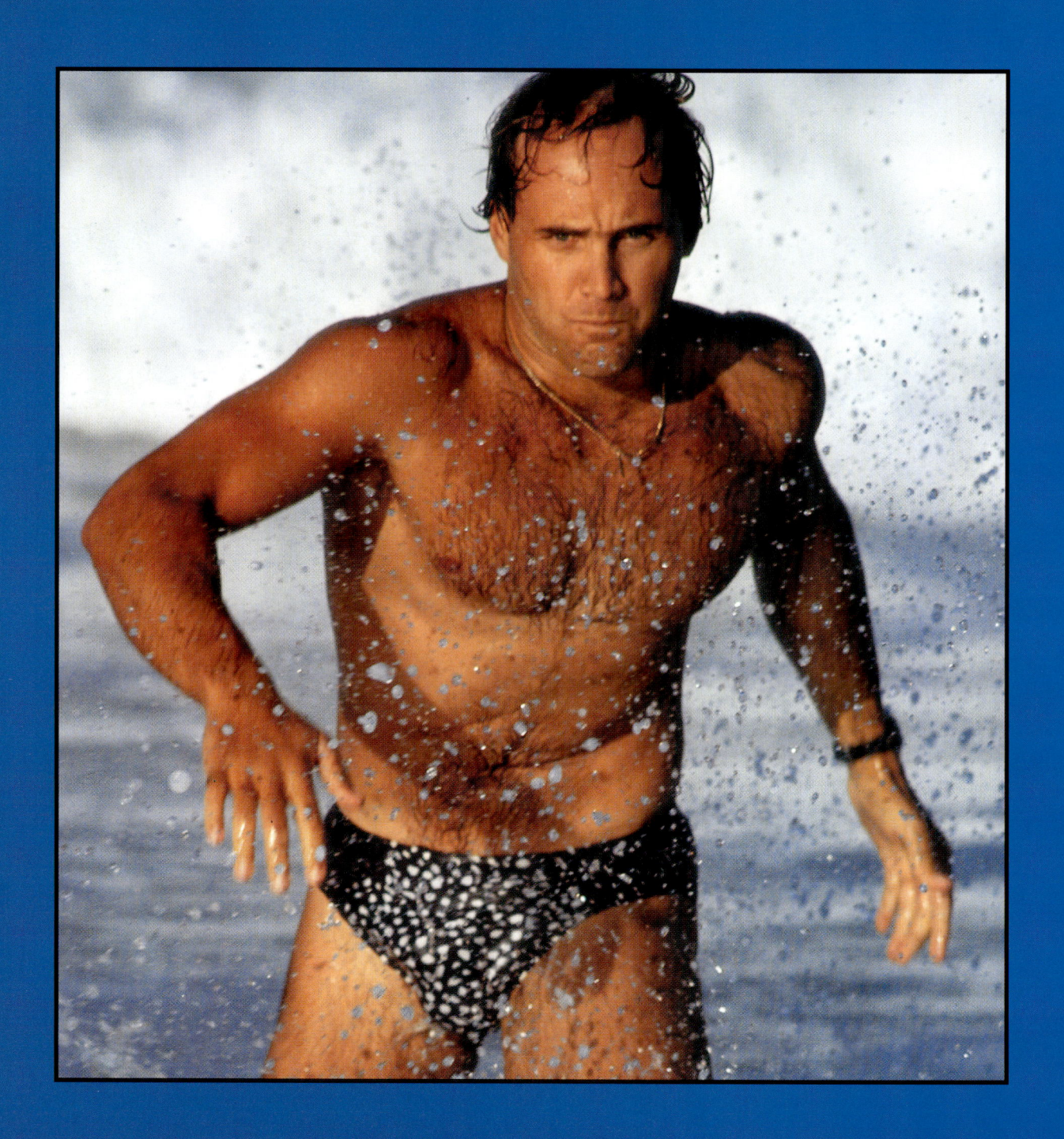

Training & Fitness

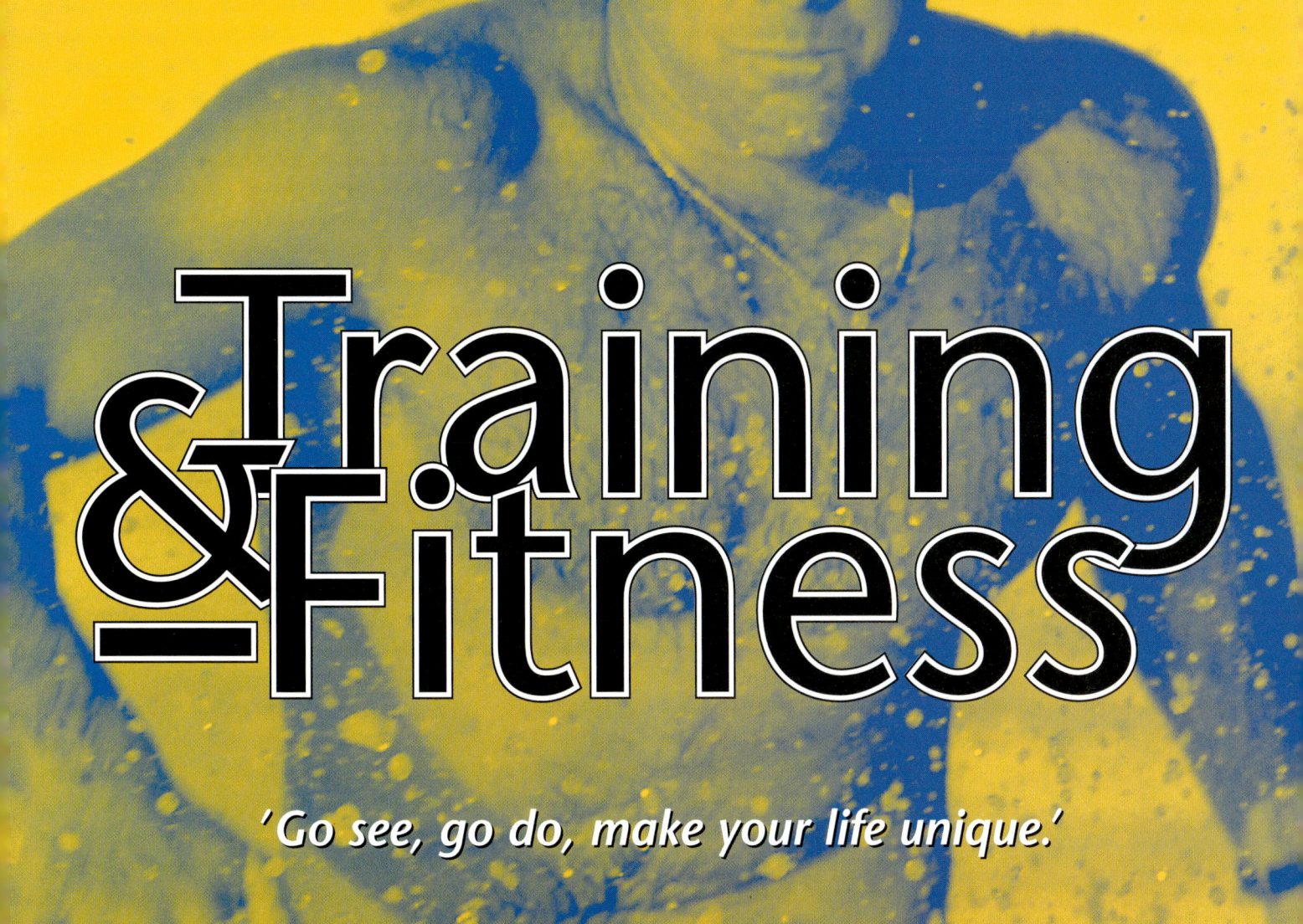

'Go see, go do, make your life unique.'

Preparing to Train

There is a difference between exercise and training. This chapter discusses what you can expect in each of the three phases of training: training to train; training to compete or improve; and training to win or get results. You will also learn the importance of posture, muscle balance, control and flexibility in any training program, as well as the value of including rest periods so as to avoid overtraining.

Exercise versus Training

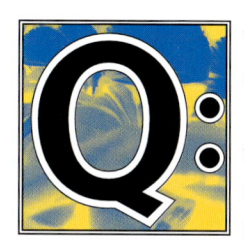

Q: What's the difference between exercise and training?

A: Exercise is any activity that causes the body to move and requires energy for these movements, which places stress on your body's systems (the heart and lungs, for example). Exercise tends to be based around enjoyment; it's usually aimed at improving and maintaining general health and fitness, is more socially structured and less competitive, and is based on how you look and feel rather than on how you perform.

Training is a form of exercise, but it is exercise performed for specific reasons in specific situations. Training is generally performed within a structured program by people who have a goal in mind for each session, and who have long-term plans centred around performance-based goals. Pure 'enjoyment' needn't come into it.

You can see how these terms can be easily confused. Exercise can be competitive and training can certainly be enjoyable.

This book concentrates more on training than exercise. Exercise may get you the results you're seeking, but for you to get *great* results, and to be certain of achieving those results, you have to start thinking in terms of training.

Preparing to Train

Everyone Who Trains is an 'Athlete'

The title 'athlete' isn't confined to professionals, or even elite amateurs. An athlete is anyone who plays sport or is involved in a committed training program which measures progress in any way, shape or form, and who spends any amount of time preparing for that activity.

```
Social            Recreational              Elite
|_____|_____|_____|_____|_____|
      Occasional            Serious        Professional
```

What Type of Athlete Are You?

The social athlete enjoys weekend tennis, golf, bowls, etc — activities where there is no pressure to train and no commitment to any program or other team members. They usually exercise where and when they like and enjoy a relaxing drink with team-mates afterwards.

The occasional athlete may train seriously for one event each year, but not constantly. They love the sense of achievement they get from competing in a fun run, triathlon, half marathon or the annual Masters Games.

For the recreational athlete, competition isn't the main emphasis. They tend to train more for enjoyment and, if they compete, they only do so because they can, not because it's vital to them.

The serious athlete is committed to fitness, training and their goals. They may not be especially talented but they get in there and have a go.

The elite athlete competes at the top level in sport but often still trains with squads and may still work or have sponsorship to cover expenses.

The professional athlete is a full-time athlete with income generated by competition — their job is their sport.

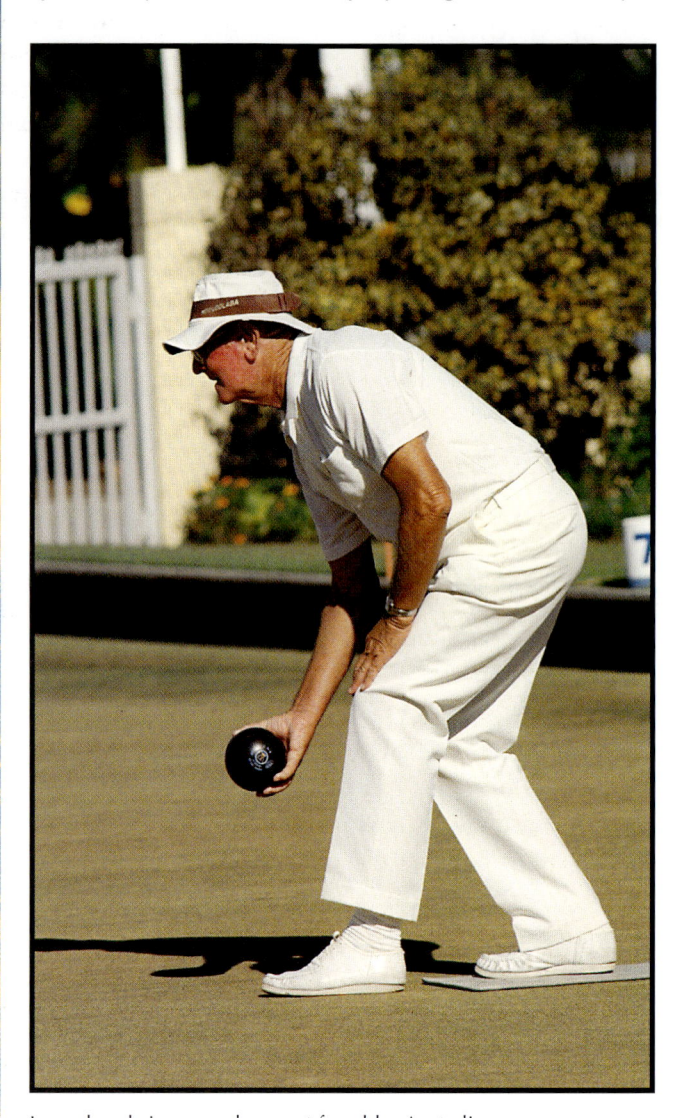

Lawn bowls is a popular sport for older Australians.

What type of athlete are you? You should be aiming to become at least a recreational athlete — where you will include training in your weekly timetable for good health and fitness and be able to work towards specific goals.

Be Properly Prepared

I can't emphasise strongly enough the importance of being properly prepared *before* you start out on your chosen training program. All too often, recreational athletes think only about getting out there and running, or about how much weight they might be able to lift in a month's time. The point is that our bodies need time to adjust to training. Treat your body well from the start and it will be there in good shape for you when you need it to perform.

How often do you hear of athletes breaking down time after time? But to suggest they might be doing something wrong, or that there might be a bad balance of training, is like waving a red flag at a bull. No matter who you are, or how good you are, the fact remains that you have to be *ready* to train and *ready* to compete.

World-renowned strength and conditioning coach Istvan Balyi believes in three phases of preparation for athletes, but they can be applied to all forms of exercise and training. Each phase will take a different amount of time depending on your previous experiences and current fitness.

Phase 1: Training to train

During this phase you need to learn how to train well. Most problems in training come from having a poor base of fitness. You should acquaint yourself with the methods of training, and learn how to do them properly.

Consider the following:

■ Learn the techniques of all the exercises you plan to include in your training program. Whether you exercise in the gym or at home, learn the techniques of all the skills you will need from a very basic level. This may involve seeking advice from an instructor, coach or personal trainer.

■ Find out how much rest you need to have each week, and how often you need to unload your program each cycle — every four weeks, every six weeks, etc. ('Unload' refers to easing off training volume, intensity or both to allow recovery.)

■ Discover what sort of progressions you feel comfortable with: do you like long, gradual increases that require time and patience, or short, small increases that instil confidence and can help to maintain motivation?

■ If necessary, get some coaching on how to move correctly — how to run, walk, cycle, swim, etc.

■ Listen to your body — learn to understand the way your body works, and why it feels the way it does after different types of training.

■ For a recreational athlete who is wanting to get fit, and possibly lose body fat and improve their shape, the 'training to train' phase will emphasise understanding what type of training will best suit your needs.

■ For a serious athlete in this phase, competition will not be your primary aim. You may still compete, but the focus will be on training, and training well.

■ If you don't learn to train well, it will be that much harder — perhaps even impossible — for you to achieve the results you want and to reach the goals you have set.

> 'Success happens whenever preparation meets opportunity.'
> — John Naber

Preparing to Train

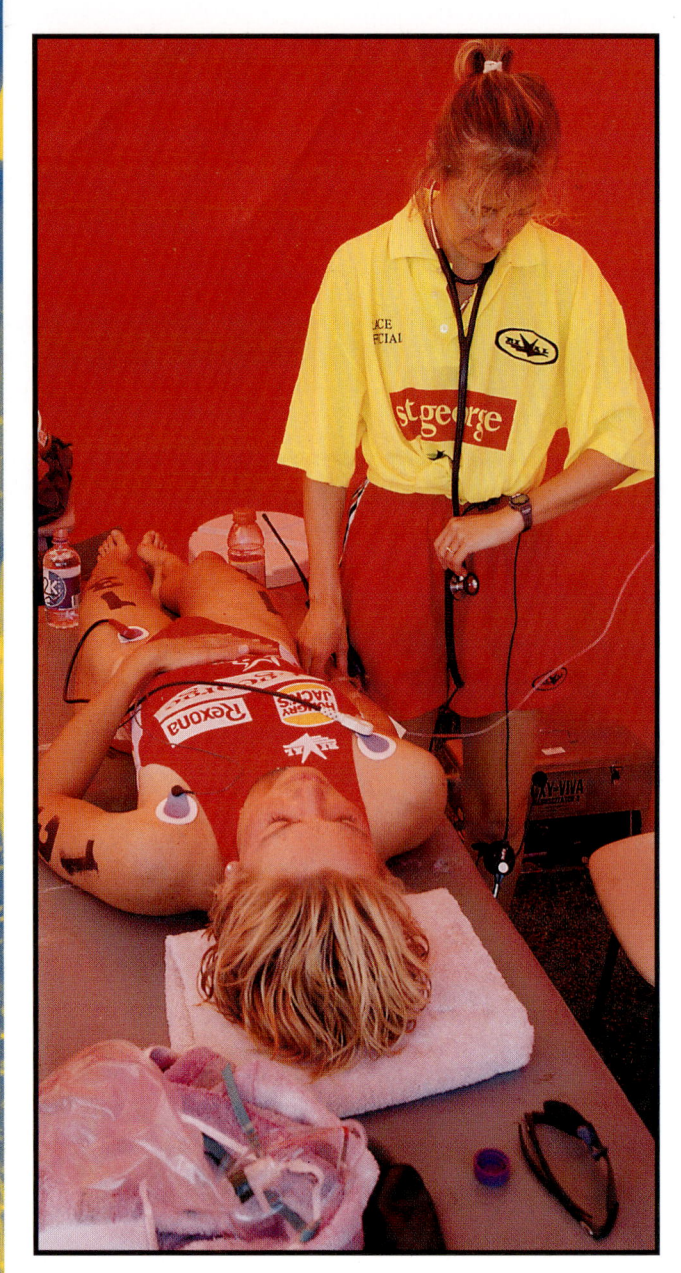

Serious athletes should never underestimate the importance of preparation. The above triathlete had suspected food poisoning on the morning of her competition. Pay absolute attention to detail and be aware of what you are eating and drinking — especially the night before competition.

Phase 2: Training to compete or improve

During this phase you should apply the concepts you learned during the 'training to train' phase, in order to develop a specific program that will work for you. During phase 1 you will have tried many different styles and types of training — some worked and some didn't. In this phase you'll modify those that worked to suit your individual needs, and you'll begin to find out what other things you need to include in your program to improve your results.

For recreational athletes, phase 2 is all about training to show improvement. Throughout this phase you'll start to notice changes in the way you feel and look and how you respond to training. You'll find that some of the results you had hoped for didn't occur, while other positive changes happened that you hadn't counted on.

Sometimes when women first start weight training, they'll see an increase in the size or girth of their thighs. For many women who experience this, it's a nightmare. Yet, it seems to occur only for the first few months; after the training has become more individual and specific to that person, the results reverse and they end up with legs they are really happy with.

By focusing on learning control and stability you'll become stronger or fitter with seemingly little effort.

In this phase you'll still be putting all your training together — planning and experimenting.

A serious athlete in this phase will be planning to compete more often. During this phase you will learn:

- how to prepare for competition;
- how to taper and plan recovery cycles;
- how to eat on the days before and after competition;
- how much of each type of training you should do in the weeks preceding competition; and
- when to stop certain aspects of training and allow your body to recover from them.

Preparing to Train

The main aim for the serious athlete is to put together a plan for your competition period. You need to have it down perfectly. Once you have designed this plan for the final two or three weeks leading into a competition, you'll need to practise it again and again until you have refined it and it works perfectly.

Serious athletes should have a routine for everything they do. Knowing what you have to do before you compete — how much you have to stretch, when to drink, when to eat, what time to start warming up, when to get your gear ready, and so on — all adds up to better preparation and a more polished performance.

Phase 3: Training to win or get results

This is the final — and best — phase. All the information you've gained from training through phases 1 and 2 will be put to use. You shouldn't need to modify too much of your program, as it's taken a long time to work out what suits you. During this phase it's time to achieve your best results.

For recreational athletes, training will really become enjoyable. Your program will be set up to suit you and only you. Every time you train you'll feel better, as you achieve small goals. You feel as if every step you take brings you closer to a better shape and greater fitness.

For serious athletes, the number of competitions undertaken in this phase should decrease as you concentrate on the major events you want to compete in. (Whether this is a local fun run or a national competition is irrelevant — whatever fits in with your goals.) You'll allow yourself time to put in place all your final taper cycles and ensure you are fully recovered and prepared for each competition. Minor adjustments can be made to your program between each competition if needed, or should you be injured or become ill.

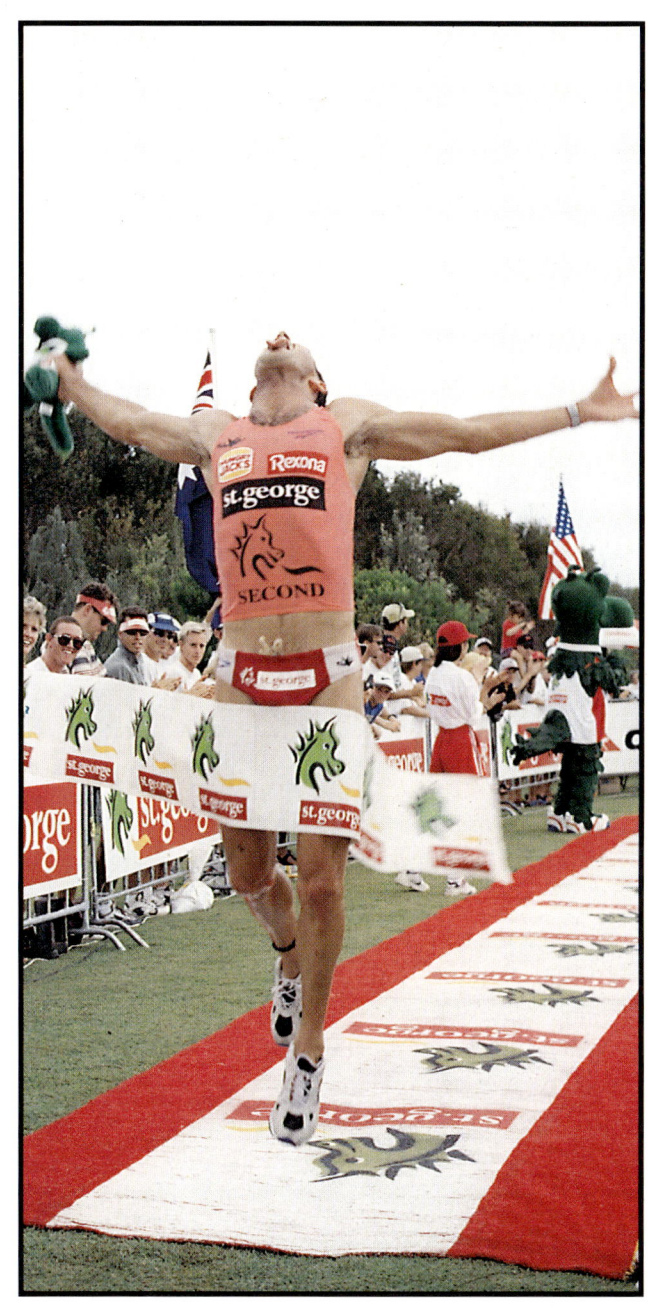

The hard work pays off. The difference between good and great athletes is that great athletes do everything right — right down to the smallest details — every session, every day, every week.

The Importance of Posture, Muscle Balance, Control and Flexibility

Our body was designed to move. It has muscles in specific areas that move bones and joints in exact ways. It's a bit like the secret to being able to rub your head in a circle while patting your tummy at the same time.

However, throughout your life certain things can happen that can change the way your muscles work, or the range of movement of your bones. This could be due to injury, illness, inactivity, incorrect technique, overtraining, excessive training of one muscle group, too much specific training, or you may have been born with minor imbalances that become worse with training.

Once you have good posture, muscle balance and control, your body will be more efficient in its movements and more effective at performing specific tasks. Activities will require less effort and less stress will be placed on your body.

Posture

Poor posture can lead to back and neck pain, decreased lung capacity, poor digestion and many other complaints.

Improvements in posture can make the difference between you getting through the day without headaches, feeling bloated or like you have to gasp for air each time you breathe. It can also mean the difference between doing a personal best in your next fun run and ending up injured after the first ten minutes. We have to watch the way we sit, stand, walk and carry our bodies while doing everyday, normal things if we are to avoid bad posture.

As part of your preparation for training, be sure to be aware of your posture and what you need to do to make any improvements. (See page 142 in the next chapter for postural tests.)

Muscle balance

Muscle balance refers to the strength and range of movement possible in muscles that work around each joint. Muscular imbalance occurs when one group of muscles becomes too strong or too tight, which can cause problems with posture as well as technique.

Many athletes have problems with technique because they have trouble getting their body into the required position. Tight muscles will make it hard to move a joint or limb into a position specific to a technique or movement. Strong muscles may pull a joint or limb out of a required position.

Common muscles in which imbalances can occur include:

Main abdominal muscles (Rectus Abdominis) — can cause hip instability and lower back problems. These problems are common, regardless of a person's fitness level.

Upper muscles of the back (Upper Trapezius) — can cause shoulder and neck problems. These problems are common to swimmers and throwers (for example, baseball players, javelin throwers and tennis players).

Outer muscles of the thigh (Vastus Lateralis) — can cause knee problems and shin splints. These problems are common to runners and can be a result of poor running technique or unsuitable footwear.

Muscle on either side of the spinal column (Erector Spinae) — can cause spinal misalignment and lower back problems. As with main abdominal muscles, these problems are common and occur, regardless of someone's fitness level.

Preparing to Train

A physiotherapist or experienced trainer can diagnose these problems and prescribe certain exercises to improve the strength of the weaker muscles while improving the flexibility of the tighter muscles. The tight muscles may have reduced the range of movement about a particular joint, and the weak muscles may have lost their ability to control a position of the joint.

Exercises to correct muscular imbalance and poor posture are probably the most critical exercises you can perform. However, many people don't treat these exercises with the respect they deserve. They are given exercises and treatment for an injury, but as soon as their symptoms disappear and they start to feel better, they stop doing the exercises and immediately resume their regular activities and exercise — which were probably the cause of the original problem! Whether you are training seriously or for social reasons, you should be including postural exercises in your training program every week.

Getting rid of the symptoms doesn't get rid of the problem. Be sure you find the time to include these crucial exercises in your daily schedule.

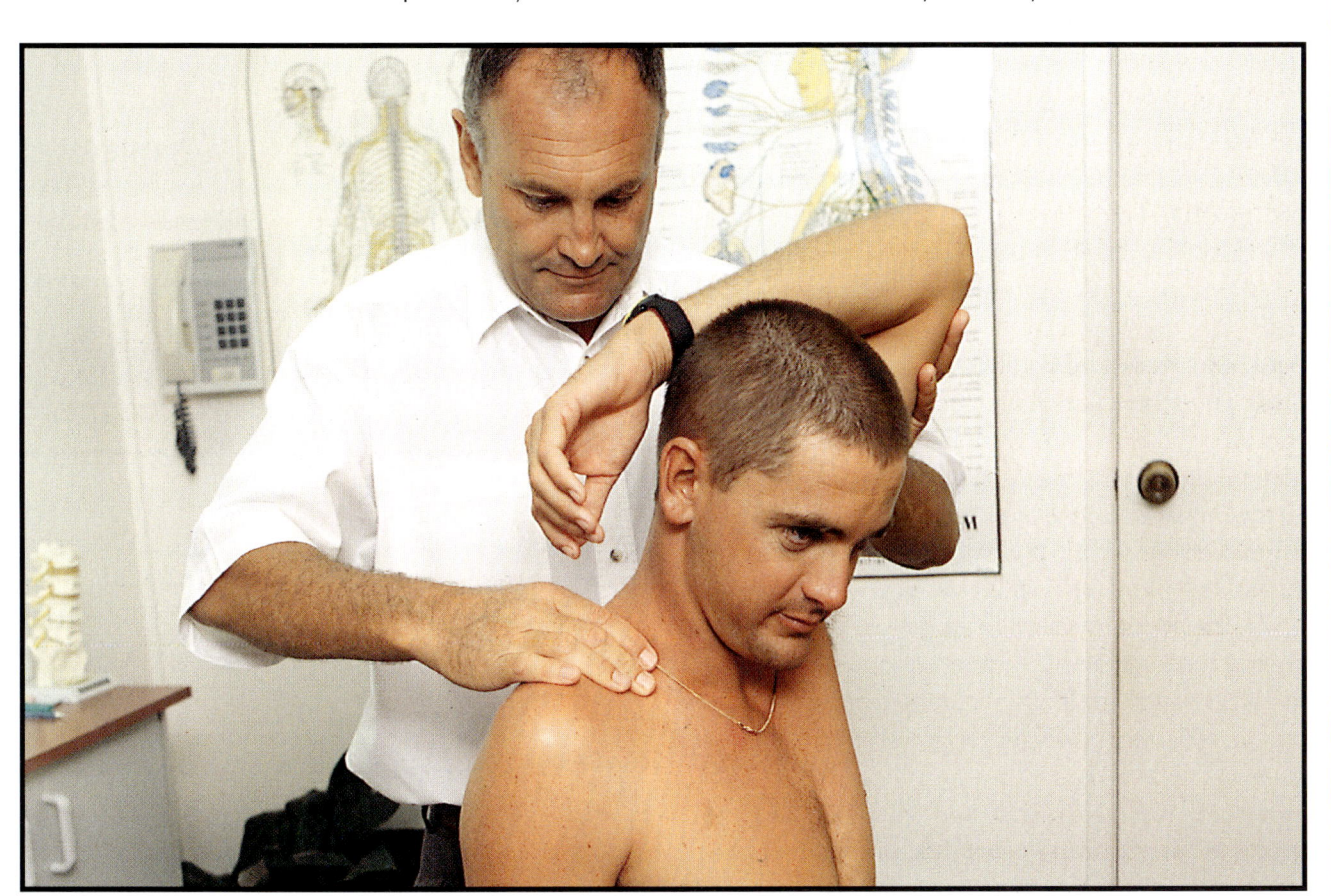

'I thought it would go away' — the most common words heard in a chiropractor's office. Keep yourself in line with regular checks.

Preparing to Train

Control

Once you have improved your posture and corrected any major muscular imbalances, the next aspect of preparing for training should be to achieve control of all your movements.

Learning how to control your body is like learning how to walk again using the correct muscles in the most efficient way. We can all walk, but we never give much thought to *how* we walk. Watch yourself walk towards a mirror. Do you throw your hips from side to side, or do you walk with no movement at all in your hips? Ideally, you should be somewhere in between. You need strong abdominals, and your hips should be square to the direction in which you're moving. Whatever your style of walking may be, it may need some work to improve flexibility and control of the muscles being used.

Abdominal muscles are another group of muscles we use poorly. For years we've had machines and exercises designed to improve our abdominal strength. Unfortunately, most of these exercises and machines have been designed to work only the major abdominal muscle — Rectus Abdominis. This is the muscle that gives you the 'washboard' look in your abdominal region. But this isn't the most important muscle in our abdominal region. This distinction is held by a smaller, lesser-known muscle called Transversus Abdominis — a muscle low in our abdominal area which is used extensively to control hip positioning when we move. A weakness in this muscle can reduce your ability to control the position of the hips during any movement that involves the hips. Neglect of this muscle is one of the reasons why people get lower back pain. Try sucking your stomach in and holding it, while continuing to breathe, walk and talk. Then let go and then see how 'laziness' contributes to your stomach sticking out. Make a conscious effort to hold your stomach in — make it a habit.

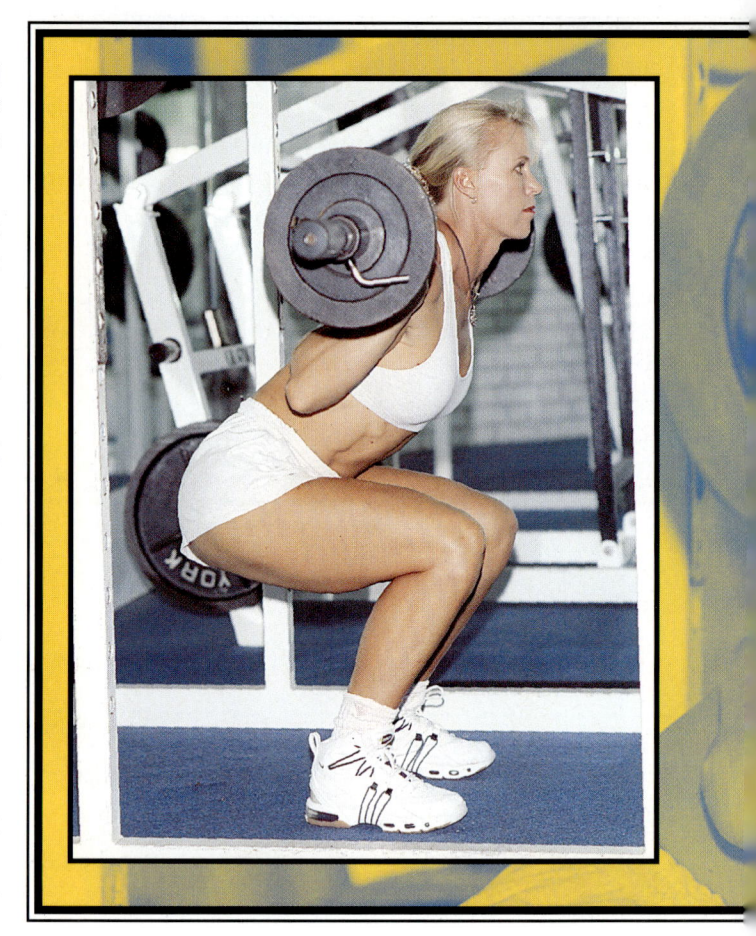

Physiotherapists and trainers have had to re-educate people about how to use their Transversus Abdominis properly to reduce back, hip and knee pain. This little muscle can be the cause of many injuries. All the abdominal exercises listed on pages 212–213 will train this muscle.

Flexibility

Flexibility is the most neglected aspect of most training programs. Commonly, you will see people finish a run or swim, hop straight into their car, go home for a shower, and then go off to work or out for dinner.

Improving My Control

Improving my control is what helped me to go from being able to squat 42.5 kilograms to squatting 80 kilograms in less than eight months — and with the correct technique. I spent 10–12 weeks on training for improved posture; I strengthened my abdominals, glute muscles and shoulder-blade stabilisers. These changes influenced and improved my muscular control. This not only improved my leg strength, but it carried over to all my other physical activities.

My 50 metres kick time in the pool dropped from 55 seconds to 41, my running improved to the point where I could run for 30 minutes continuously, which I'd never been able to do before in my life. I could bench-press 70 kilograms — more than I weighed — and my flexibility improved markedly because there was less strain on those other muscles in my hip region.

This can only continue for a short period of time. You will generally find that injury will result directly from *not stretching*. A little bit of time spent stretching can reduce the risk of injury markedly.

There are four kinds of stretching you can do:

1. Stretching as a warm-up: This is normally much lighter than all other forms of stretching because you have to be careful not to overstretch muscles too close to the time that you need to use them. Overstretching, or intense stretching, can reduce your ability to use those muscles, especially for activities where you need speed or strength. If you overstretch, your muscles will feel too relaxed and will be less inclined to respond to heavy loads or situations where a quick reaction is required (for example, a start in a swimming or running race).

2. Stretching as a means of recovery (cooling down): This can be done after an activity, during an activity, or the day after an activity, to release tension or maintain the range of movement you've developed so far. Stretching during exercise or sporting activity can allow you to carry on with more ease. It can improve the recovery time in muscles and it can be an effective way to use a rest period instead of sitting around doing nothing. Stretching the next day can ease those sore, tired muscles and free up any stiffness around a joint. Including one 60-minute session of stretching per week on top of the stretching I do after every training session has given me great results.

3. Stretching for injury rehabilitation: This is used to improve the flexibility of a muscle that may be causing a problem in movement or technique. After injury, flexibility will assist you in returning to exercise or sport more quickly, and reduce the risk of a recurrence. This stretching is generally guided by a coach or physiotherapist and will be specifically aimed at one region or joint.

4. Stretching to improve flexibility: This is the most difficult to achieve. Many people stretch to improve flexibility, but in reality they are only stretching to maintain their current flexibility. Stretching to improve flexibility requires much longer sessions and needs to be fairly structured and specific to what stretches you will do, and how long you will hold each stretch. Preferably, it will also require someone to help you.

Preparing to Train

This type of stretching can be very hard to do alone as it takes control to hold a stretch or to push it that little bit further each time to make a gain in movement.

Here are some basic rules about planning a stretching session:

- During warm-ups, stretch for as long as *you* need — don't stretch for the sake of stretching just because your friend happens to stretch for 30 minutes in his or her warm-up.
- Don't stretch immediately after a strength or speed session because this may reduce the effect of the session. However, be sure to stretch three to four hours later.
- Make time for your stretching to fit in with your normal training program so that you don't have to rush off at the end of your training session.
- As a general rule, stretch for a third of the amount of time you've been training. If your run lasted for 30 minutes, you should stretch for 10 minutes.
- Plan for at least one session of stretching each week to improve your flexibility, as well as sessions for warm-up, recovery and maintenance.

Overtraining

How many people train for an event, only to fall ill as soon as they start to rest? You must include consistent rest periods in your training program to avoid being at risk of overtraining.

I hear of so many athletes who become exhausted from overtraining. Often they are diagnosed with glandular fever, chronic fatigue syndrome or some other virus as a direct result. In such cases there has been no recognition by the coach that the particular athlete has needed more rest than they have been having. Coaches need to recognise that their athletes are individuals and need different amounts of rest.

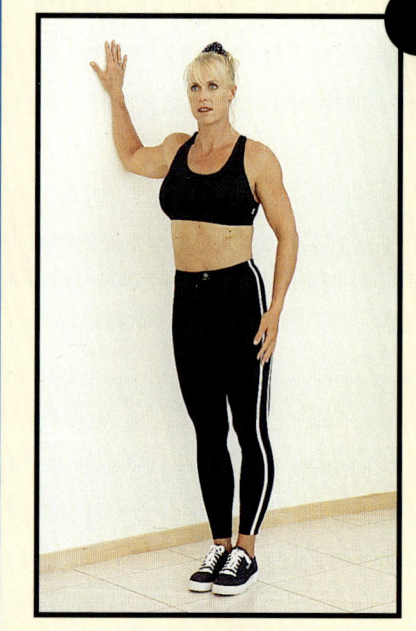

Chest
Place one arm up at a right angle against a wall, turn away from the wall and feel the stretch come into your chest and shoulder area.

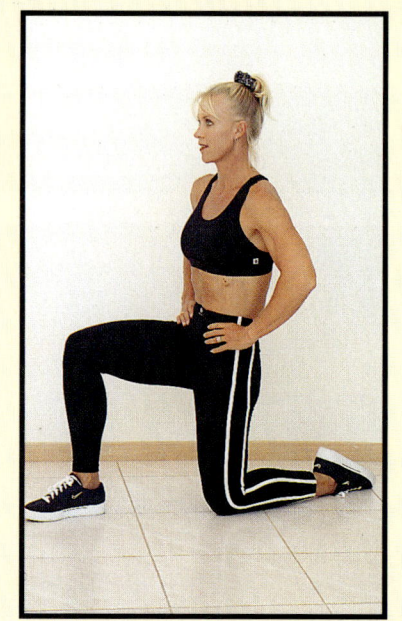

Quadriceps
Kneeling on one knee — keeping your upper body tall — suck your stomach in and tuck your bottom under and feel the stretch in the front of the thigh you're leaning on.

Preparing to Train

Five All-over Body Stretches

Use these five stretches
- after a light warm-up (15-30 secs)
- after a cool down (30-45 secs)
- as a stretching maintenance session (30-60 secs, 3 x week).

- Do these stretches while watching TV or after a warm bath/shower. Remember to change sides. Breathe and relax deeper into the stretch.

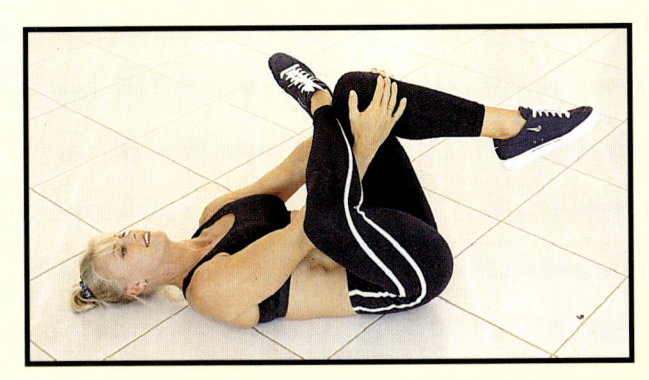

Glutes
Cross your right ankle over your left knee and pull your left knee into the chest. You'll feel your right hip and bottom stretch.

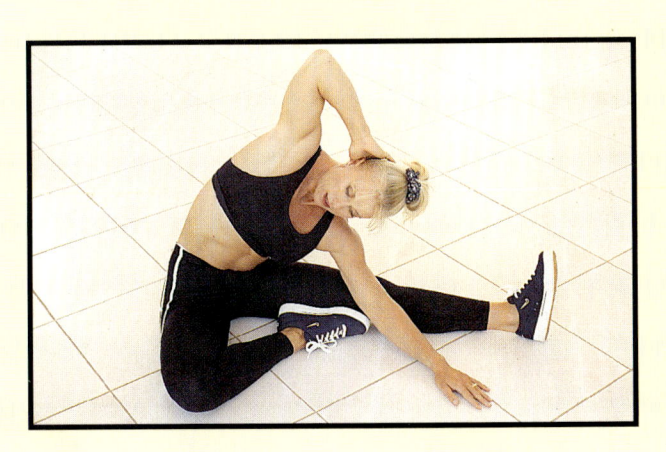

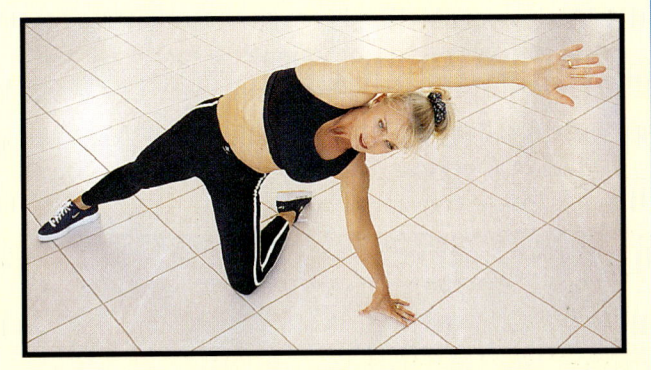

Lats/shoulders/hips
Kneeling on one knee with your other leg stretched straight out to the side, stretch the same arm as your outstretched leg over your head and slowly arch your body up so that your hips lift to the roof. You'll feel the stretch under your shoulder, and in your side and hip.

Hamstrings/back
Sit down with your right leg tucked in against your straight left leg. Place your right hand on your head and lean forward. Try to place your left shoulder on your left knee and keep your right elbow high. You will be stretching your right side and left hamstring.

Training & Fitness

Get UP&GO!

Preparing to Train

When you combine training with school work, college or uni, work, parenthood or any other major part of your life, those factors other than training must be accounted for in your training program. Failure to do this will almost certainly result in overtraining — which can involve fatigue, stress, depression, illness and/or injury.

Take it upon yourself to decide when you need to rest. Don't make excuses for missing training, but if you truly need a rest, then take it. You won't lose any conditioning by taking two or three days' rest; however, after three days of no training your body will start to 'detrain'. Parents also need to make decisions based on how they see their child coping with training — make sure they get enough rest periods.

If you rest straight away, you may only need to miss a day or two of training. If you continue to push yourself, you'll end up having to have a week off or, worse still, several months.

Watch out for these symptoms of overtraining:

- feeling constantly tired and irritable or aggressive; insomnia;
- an elevated morning pulse (that is, your pulse is ten or more beats higher than normal — make sure you know what 'normal' is) for several days in a row;
- consistently elevated blood pressure (visit your doctor to have your blood pressure checked);
- aching or a heavy feeling in your legs;

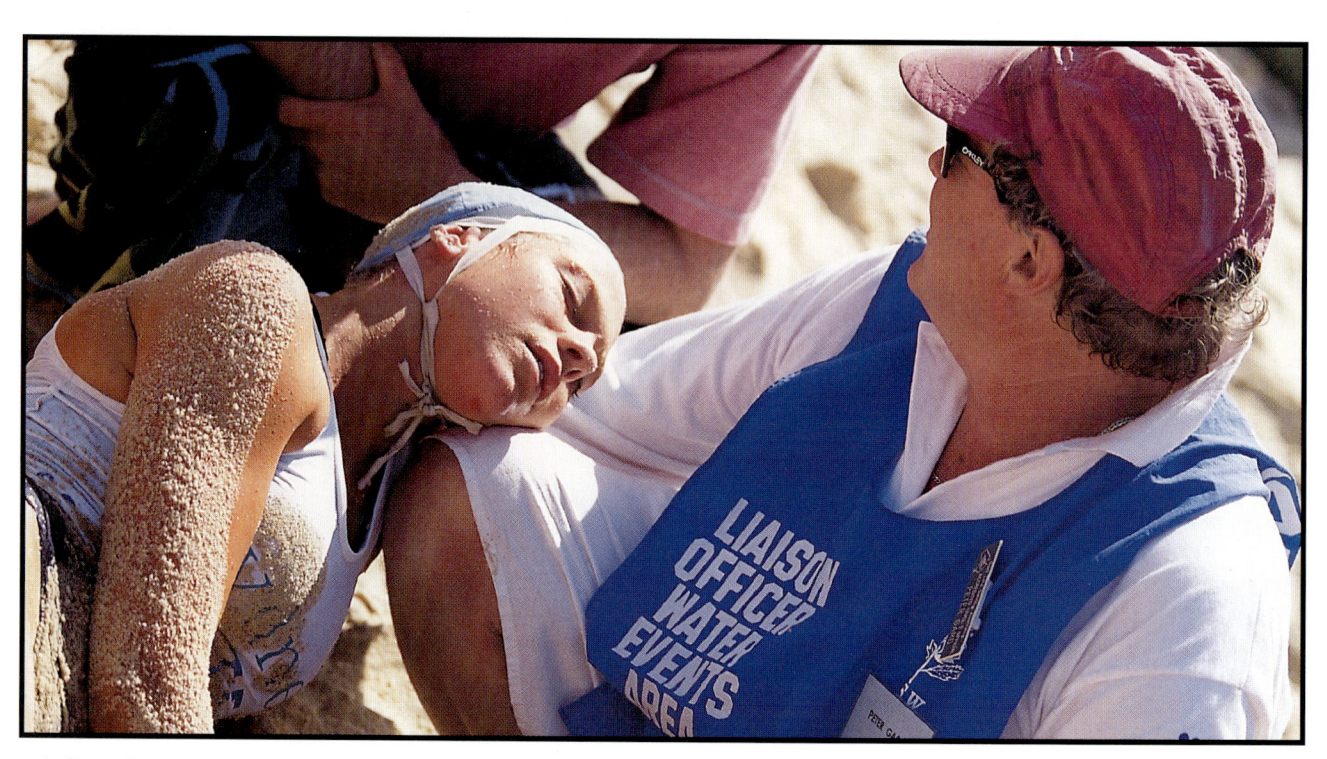

A well-conditioned and smartly trained athlete will be fresh, energetic and motivated. These athletes can back up race after race with a very high standard of performance. Failure to observe overtraining symptoms can result in illness, injury and exhaustion.

Preparing to Train

- loss of appetite; developing poor eating habits; loss of body weight;
- depression; low self-esteem; lack of concentration;
- loss of motivation to exercise;
- increased frequency of colds and flu;
- increased frequency of injury;
- decrease in performance;
- amenorrhoea (the absence of menstruation);
- low iron levels; and
- physical symptoms such as dry, loose skin, poor hair condition, loss of muscle tone, excessive looseness or tightness in muscles.

How to prevent overtraining:

If at any stage you think you might be suffering from overtraining, rest immediately and modify your training program. Try some of these suggestions:
- Take one to three days off training. Only do very light walking, or very light work of your particular sport. Have a massage, go to the movies, go surfing, play tennis — do something different and enjoyable, or do absolutely nothing.
- Get to bed earlier for a few nights, and nap during the day. If you can't sleep during the day, try lying down and listening to some relaxation music — think of nothing and relax.
- Eat really well and drink plenty of water — cut out all junk food.
- Have a blood test. Record your results so that you can monitor your health further down the track.
- It's time to go back to training when you start to feel human again and are itching to get back. These are good signs that you are freshening up. Give your body a chance to gather the strength it needs.
- Plan your training program carefully and precisely.
- Include variety in your training program.
- Include regular rest and recovery periods.

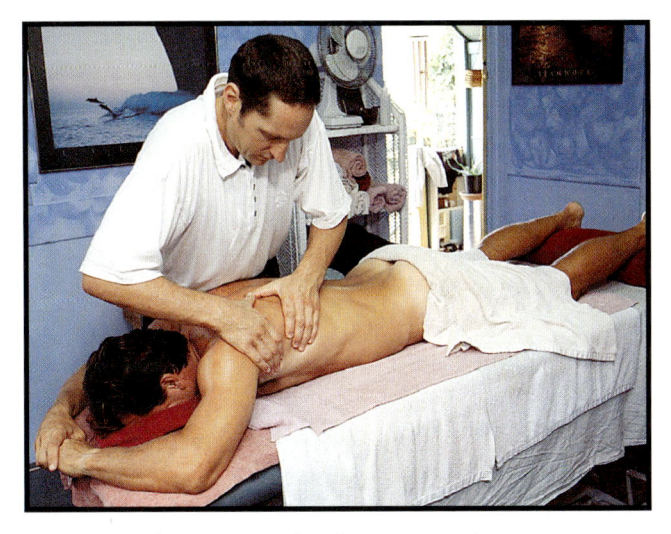

Use massage for recovery, relaxation or stress release. Next time you have to buy someone a present buy them a massage — it feels wonderful!

- Test your progress on a regular basis.
- Maintain an awareness of your attitude to training and the attitudes of those around you.
- Regularly monitor your recovery from training — for example, record your resting heart rate after training and note how much sleep you need. Look in the mirror — how does your face look? Bright or dull? How do your eyes look? Red and puffy, or clear and bright? How does your tongue look? Coated or normal?

■ ■ ■

The most important point to consider is that what you've been doing up until now has probably not been what's best for you. Go back to the basics and learn how to train properly *now* — it will pay off later.

In the next chapter, we'll test your fitness so that you'll have a starting point from which to begin planning your own training program.

Test Your Fitness

Don't just rush out and start exercising. You could do yourself
a lot of damage, or waste your effort by exercising incorrectly, making
your goals much more difficult — even impossible — to achieve.
You must have a starting point from which you can both set and measure
your goals. This chapter shows you how to test your current level of fitness
and identify which areas of your body need special attention.

[Where Are You Now?]

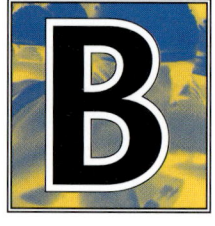

Before starting any new training program, you should first establish where you are now. Do your feet hit the ground running at the mention of exercise, or would you rather stay in bed? How much time are you prepared to allocate towards exercise and training? What kind of training do you like?

The following questionnaire will help you to establish your attitude towards exercise and training. After you have answered all ten questions, add up your score and check your results.

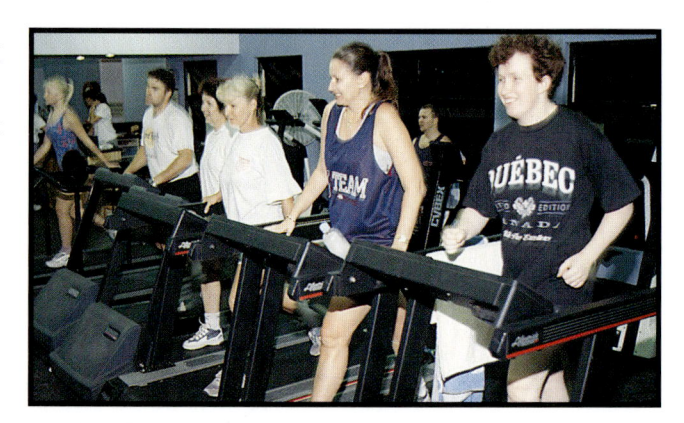

Treadmills can be custom-programmed to suit your individual fitness level and exercise requirements.

Test Your Fitness

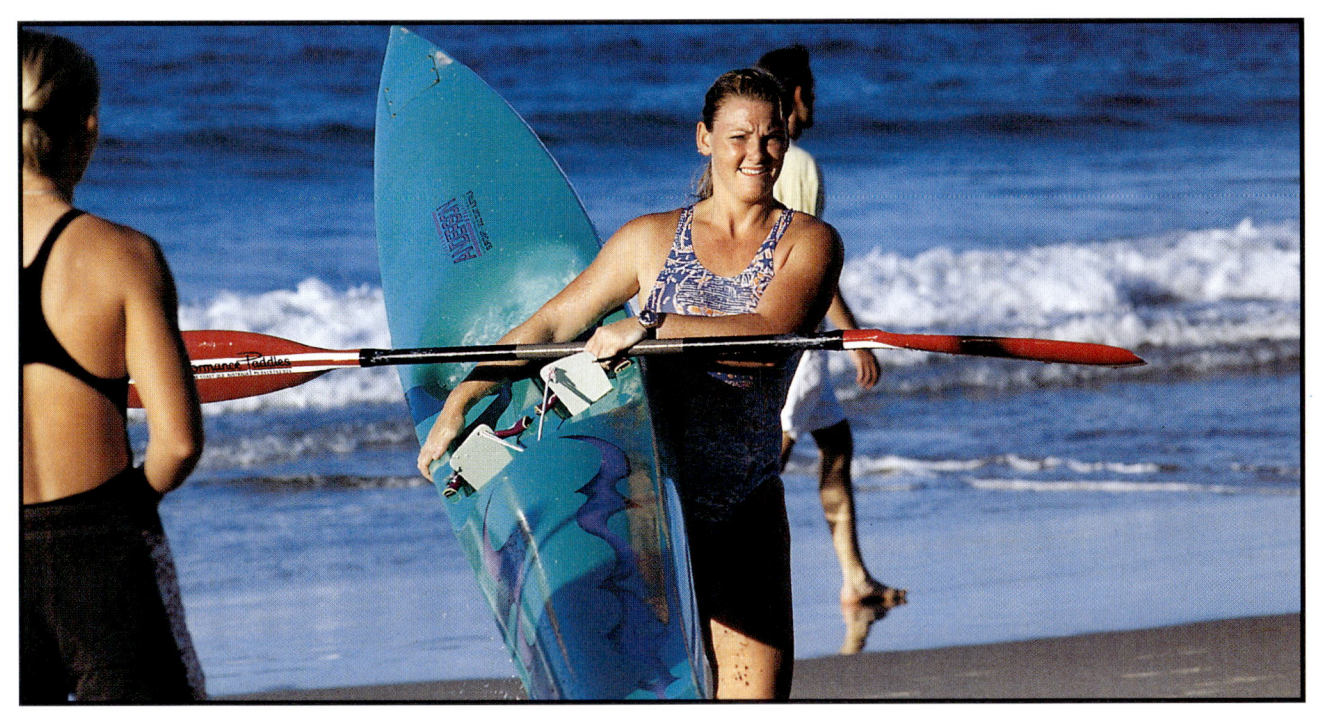

Surf lifesaving offers a wide range of activities for the whole family.

1. Training History

I have never really exercised. 5
I have yet to take on an exercise program fully and have only dabbled in the past.

I have been regular with my fitness recently. 3
I have been training regularly for between six months and two years. During this time I've been involved in a number of different training activities and I've had reasonable success with each one, but not really great results.

I was born with cross-trainers on my feet. 1
I have been training for more than two years and I've had periods of great intensity and seriousness, and have been involved in a number of different training methods.

2. Motivation

I love my bed/chair/spa. 5
Don't wake me in the morning, I need my sleep!

I enjoy some activity. 3
When the mood is right, I can be very active.

When's the next workout? 1
Just mention the word 'exercise' and my feet hit the ground running.

Get **UP&GO!**

3. How Often Do You Exercise?

Never or occasionally. 5
I do no exercise or only one session a week.

I'm fairly regular with my exercise. 3
I do two to three sessions a week.

I'm committed to exercising regularly every week. 1
I do four to five sessions a week.

4. Preferred Training

I only want to walk or swim or run, etc. 5
I really only want to concentrate on one activity at present.

I want to do a number of different training activities. 3
I'm keen to cross-train to add some variety to my training.

I try to do a little bit of everything — gym, run, swim, cycle, etc. 1
I want to make the most of all my training options

5. Time Available To Train

I have only limited time each week. 5
I'm able to commit to one or two sessions each week.

I can train fairly regularly. 3
I can train at least two or three times each week.

I can train anytime, anywhere. 1
I can train daily if I need to.

6. Injuries

I have a few injuries I need to be careful with. ... 5
I'm carrying a few niggling problems that cause me concern.

I have had a few injuries in the past. 3
But that was then — I seem to be fine now.

I have never had any injuries. 1
I'm free of injury and pain.

7. Training Routine

I would like a very general training routine that's easy to follow. 5

I would like an individual program, but not too complicated. 3

I have a very specific exercise program. 1

8. Postural Considerations

When I look in the mirror I see someone who is slightly stooped, with head leaning forward or to one side, abdomen protruding and arms hanging in front of my thighs. 5

When I look in the mirror I see someone who has slightly uneven shoulders, slight abdomen protrusion and is slightly hollow in the lower back area. 3

When I look in the mirror I see someone who stands very tall, square shoulders, head held straight, arms hanging straight by the side and abdomen tucked in, not protruding. 1

9. Medical Considerations

I have a medical condition which limits my activities. 5

I have no medical conditions at present, but I have to be wary of doing certain exercises which have caused problems in the past. 3

I have no medical conditions that will limit my activity. 1

10. Nutritional Considerations

I eat and drink anything I like whenever I like. . . . 5
I often miss meals, and takeaway food often gets me through the weekends. As for vegetables, well . . .

I think my diet is healthy. I don't eat much junk food and I try to be careful about my fat intake. 3
After keeping a food and fluid diary for a week I wasn't so sure — I found I was eating too much of some food groups and not enough of others.

I try to eat a healthy, well-balanced diet. 1
I enjoy eating plenty of nutritious carbohydrates, moderate amounts of meat (or meat alternatives) and I only use mono-unsaturated and polyunsaturated fats carefully. After keeping a food and fluid diary I found I was a little careless in some areas of my diet, and I need to change when I eat and drink to improve my training performance.

> 'Only you can make that decision to get out and change your life.'
> — Mark McKean

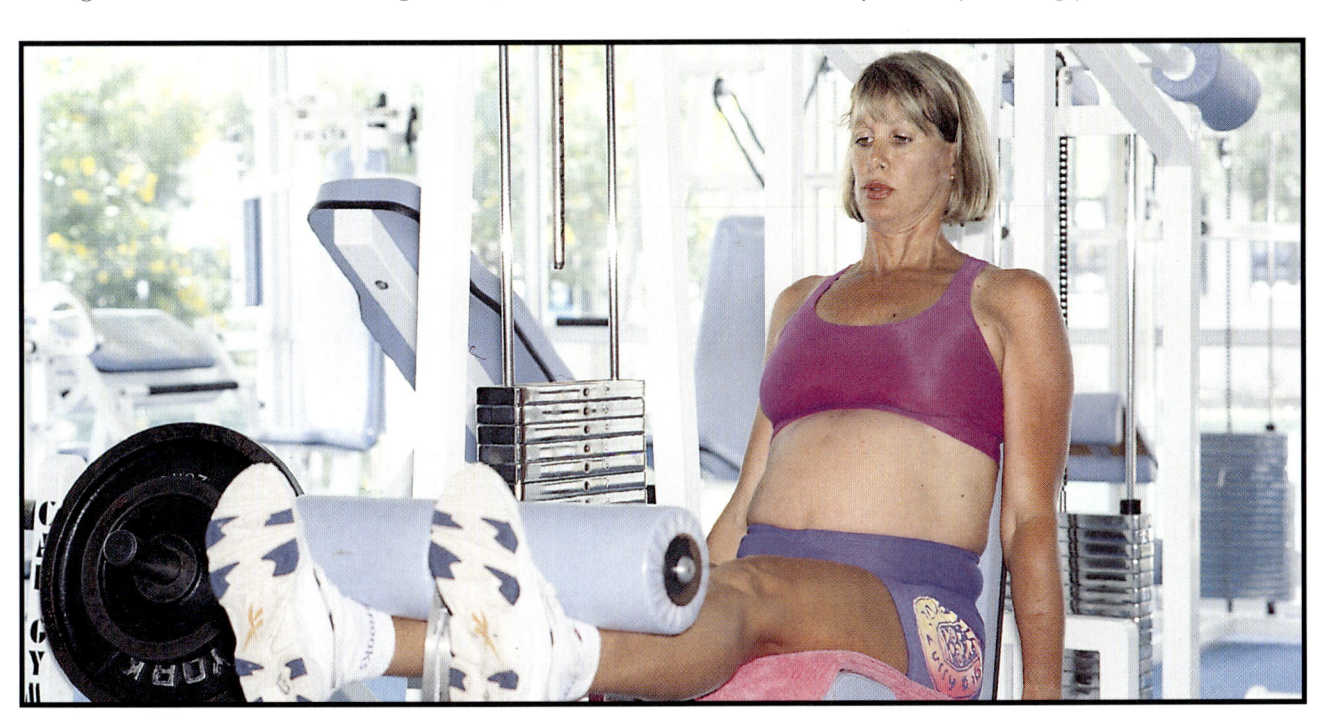

Keeping fit is a long-term commitment, whatever your shape.

Test Your Fitness

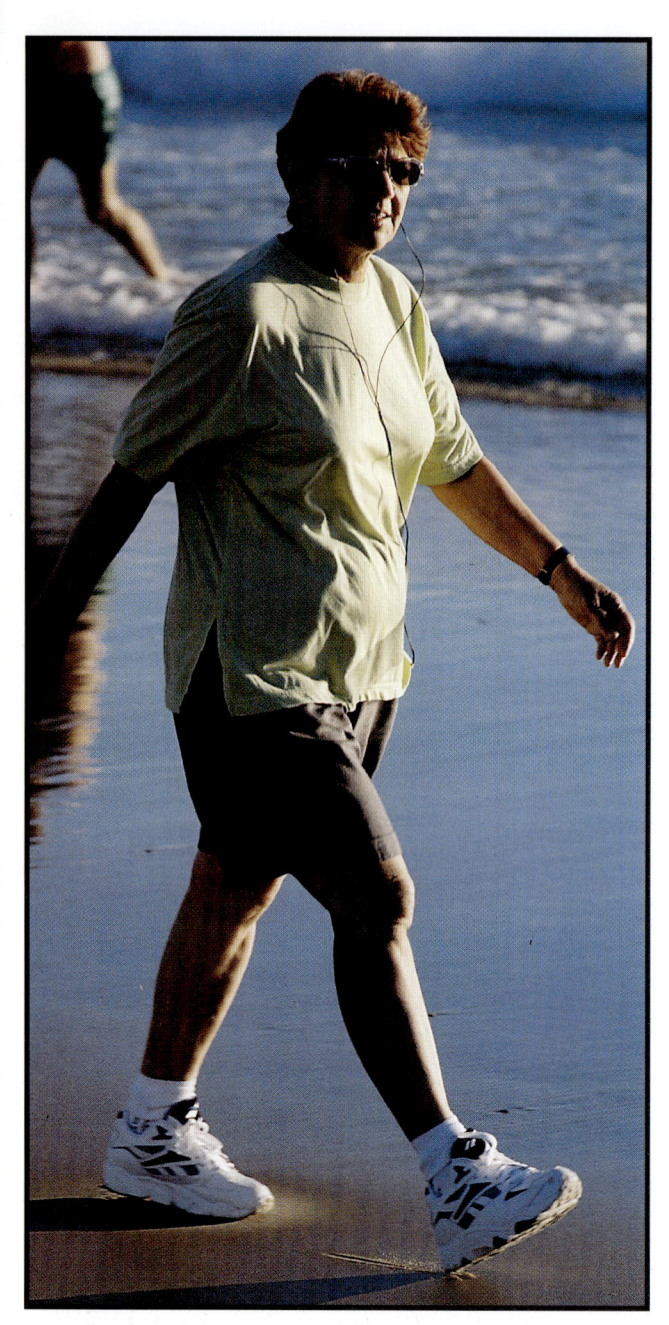

So many people run or walk on beaches. Early morning and late afternoon are great times to enjoy exercise and watch beautiful sunrises and sunsets.

Your Score

41 to 50 points:

You haven't been active lately so you'll need to be extremely careful in your choice of activity and the level at which you do it. Make sure you get a medical clearance and have a fitness professional do a full analysis on your current fitness level before starting. Initially, you'll probably find exercise difficult (and naturally so — don't be afraid or disillusioned). Set yourself smaller goals spread over a period of time and build on your success. Set goals for every level of activity: body-fat changes, how your clothes feel, how your skin looks, how your energy levels improve. Be more concerned initially with the fact that at last you are exercising rather than how much you do and how hard you do it.

31 to 40 points:

You have probably done some exercise recently and find that you go through periods of extreme keenness and periods of absolute boredom. Often things get in the way of a real commitment to fitness and health — other areas of your life may take priority; you might put your work, family and hobbies before your health and fitness. Exercise may not seem to be doing much for you; however, when you do exercise you notice a different level of wellbeing and it does improve your ability to get through each day. You might have some conditions that may cause problems but you can overcome them when you want to. You'll need to find an activity you really enjoy or you simply won't do it. The more you like it the more quickly you'll get results and the better you'll feel about taking time out to do it.

21 to 30 points:

You enjoy exercise and you make time to include it in your life. There will always be times when you have to

Test Your Fitness

put your training program on hold, but generally you can get back into it easily and have been doing so for some time. You may not yet have had the results you wanted, but you feel pretty good doing it and this is just as important to you. You have been successful in organising your time and balancing your exercise with other aspects of your life. However, you have possibly been frustrated by not achieving what you really wanted and haven't been prepared to put more into working at it. The good news is that you don't need more time — you just need a more suitable program.

11 to 20 points:
You almost have the ideal attitude to exercise. You have probably been keen on exercise for some time and generally enjoy yourself. You feel you need just a little guidance to make the crucial difference that will lift you to the next level. Generally, you find that most exercises and activities are okay, but some of them don't get the results you want, and this is where you need help in identifying more options. Your health is generally good, but there are occasions when you feel a bit low or lethargic. The type of exercise you need to do should be based on your specific needs. General exercises will no longer give you the results you're after; you need to find out what it is *exactly* that will get you those results.

0 to 10 points:
You are a very organised person who has total control over your lifestyle. You could be termed fanatical — but in the nicest sense, of course. You have probably dealt with all areas of fitness and health and have had success. All options have been considered and sorted out, and your exercise level suits your time and needs. You may not have achieved all your goals, but you're probably steadily working towards them. When you encounter difficulties, you will generally seek professional help, or spend time reading about how to improve things. You may feel you need reinforcement to make sure you're doing it properly and doing it well. Most concerns about your fitness revolve around the concept of overall planning for the year.

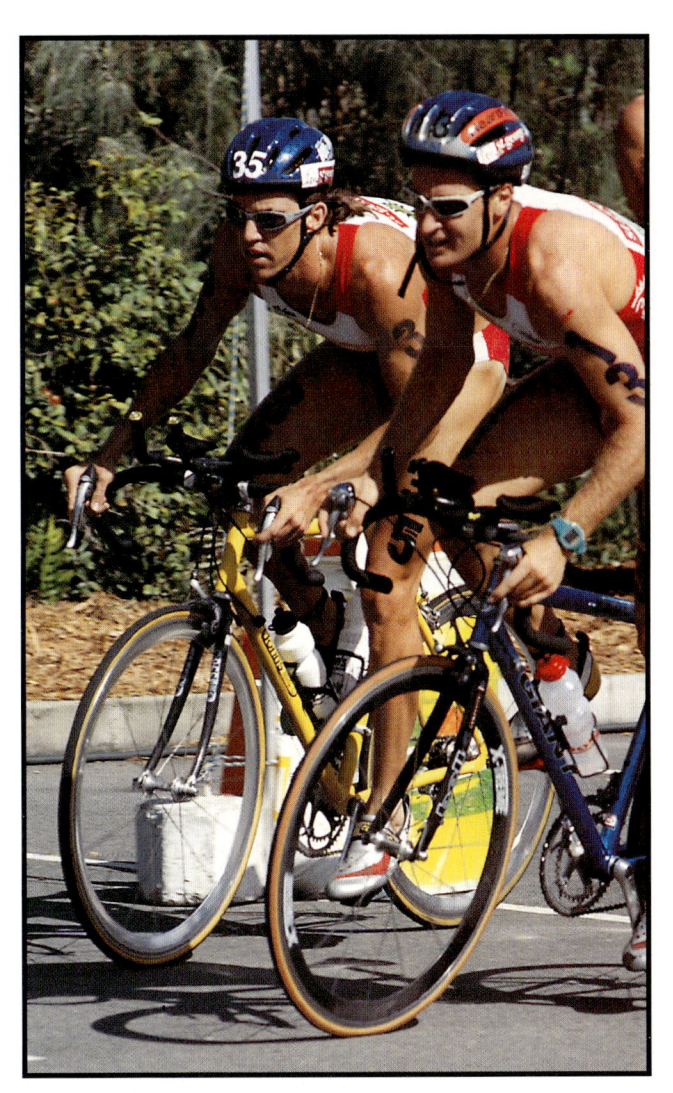

Who wants it more? Who is prepared to hurt themselves more? Who has been the better prepared? The finish line will tell the story.

Training & Fitness

Get UP&GO!

Test Your Fitness

> ### Warning!
> Fitness testing can be dangerous if it's not done properly. Make sure you get a medical clearance before performing any of the fitness tests outlined below. If, at any time during the tests, you feel unwell, faint, lightheaded or nauseous, or you feel tingling or numbing pain anywhere in your body, you should stop immediately and check with your doctor or a qualified trainer before starting again.

Test Your Fitness

The following tests will gauge your current abilities in several areas so that you'll know exactly where you are now and can measure and enjoy your success in the future.

We'll be looking at your:
- heart rate;
- aerobic fitness;
- strength and muscular endurance;
- girth measurements; and
- posture.

General rules for testing

Each test has a set of procedures relating to how it should be conducted and measured. Make sure you use these protocols and adhere to them strictly. By failing to follow these rules your results are open to questioning and can not be considered reliable tests of performance for now or for comparison when further testing is carried out.

1. Maintain accurate records of results so that you can easily measure your improvement and relate it to the goals you have set for yourself.
2. Only test yourself if you're going to do something with the results.
3. Repeat the test exactly as you did it the first time in order to accurately measure your progress.

Resting heart rate

Your resting heart rate is a measure of your heart's rate of pumping while you are inactive, which can be used to measure stress or the rate of recovery from exercise. Your resting heart rate can also be used to set training intensities. The average resting heart rate is 72 beats per minute (bpm). As your fitness level improves, your resting heart rate will drop.

After you have been seated for at least three minutes in a relaxed state, take your pulse. To take your pulse, place your first and second fingers on your carotid artery — just behind your windpipe in your neck — and count the number of beats for 60 seconds. The number of beats you count will give you your heart rate as measured by beats per minute. Remember not to use your thumb to monitor your pulse because your thumb has its own pulse.

Aerobic Fitness

Your aerobic fitness is a measure of the efficiency of your heart and lungs in providing oxygen and blood to working muscles and aiding recovery.

The 12-minute run/walk test

Go to an oval or athletics field where you can measure the distance. If you don't have access to a field that has distances marked you could record the point you reached and when you come to re-test, see if you get any further. If you choose to run, you may switch to walking at any time during the test; however, you should only walk during the walk test. You should note that continuous activity is best. After 12 minutes, record your heart rate and the distance you completed. After you have completed a period of time on your training program, repeat the test and see if your results have improved. You may be able to cover a greater distance with a lower heart rate, be able to walk or run further in 12 minutes, or perhaps you will notice that you can walk or run continuously for the 12 minutes and it begins to feel easier than the last time you took the test.

The 12-minute swim test

This is done by swimming as far as you can in 12 minutes. It's best to have someone else help you with this test by timing you and recording your results. Alternatively, you could invest in a sports watch and set your alarm for 12 minutes. You may switch strokes or stop at any time, but continuous freestyle is the best choice for an accurate assessment.

Use the guide on page 132. Find your age group column and look down until you find the distance you were able to cover in 12 minutes, then look across to the fitness level column to gauge your level of fitness.

> 'The greatest pleasure in life is doing what people say you cannot do.'
> — Walter Bagehot

The 12-minute Run/Walk Test

Fitness level	Sex	Age group					
		13—19	20—29	30—39	40—49	50—59	60+
		Distance taken to complete the 12-minute run/walk test					< less than > more than
Poor	Men	<2.09	<1.96	<1.90	<1.83	<1.66	<1.40
	Women	<1.61	<1.54	<1.51	<1.43	<1.35	<1.26
Below minimum	Men	2.09–2.20	1.96–2.11	1.90–2.10	1.83–2.00	1.66–1.87	1.40–1.65
	Women	1.61–1.90	1.54–1.79	1.53–1.70	1.43–1.58	1.35–1.49	1.26–1.39
Minimum	Men	2.21–2.52	2.12–2.40	2.11–2.34	2.01–2.24	1.88–2.10	1.66–1.94
	Women	1.91–2.08	1.80–1.97	1.71–1.90	1.59–1.79	1.50–1.70	1.40–1.52
Good	Men	2.53–2.77	2.41–2.64	2.35–2.52	2.25–2.47	2.11–2.32	1.95–2.13
	Women	2.09–2.30	1.98–2.16	1.91–2.08	1.80–2.00	1.71–1.90	1.53–1.76
Excellent	Men	>2.78	>2.65	>2.53	>2.48	>2.33	>2.14
	Women	>2.31	>2.17	>2.09	>2.01	>1.91	>1.77

Modified from B. Leelarthaepin & J. Schell, *Physical Fitness Assessment in Sport and Exercise Science*, 2nd ed. (Leelar Biomedisience Services, Sydney, 1994.)

Test Your Fitness

The 12-minute Swim Test

Fitness level	Sex	Age group					
		13—19	20—29	30—39	40—49	50—59	60+
		Distance covered in 12 minutes (in metres)					< less than > more than
Poor	Men	<545	<440	<385	<330	<275	<275
	Women	<440	<330	<275	<220	<165	<165
Below minimum	Men	545–655	440–545	380–490	220–330	275–380	275–330
	Women	440–545	330–440	275–380	220–330	165–275	165–220
Minimum	Men	655–765	545–655	490–600	440–545	380–490	330–440
	Women	545–655	440–545	380–490	330–440	275–380	220–330
Good	Men	765–875	655–765	600–710	545–655	490–600	440–545
	Women	655–765	545–655	490–600	440–545	380–490	330–440
Excellent	Men	>875	>765	>710	>655	>600	>545
	Women	>765	>655	>600	>545	>490	>440

Adapted from Joseph E. McEvoy, DPE, *Fitness Swimming Lifetime Programs* (Princeton Book Company, 1985)

Strength and Muscular Endurance Tests

The following tests will measure your ability to lift a certain amount of weight and the number of times you can repeat the movement before exhaustion sets in.

The push-up test

This test measures the strength and endurance of your upper body, particularly your chest, shoulders and arms. One push-up involves lowering your body until your chest comes in contact with the floor and extending your arms back up until you reach the start position again.

The push-up test for men is different from that for women. Men use the standard push-up position with the body straight off the floor, on hands and toes only. Women use the 'modified' push-up, with legs bent, knees on the floor, and with the body straight and supported by the arms. Hands should be shoulder-width apart and the body should be kept rigid.

Perform as many push-ups as you can without rest, then compare your score with the chart below. Find your age group column and look down until you find the range that covers the number of push-ups you were able to complete, then look across to the fitness level column to gauge your level of fitness.

Test Your Fitness

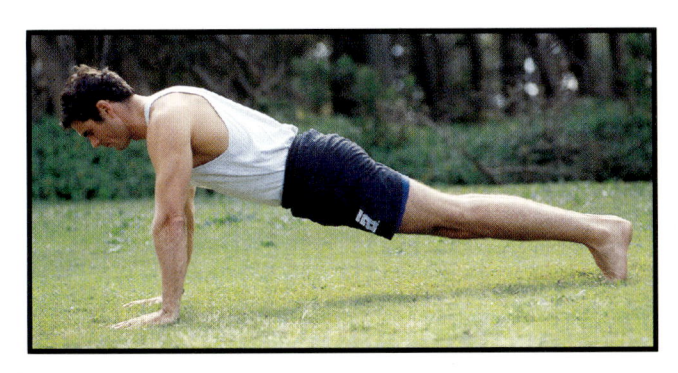

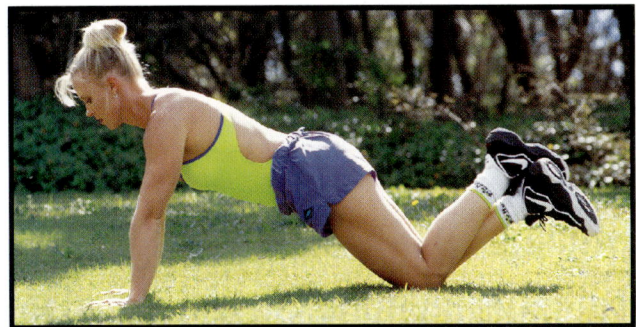

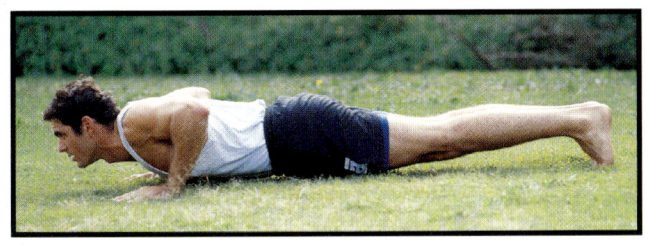

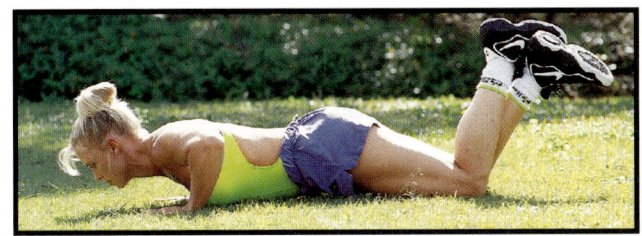

The 'standard' push-up position.

The 'modified' push-up position.

The Push-up Test

Fitness level	Sex	Age group					
		13—19	20—29	30—39	40—49	50—59	60+
		Number of push-ups completed				< less than > more than	
Poor	Men	<3	<3	<1			
	Women	0	0	0	0	0	0
Below minimum	Men	4–18	4–16	2–12	1–10	0–8	0–5
	Women	0–10	1–11	0–9	0–7	0–6	0–4
Minimum	Men	19–34	17–29	13–24	11–20	9–17	6–16
	Women	11–20	12–22	10–21	8–17	7–14	5–12
Good	Men	35–50	30–42	25–36	21–30	18–27	17–26
	Women	21–31	23–32	22–33	18–27	15–22	13–20
Excellent	Men	>51	>43	>37	>31	>28	>27
	Women	>32	>33	>34	>28	>2A	>21

Modified from B. Leelarthaepin & J. Schell, *Physical Fitness Assessment in Sport and Exercise Science*, 2nd ed. (Leelar Biomediscience Services, Sydney, 1994.)

Training & Fitness

Get UP&GO!

Test your Fitness

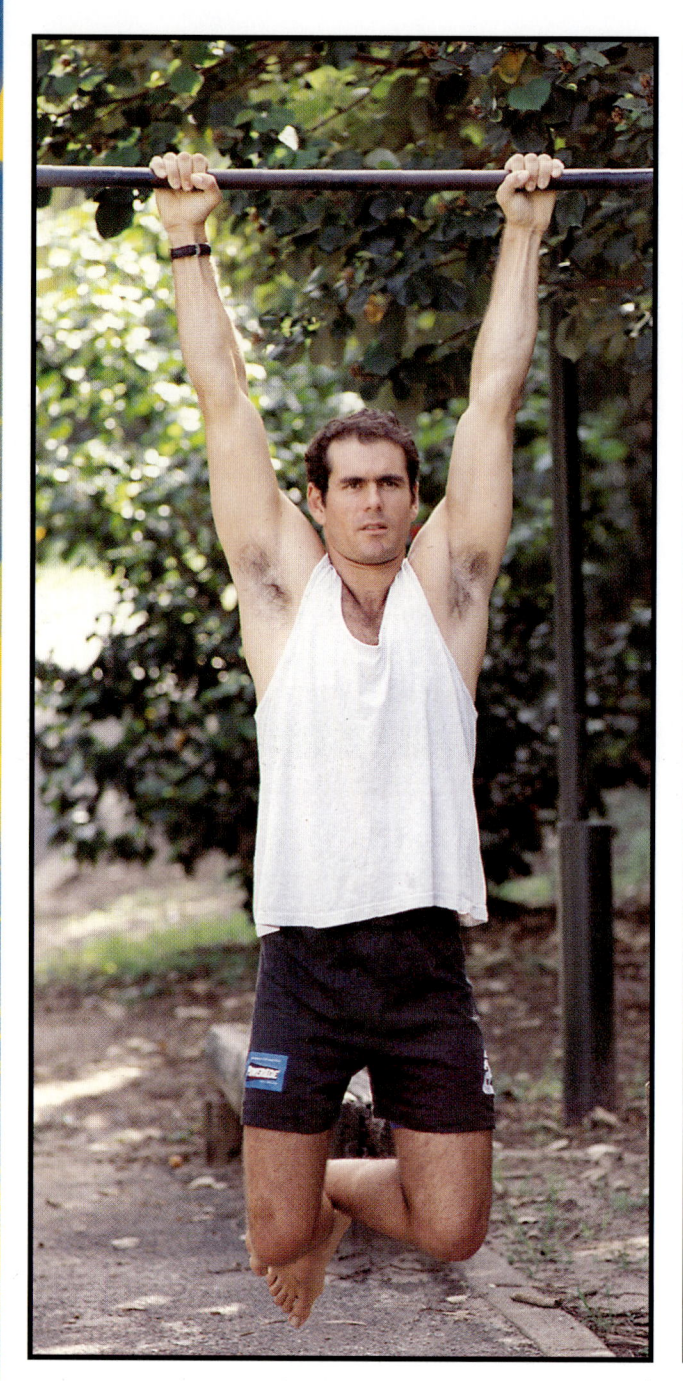

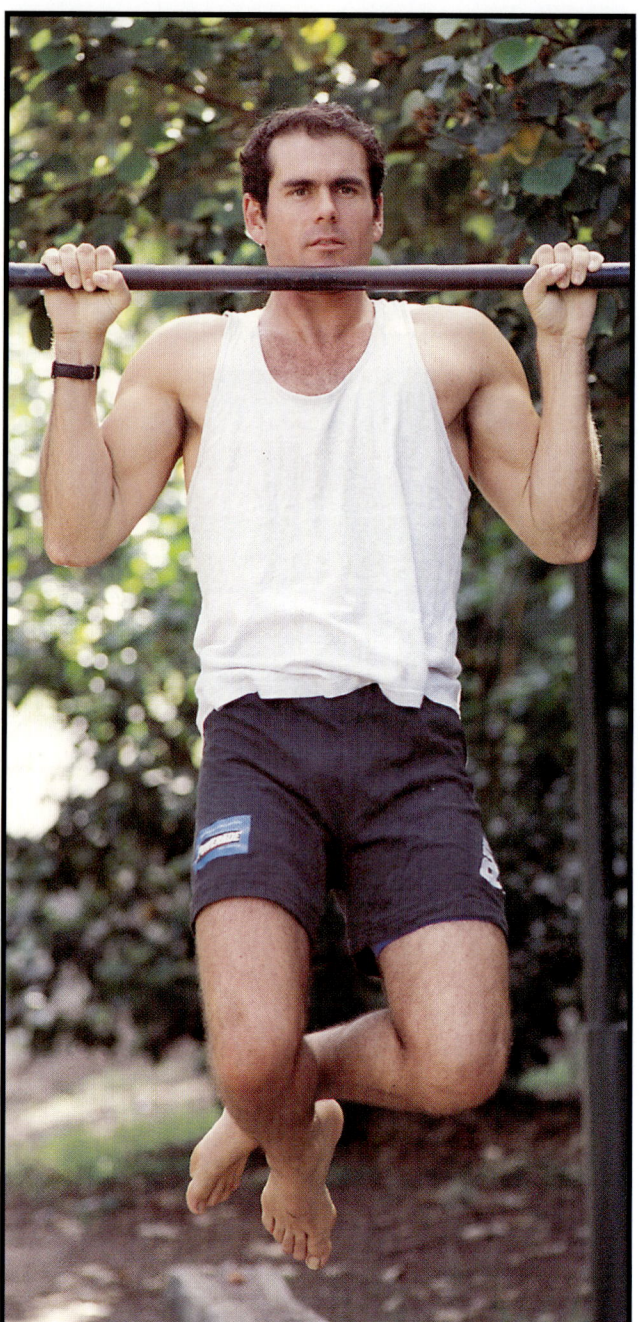

Men use the medium-grip width position, with palms facing outwards.

Test Your Fitness

The chin-up test

This test measures the strength and endurance of your upper body, particularly your back, shoulders and arms. One chin-up involves raising and lowering your body until your chin comes to the same level as the bar. At the bottom of each chin-up you should be fully extended.

As with push-ups, the chin-up for men is different from that for women. Men use the medium-grip width position, with palms facing away from them. Women use the reverse-grip position, with palms facing towards them and with their hands shoulder-width apart.

Perform as many chin-ups as you can without rest, then compare your score with the chart below. Find your age group column and look down until you find the range that covers the number of chin-ups you were able to complete, then look across to the fitness level column to gauge your level of fitness.

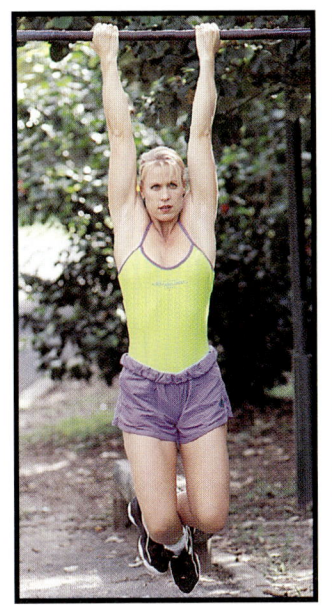

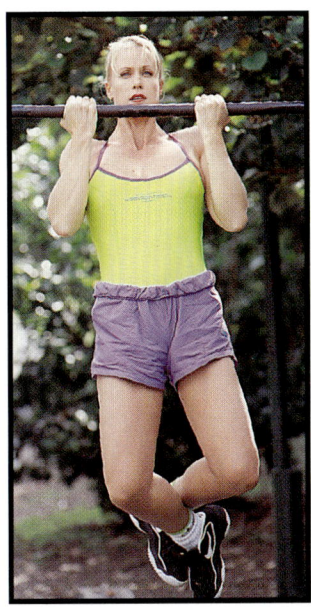

Women use the reverse-grip postion, palms facing inwards.

The Chin-up Test

Fitness level	Sex	Age group					
		13—19	20—29	30—39	40—49	50—59	60+
		Number of chin-ups completed					
Poor	Men	1	2	2	2	1	0
	Women	0	0	0	0	0	0
Below minimum	Men	2	4	3	3	2	1
	Women	0	1	1	0	0	0
Minimum	Men	4	7	7	5	3	2
	Women	1	3	2	1	0	0
Good	Men	7	11	10	7	5	3
	Women	3	5	4	2	1	0
Excellent	Men	12	15	12	9	8	4
	Women	5	8	6	3	2	1

Modified from B. Leelarthaepin & J. Schell, *Physical Fitness Assessment in Sport and Exercise Science*, 2nd ed. (Leelar Biomediscience Services, Sydney, 1994.)

Test Your Fitness

The abdominal strength test

This test measures your relative abdominal strength on a scale from 1 to 7. Ideally, you should have a score of at least Level 4. Complete the test and compare your scores with the chart below. Movements should be slow and controlled — don't throw yourself up. You should only do one of each in the test.

Start at Level 1 and try to do one rep, keeping the movement slow and controlled.

If you can do one rep on Level 1, try to do one on Level 2 and so on. You score yourself on the highest level you can do one of successfully.

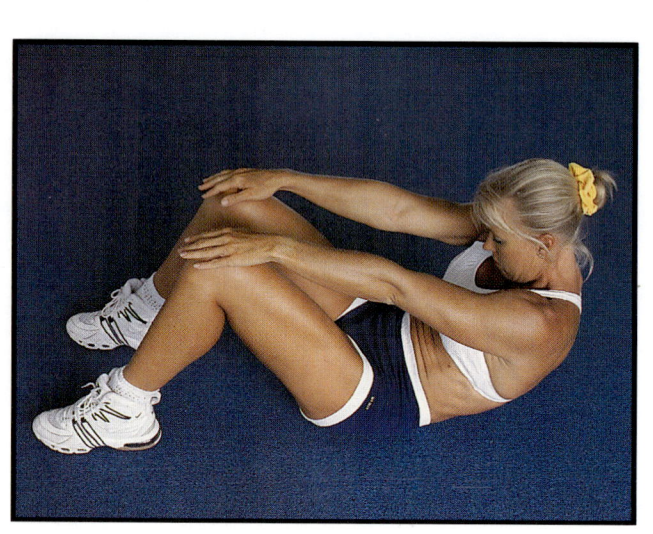

> 'Good abdominal strength is like solid foundations in a house. Without good foundations, eventually you or your house wiil have problems.'
> — Mark McKean

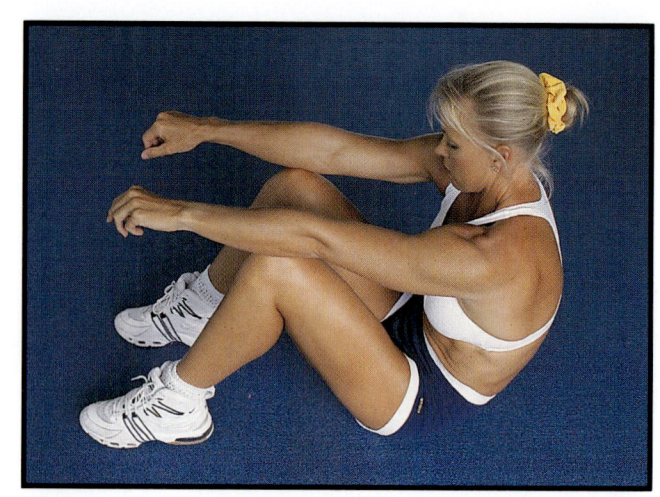

Level 2

- **Start** — Arms straight, hands resting on top of thighs
- **Finish** —Arms straight, elbows touching the kneecap

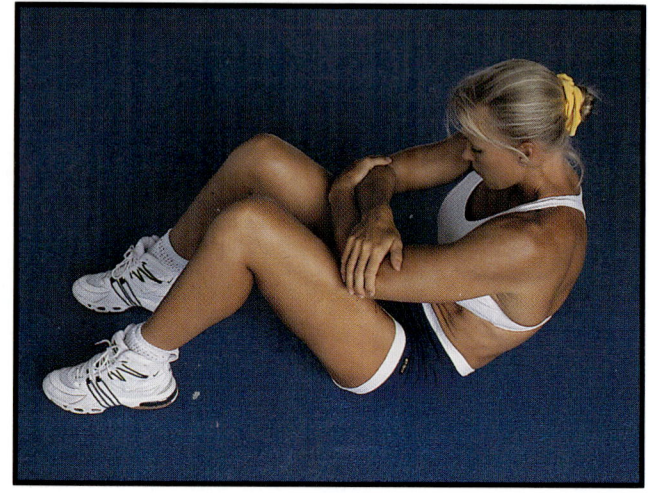

Level 1

- **Start** — Arms straight, hands resting on top of thighs
- **Finish** — Arms straight, fingertips touching the kneecap

Level 3

- **Start** — Arms across abdomen, hands gripping opposite elbows
- **Finish** — Forearms touching thighs

Get UP&GO!

Test Your Fitness

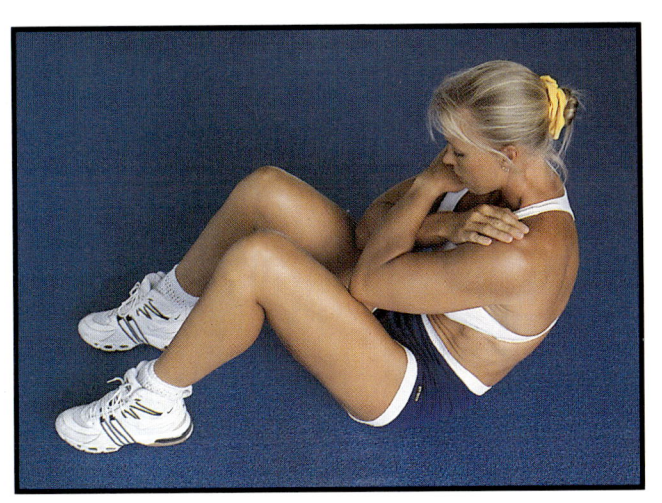

Level 4

- **Start** — Arms across chest, hands gripping opposite shoulders
- **Finish** — Forearms touching thighs

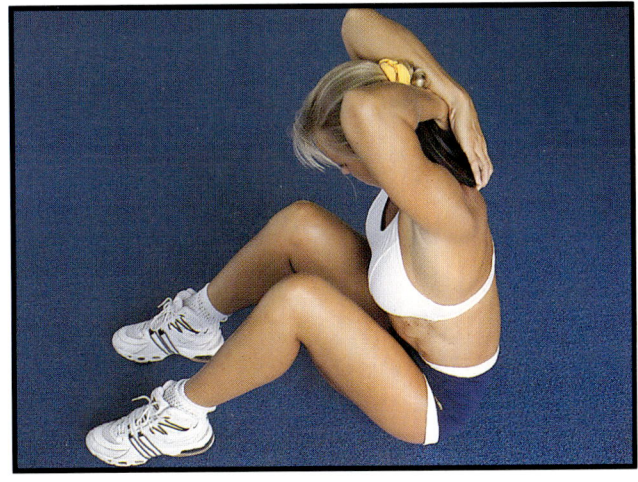

Level 6

- **Start** — Arms flexed behind the head, hands gripping the opposite sides of a 2.5kg weight
- **Finish** — Chest touching thighs

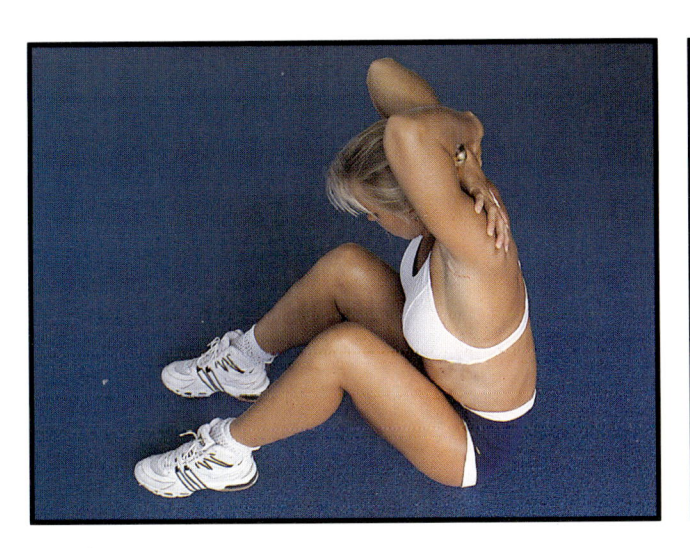

Level 5

- **Start** — Arms flexed behind the head, hands gripping opposite shoulders
- **Finish** — Chest touching thighs

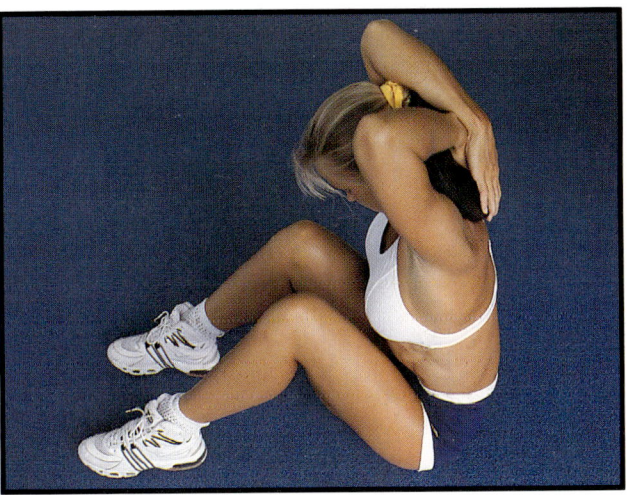

Level 7

- **Start** — Arms flexed behind the head, hands gripping the opposite sides of a 5kg weight
- **Finish** — Chest touching thighs

Training & Fitness

Get UP&GO! 137

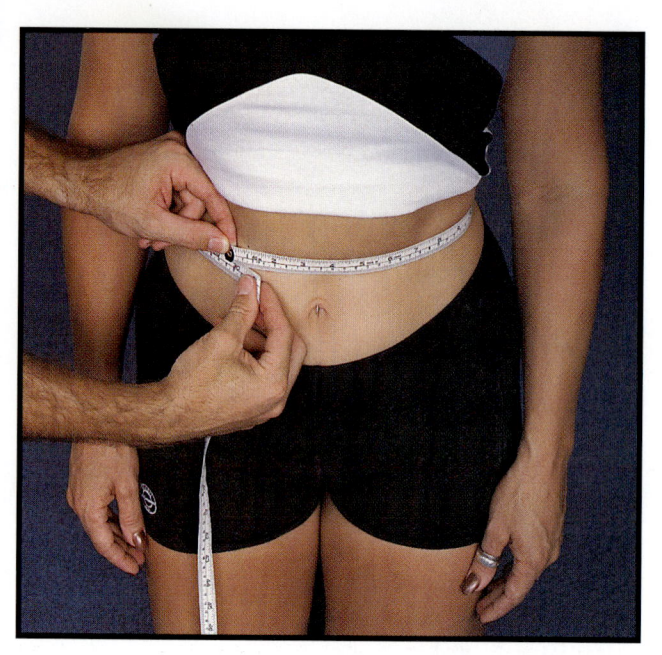

Test Your Fitness

Girth Measurements

Your girth measurements are the circumference of specific areas of your body — your hips, thighs, waist, arms, chest, etc. To ensure accuracy, you should take each measurement twice and get someone to help you.

Arms: This measurement should be taken at the widest part of your upper arm with your elbow bent at 90 degrees with your biceps flexed, arm held at the same height as your shoulder.

Shoulders: This measurement is taken around the widest part of your shoulder or deltoid muscle.

Chest: This measurement should be taken at nipple level of your chest with your chest relaxed.

Waist: Women should take this measurement at the narrowest part of their waist and men should take it at navel level.

Hips: Take this measurement at the widest part of your bottom. It can be a mistake to take this too low and use the wider thigh region as a point to measure. Remember, the widest part of your gluteals (muscle at back of bottom) is more accurate measured from the side.

Thighs: Take this measurement at the widest part of one of your thighs. Look for the wide region both on the outside and inside thigh and use these as points to measure around. You can do this standing with one foot up on a chair and with your leg relaxed.

Calf: Take this measurement around the widest part of the calf while the person is standing evenly on both feet.

Women take this measurement at the narrowest part of their waist.

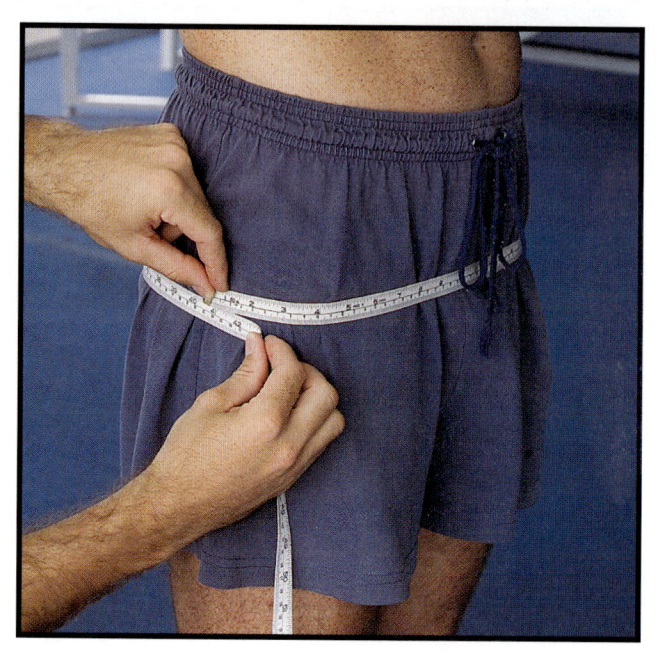

Take your hip measurement at the widest part of your bottom.

Body-fat Measurements

Throw away your scales — the reading you get on the scales is a measure of the total weight of your bones, organs, muscle, body fluids, hair and body fat. Over the long term — several months — the scales will show a decrease in body mass, but not always in the short term.

Muscle tissue is more than twice as heavy as fat, so a muscular person will weigh more than someone of the same size who has a lot of body fat. It's for this reason that, if you're exercising and increasing your muscle mass as you lose body fat, you may not see a weight change on the scales. It is body fat and its distribution that's important.

There are a number of ways that you can measure body fat — we'll be looking at the waist–hip ratio method and skinfold measurements.

Waist–hip ratio

Your waist–hip ratio is determined from your waist and hip girths. After taking your waist and hip measurements (as explained previously in 'Girth Measurements'), divide your hip measurement into your waist measurement. For example, if your waist measurement is 90 centimetres and your hip measurement is 109 centimetres, your waist–hip ratio would be 0.86 (90÷105=0.86). This measure is an indication of the fat stored on the stomach and around the internal organs relative to fat stored on the hips and is used to identify distribution of body fat.

Research has shown abdominal and upper body fat poses a greater risk to health than hip and thigh fat. There is a greater health risk when:

- men have a waist–hip ratio greater than 0.9 or a waist measurement greater than 95 centimetres; or
- women have a waist–hip ratio greater than 0.8 or a waist measurement greater than 80 centimetres.

If you're already within these guidelines and are looking at lowering your body-fat level, monitor your girth measurements on a monthly basis. Also, check how your clothes fit — this is usually a good indicator of shape change.

Skinfold thickness measurements

These measures are taken at specific body sites using special callipers. The sum of the measurements is a guide to body fatness. Traditionally, this method was used to measure fatness in elite athletes.

If you are attending a gym, have a personal trainer take the measurements. It's important that a skilled person do the measurements, and the same person uses the same callipers each time for accuracy. These measures are useful for people who are moderately overweight and for athletes. There are several formulas for converting the sum of the measurements to percentage body fat, but this isn't accurate — stick to the sum total. As you lose body fat you'll see your sum total figure drop and your girth measurements change. In a well-planned training program, you'll see a decrease in all the areas measured.

Each measurement should be taken on the right-hand side of your body. Grasp the fold of skin between the thumb and first finger and place the callipers on the fold one centimetre below the fingers. Hold the callipers on the spot for three seconds and then take the reading. Make sure you keep holding with your fingers while you take the reading. Take each measurement twice and record the average of the two measurements.

Acceptable totals for sum of eight measurements are 90–100 millimetres for males and 120–130 millimetres for females. Ideally, though, for younger or active people the measurements should be in the vicinity of 85 millimetres for males and 95–105 millimetres for females.

Test Your Fitness

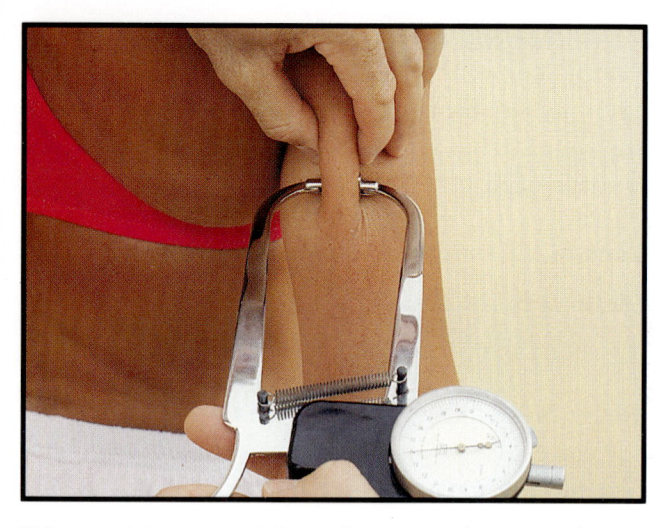

Triceps: Measure midway between the top of your shoulder and the elbow at the back of your upper arms while they are in a vertical position.

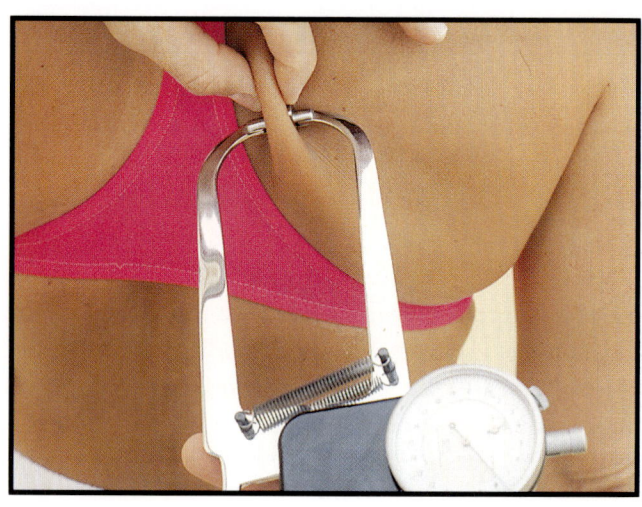

Scapula: Find the inside edge of your shoulder blade closest to your spine, come down 2–3 centimetres diagonally and take your fold at the same angle as the bottom edge of the shoulder blade.

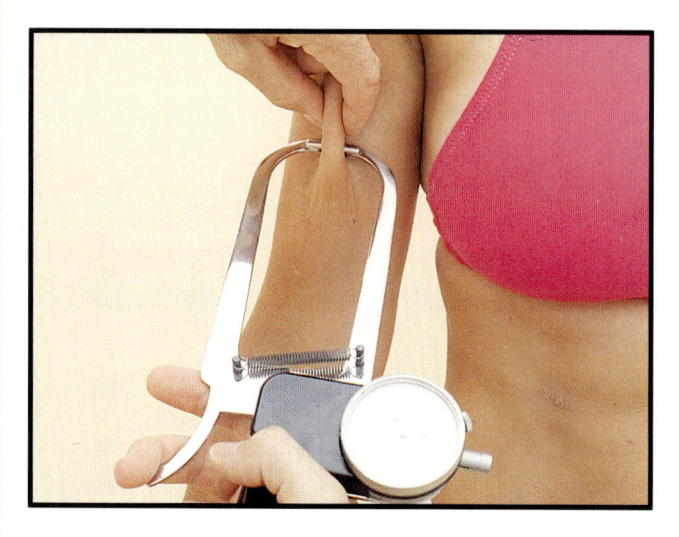

Biceps: Measure midway between the front of the top of your shoulder and the bend in your elbow while your arms are in a vertical position.

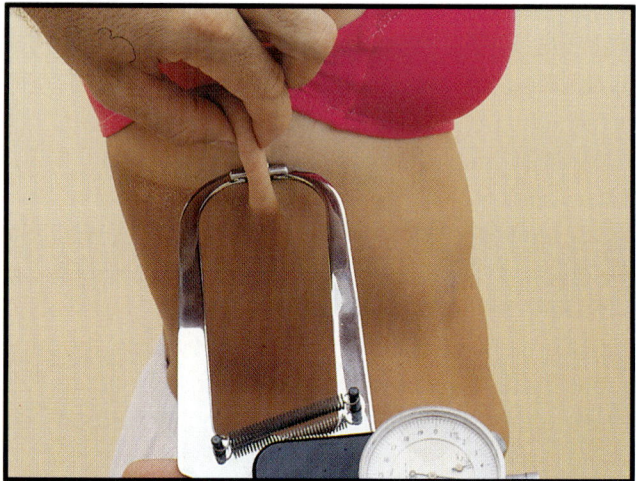

Axilla: Find the bottom of your sternum and follow a line around to the side of your body until you have a point level with the bottom of the sternum and directly under your armpit on the side of your ribs.

Test Your Fitness

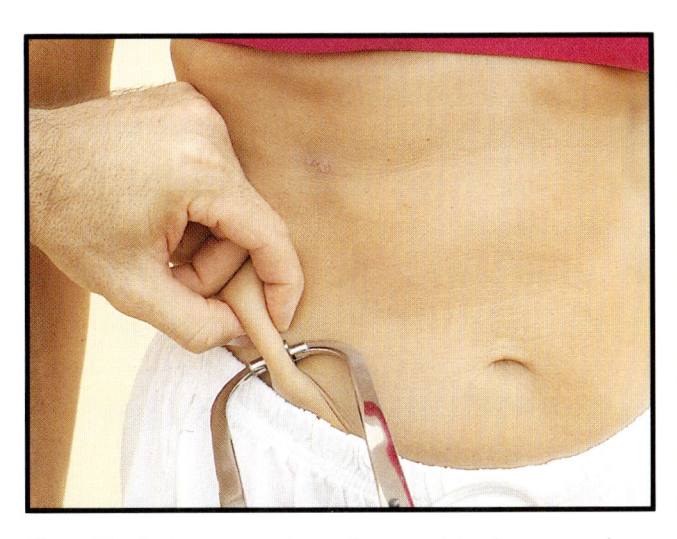

Iliac: Find the top edge of your hip bone and go directly towards your navel for 3–4 centimetres. Take a fold of skin at the same angle as your hip bone, slightly lower at the middle of the body and higher at the outside part.

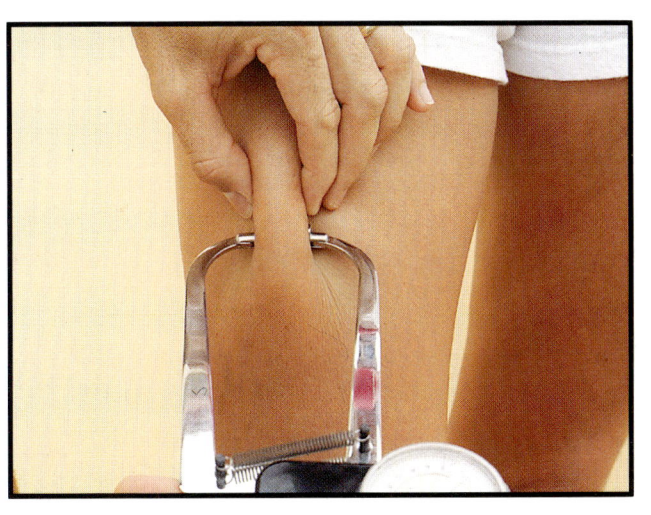

Thigh: Take a vertical fold midway between the hip bone at the top of your thigh and the kneecap.

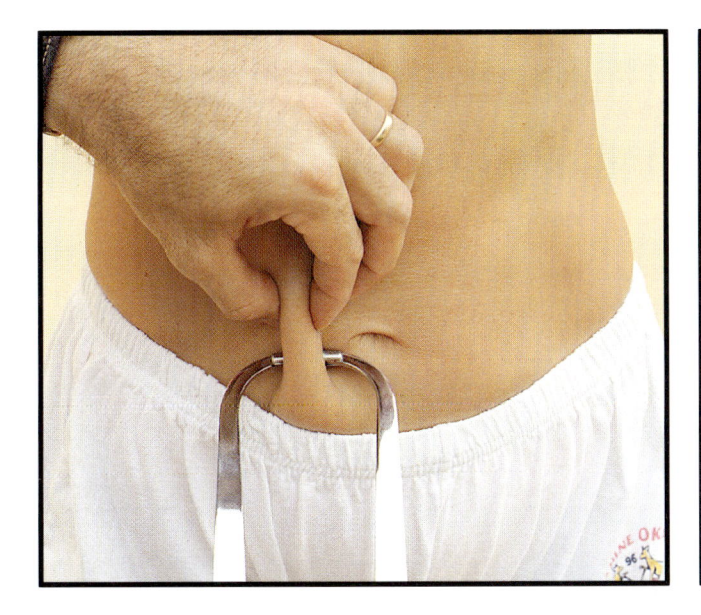

Abdominal: From your navel, come 4–5 centimetres to the right side of your body and take a vertical fold.

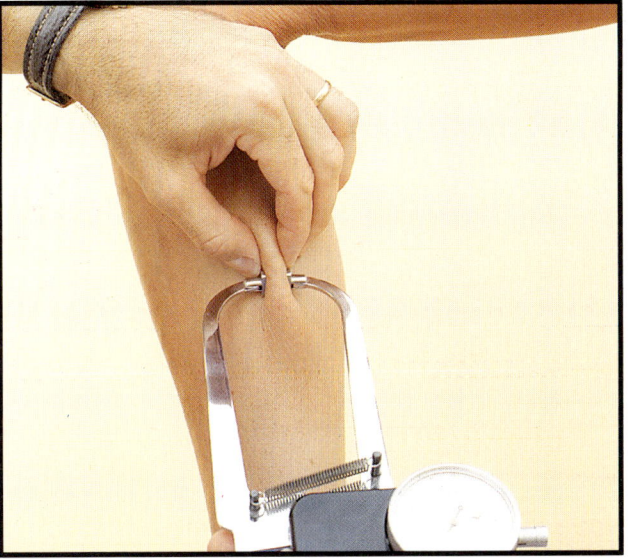

Calf: Find the inside of your calf muscle in the middle of the fleshiest part of the muscle and take a vertical fold.

Training & Fitness

Get UP&GO!

Test Your Fitness

Postural Tests

1. Arm position: Stand facing a full-length mirror with your feet shoulder-width apart.

Ideal — Arms hanging by your side with palms facing hips.

Not so good — Arms hanging slightly to the front of your side.

Needs work — Arms hanging at the front of your thighs with your palms facing the front of your thighs.

2. Shoulder position: Stand facing a full-length mirror with your feet shoulder-width apart.

Ideal — Both shoulders are at the same level.

Not so good — One shoulder is slightly lower/higher than the other shoulder.

Needs work — One shoulder is at a very different height to the other shoulder.

3. Abdominal position: Turn sideways to the mirror.

Ideal — Abdomen sits in below rib cage and doesn't protrude.

Not so good — Abdomen protrudes slightly past ribs and hips.

Needs work — Abdomen hangs out past ribs and belt line of hips.

4. Upper back position: Turn sideways to the mirror.

Ideal — Upper back is very straight.

Not so good — Upper back is slightly curved forward, with a roundish appearance.

Needs work — Upper back is curved forward noticeably, and is round.

5. Lower back position: Turn sideways to the mirror.

Ideal — Lower back is only slightly curved inward or hollow.

Not so good — Lower back is curved inward, giving a more hollow appearance through the lower back.

Needs work — Lower back is very swayed and there is a noticeable inward curve.

6. Neck position: Turn sideways to the mirror.

Ideal — Neck is quite straight and in line with your shoulders and trunk.

Not so good — Neck is slightly curved and sits slightly forward of the straight line of your back.

Needs work — Neck is noticeably curved, dropping forward from your shoulders with your head hanging forward.

7. Shoulder position: Lying flat on your back on the floor.

Ideal — Shoulders rest almost on the floor.

Not so good — Shoulders sit just off the floor.

Needs work — Shoulders sit well above the floor.

■ ■ ■

Be sure to record your results accurately. You should do these tests about every three months to check your progress and see if your program needs to change to work on any specific problems the tests may highlight.

The next chapter will help you decide what exercises you will include in your training program.

Smart Training

If you want results from your training, you have to learn how to train smart. Smart training is about knowing what will result from the different types of exercise you include in your training program. This chapter explains the basic principles that need to be considered in any training program and outlines various exercise options — including their results and benefits — to help you train smart.

[Smart Training for Results]

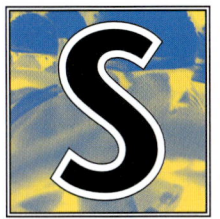

Starting a training program means you are serious about what you're doing and that you're committed to achieving your goals, but it doesn't guarantee success. If you are training inappropriately it won't get you what you want. If you want success, you have to train *well* and you have to train *smart*.

Training doesn't always give you what you might expect: you might train for fat loss and see a huge gain in strength, or you might train to run faster and end up losing fat. Knowing what will result from each form of training will make the difference between success and failure.

The world is full of people who take up training because they think that with a few weeks' effort they'll look like a Greek god or goddess. How many people do you know who joined a gym to get fit and ended up giving it away after two or three months? Three months seems to be the time most people give themselves to get fit, or at least to see something happening. They think that if it hasn't happened by then, it's not going to happen. The big mistake they make is thinking nothing has happened, when actually quite a lot has been achieved.

If you look beyond this negativity, you might realise that you have more energy and feel more active during work or study. You're too busy bemoaning the

Smart Training

fact that you haven't yet got the legs of a supermodel to notice all the positive things that are happening. After three months you should just be getting to the point where you start seeing physical changes, instead of just feeling better.

You'll fail only when you stop working towards your goals. You have to be realistic and give yourself longer than three months to achieve such important goals. The results will come if you eat well and train well, but they won't come overnight. Success is all about long-term self-management of your lifestyle.

Set up your plan for a minimum of 12 months. Give yourself time to find out what you enjoy and what works for you. Results will only happen if you put it all together and spend time doing it smart.

The FIT Principle

With so many different types of people wanting to achieve so many different goals, the possibilities for training program combinations are endless. However, there are a few basics that allow you to control what you are doing and when you are doing it.

These basics are known as the FIT principle:

F — frequency of training;

I — intensity of training; and

T — time you train for.

It's the manipulation of these three variables that underlies every training program you will ever undertake.

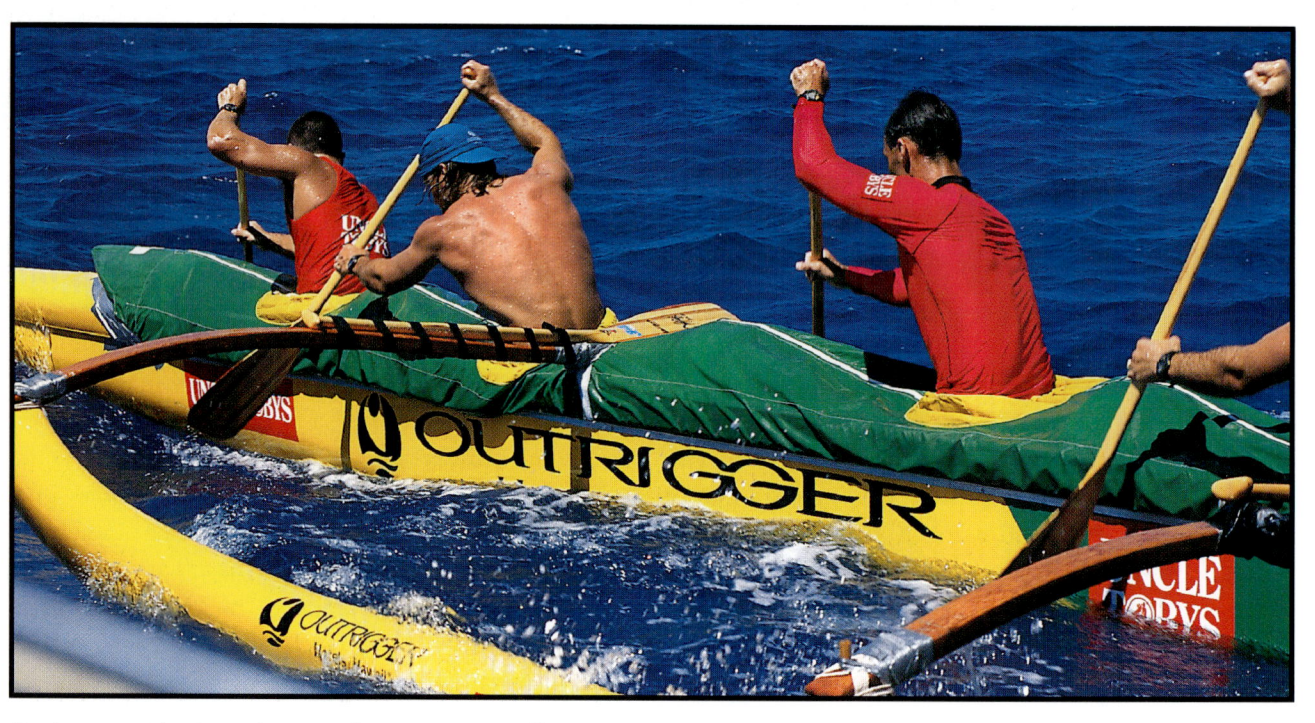

Outrigger canoeing is another sport that is growing rapidly in Australia. It doesn't matter who you are or what sporting background you have, outrigging is easy to learn. However, you must be a competent swimmer, as it is an ocean sport. Australia is currently the best in the world in both women's and men's outrigger competition.

Smart Training

Frequency

Frequency refers to how often you train. We can use this information to see if you are training too much or too little. Two sessions per week of walking isn't enough for fat loss, but two sessions of weights is enough to increase your strength. Some types of training need more sessions than others.

Intensity

Intensity refers to the level of effort that you put into each session. Intensity varies from aerobic activities such as swimming and walking to strength training. To monitor the intensity you are working at during aerobic activity, you'll need to take your pulse regularly while you are training (see page 130 to learn how to take your pulse) or, alternatively, you could buy a heart-rate monitor. Heart monitors are simple to use and make monitoring your intensity easy.

Your training heart rate (your heart rate while you are exercising) is what you use to monitor intensity. To calculate what your training heart rate should be, use this formula:

220 minus your age, multiplied by the percentage of effort you wish to use.

As a guide to working out what percentage of effort you should be choosing, for increasing your aerobic fitness, follow these ranges:
For example, for a 40-year-old beginner with a below minimum fitness level, the equation would look like this:

220 minus 40 multiplied by 60 per cent = ideal training heart rate.

220 − 40 = 180
180 × 0.6 = 108 beats per minute.

Estimated fitness level	Percentage of effort you should be training at
Poor	60 or below
Below–minimum	60–65
Minimum	65–70
Good	70–75
Excellent	75–80

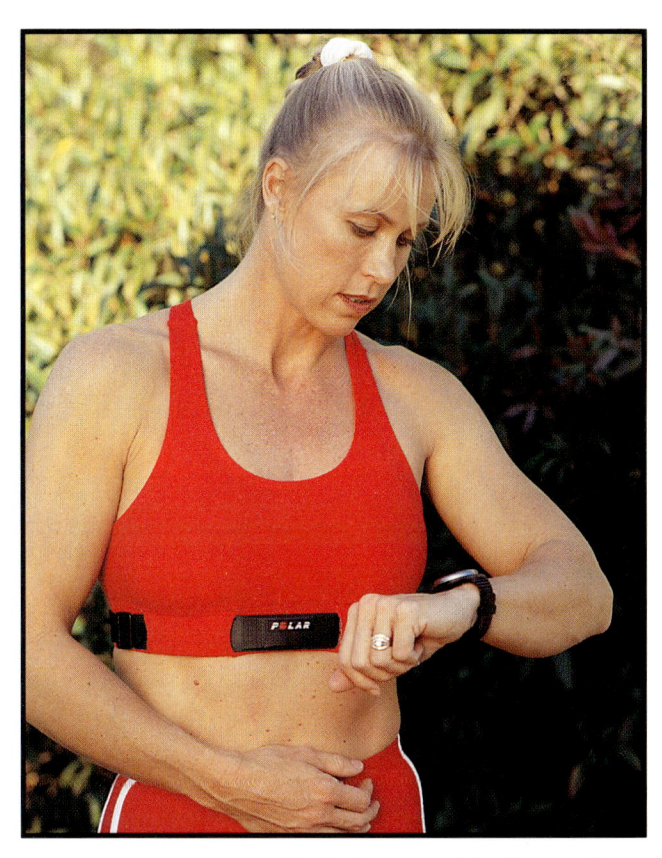

Heart-rate monitors are used by beginners, social athletes and professionals. The transmitter belts fit snugly around the chest and even come built into sports tops for women.

Smart Training

Time

Time refers to the amount of time you need to spend to complete a drill, set, effort or session. Some sessions can be too long and others too short. For aerobic fitness, 40 minutes is the preferred amount of time you should spend training, while skill sessions in field sports can last between 10 and 60 minutes, depending on how much fitness is built into the exercise. The time you need to spend will vary depending on the activity you choose and the goals you set.

Training considerations

Generally, when you start training the frequency will be low (two or three sessions per week), as will the intensity (around 60 per cent), and the sessions will be short (between 20 and 30 minutes). As your fitness improves, these variables will change.

It's always best to be a little conservative when determining the level at which you should start training. It's easier to increase your training slowly and feel positive about your ability to handle it, than to have to back off because it's too hard, and you end up feeling disappointed.

As your training progresses you'll see that there are other factors that need to be considered. These allow you to bring in more variety to your training and make it more suited to the goals you've set for yourself.

	Description	Example of training
Volume	Volume indicates the total amount of training you have done in a given period, session, week or block — that is, frequency multiplied by time. For example, four sessions multiplied by the 4 kilometres you ran each session equals a volume of 16 kilometres.	For speed training the volume needs to be low, for aerobic endurance training the volume needs to be much higher. For building muscle, the volume also needs to be high. Volume can be written in kilometres, kilograms, minutes, hours etc.
Specificity	Training needs to be specific to the goal intended.	If you lift heavy weights twice a week you'll get strong; if you run 5 kilometres twice a week you'll get fitter. The result is specific to the goal.
Overload	To get a gradual improvement in results or performance you must apply the principle of 'overload'. Small, gradual increases in frequency, intensity, time or volume will create an overload effect on your body.	Generally you should only increase one of these at any one time. Any more will induce overtraining. In swimming you might do the following: weeks 1–2: 300 metres; weeks 3–4: 400 metres; weeks 5–6: 500 metres; and so on. This is gradual overload. This principle can be applied to all areas of training.

Smart Training

	Description	Example of training
Reversibility	Once you stop training, the effects or results you have achieved will return to their original level. Each person is different. Generally the longer you have trained, the less you lose.	Aerobic fitness drops from its peak level very quickly and then levels off. The last bit of fitness you gain is always the first to go. The longer you maintain your fitness, strength or speed, the longer you'll keep it after you stop training.
Recovery	This is the time spent in regenerating your energy reserve before the next bout of training. It can be between reps, between workouts, between days of training, and between cycles or blocks of training.	Strength training for bulk may involve a rest of 60–90 seconds between each set of an exercise in the gym. Marathon runners may spend up to four weeks recovering from a race before they return to activity. Recovery influences your performance quite considerably. This is the most overlooked aspect of training.
Individuality	A program is only as good as the person it was designed for. This relates to any form of training. Each person must find out the combination of frequency, volume, time, intensity and recovery that suits them.	If two different people wanted to race in a triathlon and one was a good swimmer while the other was a good runner, the first would concentrate less on their swimming so they could try to improve the run and cycle leg of the race while the second person would concentrate more on swimming and cycling. Both might still do approximately the same time, but they will have achieved that result by focusing on their individual needs.
Variability	Variability is the changes made to each program based on keeping you motivated and differences in each day of your training. Each program needs to be slightly different to the one before. Changing the FIT regularly will create variability.	When walking for fitness you might walk hills on Monday, soft sand on Wednesday and flat roads on Friday. Every fourth week you might add an outdoor circuit to the program by reducing your walk by 20 minutes and completing the circuit at the end. This is variability

To be effective, all training programs must take the FIT principles into account and allow for the above considerations.

Smart Training

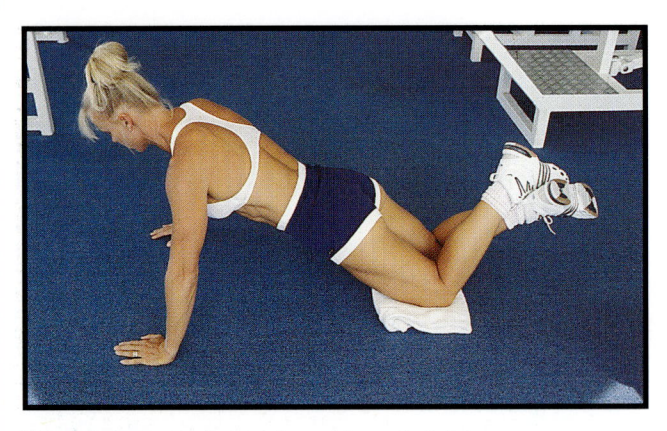

Develop correct technique in resistance training. Remember it takes time to change old habits, but it can be done.

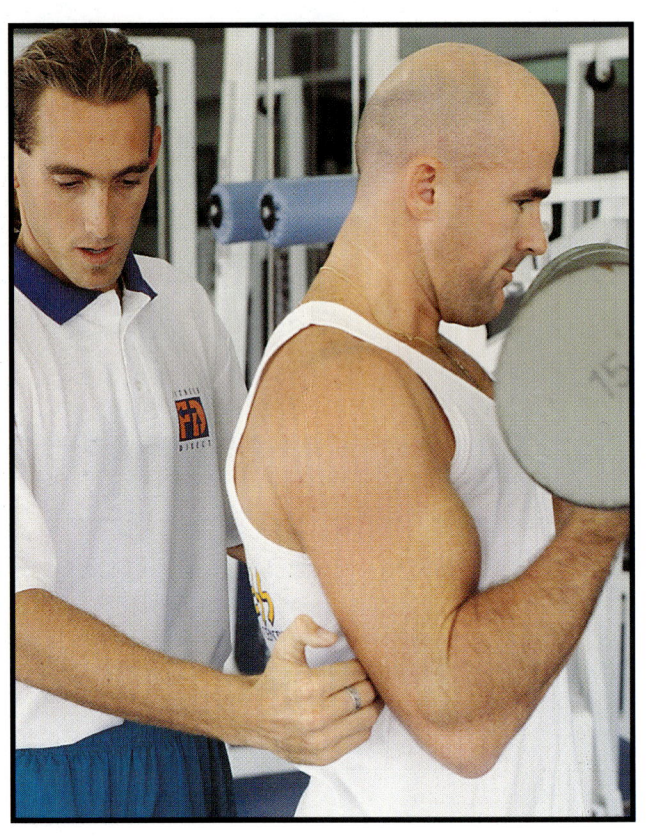

Working with a personal trainer can be of great benefit. Find one that you are comfortable with and see them on a regular basis.

Exercise and Training Options

Constructing your training program will be up to *you* — it will need to be put together by *you* to suit *your* individual needs and goals. Selecting the type of exercises you want to include will take a lot of thought and planning. You must choose exercises that will give you the results you want but that you will also enjoy. The good news is that your exercise options are many and varied — some of your options have been described in detail below, with an explanation of some of the results you can achieve from each activity.

Resistance and weight training

Many people are confused about the difference between weight training and resistance training, and understandably so. Weight training is a form of resistance training, but it specifically uses external loads of weights — either machines, bars or plates — to add to your body weight for certain exercises — bench-presses, for example. Resistance training can be done by using your body weight for exercises — for example, push-ups and chin-ups — or it can involve activities such as carrying dumbbells when you walk, towing a drag sled when you're running, towing a piece of foam on a rope when you're swimming, or even towing a tennis ball behind a kayak. When someone is discussing resistance training, it may or may not involve equipment; however, when discussing weight training, it means using weight-training equipment at home or at the gym. As with all the programs you might consider, decide what you want to achieve and get the right advice before you begin training.

The main point about weight training is that it must be done correctly, and your weights program must be written to suit you. Home gyms are great and there are some excellent pieces of apparatus available, but, again, make sure you get the right advice before you commit to purchasing anything. You can often find home gyms for sale in your local newspaper offered by people who started off with the best intentions but got frustrated or bored, and gave up because they weren't doing things properly.

Results possible:

All sorts of things are possible with weight and resistance training. You can train for fat loss, to improve your muscle tone, to change your body shape, or to increase lean muscle mass, strength, power or muscle endurance. You can also use it for rehabilitation from injury, to improve posture and deportment, and to prevent injury from work or exercise. The common mistake made here is to believe that one program suits all: your program should be set up to suit *your* needs and goals.

Too often in the past, people have been put off weight training because they have related it to images of muscle-bound strongmen and extraordinarily masculine-looking women. It sometimes appears like an activity confined to professional athletes, footballers and heavyweight boxers — not your 'everyday' person. But today's gyms are filled with a vast range of people — both male and female, young and old — from all walks of life.

Benefits:

- You can target specific areas that other sports or activities can't.
- Helps to strengthen muscle and connective tissue that protects joints, and improves abilities in other sports and activities.
- Equipment is available for use in the home, or you can choose to go to a gym.
- Suitable for men, women and children of all ages, so long as it's properly organised.

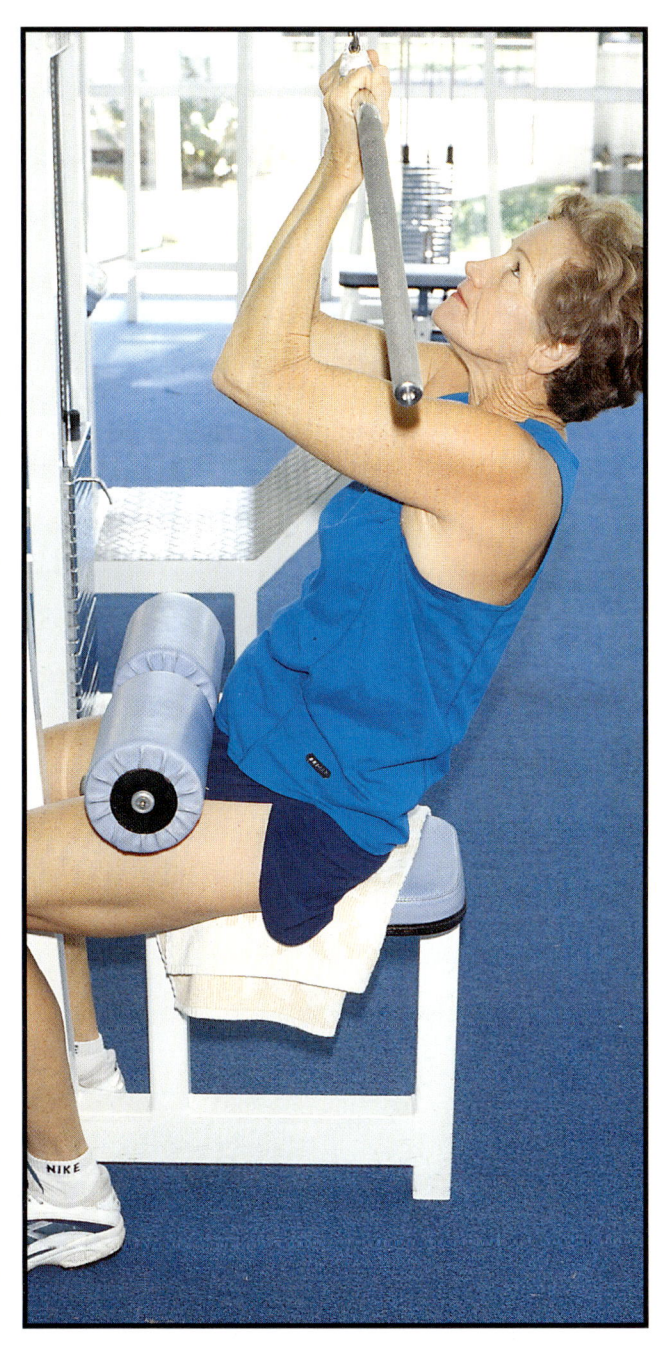

Weight training is a good training option for older men and women who want to improve muscle strength.

Smart Training

Walking

The great thing about walking is that you can do it just about anywhere, anytime. All you need is a good pair of walking shoes, suitable clothing, and perhaps sunscreen and a hat. Walking has been supported by the medical fraternity as the best form of exercise for everyone, and this is probably true for those people who don't have access, for whatever reason, to other forms of exercise. It's certainly a great activity to get you into the habit of exercising, and when you feel like you need to progress, you can vary your walking program. For example, you might choose to walk on sand or take on the challenge of hills.

Results possible:

Walking is aimed at aerobic fitness — walking for a set period of time at a constant rate, gradually improving your speed and the distance you walk over time. Aerobic activity can help to reduce body fat, improve lung and heart efficiency, increase mobility and promote your general wellbeing. Walking is one of the most common activities suggested for cardiac rehabilitation patients after they have received the all-clear to exercise.

Benefits:

- Helps you to maintain weight and fat levels, increase muscle endurance and strength, improve

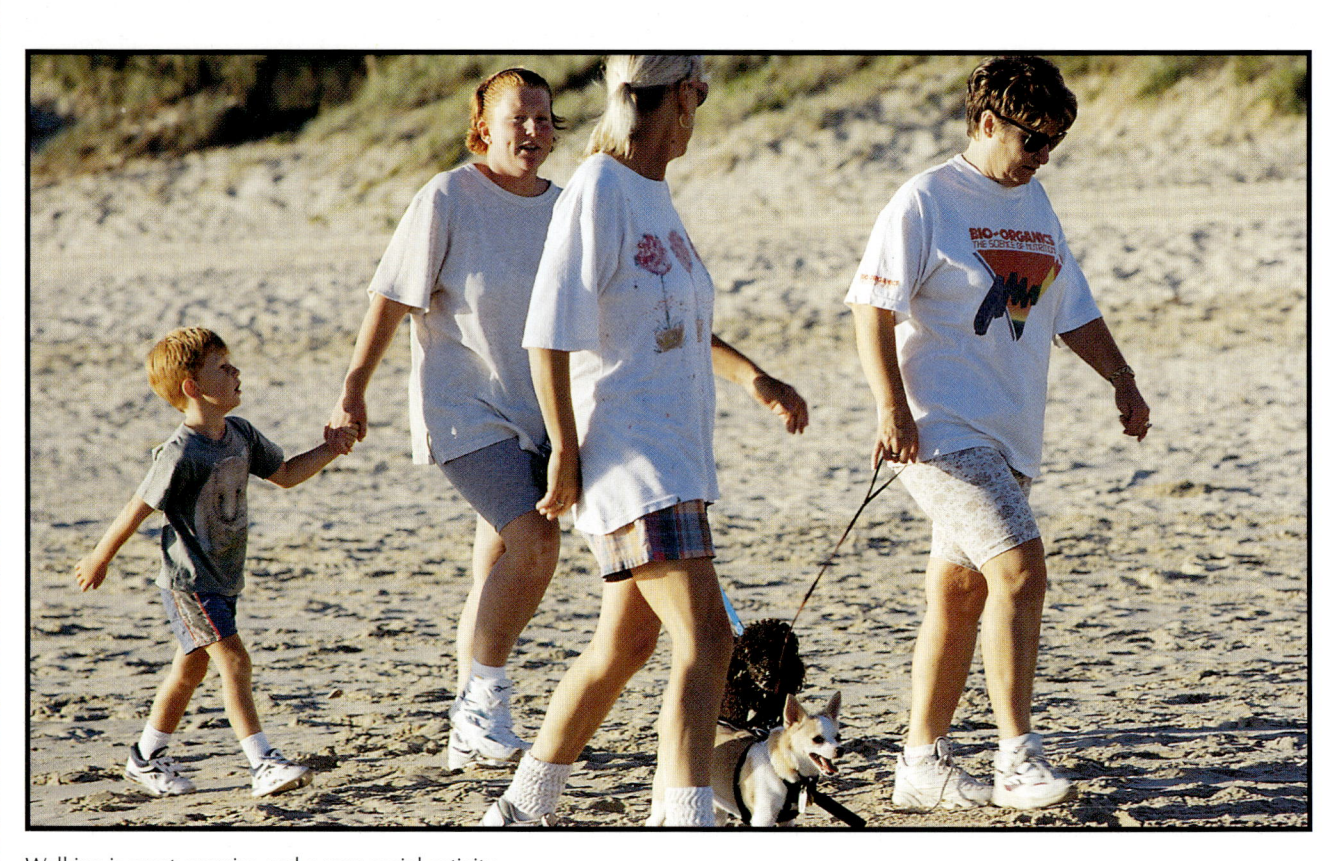

Walking is great exercise and a very social activity.

Smart Training

tone in legs, maintain bone density and improve your general fitness.
- Accessible to people of all ages and in all places.
- Requires no equipment and minimal instruction.

Running

Running is a natural progression from walking. Under certain conditions, for certain people, running can be the next step on the road to fitness. Not everyone should take this step, but for some it's one of the best exercises for aerobic fitness. Our bodies are designed to run, but problems occur when we overdo it, run with poor technique, or wear poor-quality running shoes. Technique is critical, and a few training sessions with a running coach or a running squad would be helpful.

The main problems with running revolve around poor preparation. You shouldn't make your first fitness session for ten years a 10-kilometre run. Build up your fitness first, learn how to run over short distances and increase this up to a point that begins to benefit you. While you're going through the learning phases, keep up some other form of activity, such as walking, to maintain your fitness.

Results possible:
Similar to walking, aerobic fitness is the main benefit of running — fat loss, lung/heart efficiency, general wellbeing and mobility are all also improved. And, if you take it to the next level, you can improve your speed, endurance and acceleration, too. Many people who play sport include running as an integral part of their training, especially through the off-season and pre-season.

Benefits:
- Helps you to maintain or lose body fat, improves general fitness, muscle strength and endurance in the lower legs, and benefits heart and lung efficiency.
- Requires no equipment and minimal instruction.

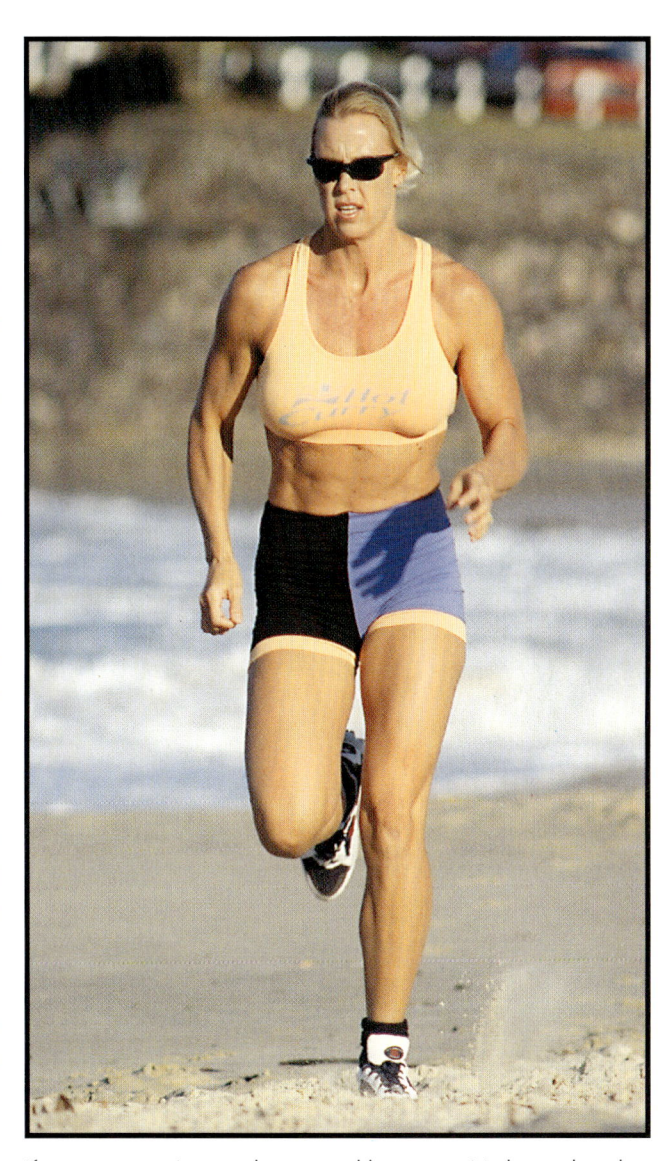

If you want to trim your bottom and legs — run! I always thought running was boring and too hard, but after learning how to push myself more with the help of a running group, I now run a lot better and really enjoy it.

Smart Training

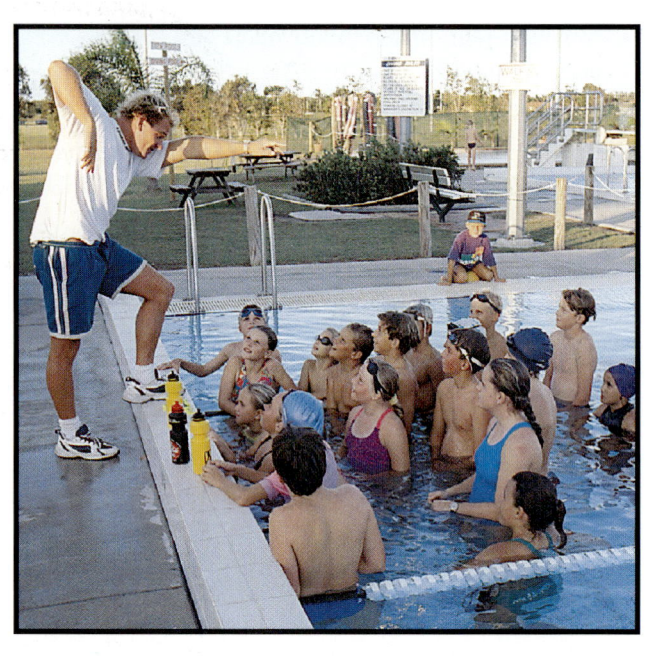

A good coach will make training challenging and fun. It makes me sad to hear of athletes dropping out of sport because they don't enjoy it anymore. Variety and smart training techniques is the responsibility of the coach. When you love what you do, hard work seems easy.

Swimming

For many Australians, swimming has always been a part of life. With so many beaches and pools at our disposal, most Australians have had a swim, or at least a dip. Swimming can be an organised activity, or simply a leisurely splash with the kids in a backyard pool. Swimming utilises many different strokes, and some are much easier than others to master. From dog-paddling to breast stroke, right up to the most difficult stroke, butterfly, everyone can be taught to keep their head above water. Some people have a natural ability to float, while others tend to sink. People with higher body fat levels may float more naturally, and this might be why many swimmers have more body fat than you would normally expect in elite athletes.

Results possible:

Swimming for fitness requires good technique and you should consider spending some time being coached if this is going to form the basis of your training program. Good technique will make it easier to complete the number of laps or time in the water required to achieve your goals.

Swimming is similar to running in that you can improve your aerobic fitness, speed, endurance and acceleration if that's your aim. Learn-to-swim classes are run for children as well as for adults, so anyone can make a start. I get my best fitness results when I include swimming in my training program along with running and gym work.

Benefits:

- Improves and maintains general fitness, making you use virtually every muscle in your body.
- A non-impact activity which can also be relaxing and stress-relieving due to its solitary nature.
- Ideal for overweight people, pregnant women, and those with injuries or some disabilities.

Cycling

Cycling is another multifaceted activity that can be used to achieve many fitness goals. Unfortunately, in most places in Australia there are few organised cycle tracks, so we have to take our chances on the roads. Social cycling may involve casual riding with friends just to be active and outdoors. Including cycling in your fitness program can be thoroughly enjoyable — but challenging and hard work, too.

When you buy your bike make sure you speak to a specialist who can help you to make the right choice for your needs and set it up for your leg length and body position. Make sure you also buy — and wear — a helmet.

Smart Training

Cycling on an exercise bike can be just as effective as outdoor cycling, as long as you have something to occupy your time. Outdoor cycling is more varied, but there is a greater risk of injury.

Results possible:

Enjoyment and fitness benefits can be achieved by riding socially, and extremely high aerobic fitness can be achieved by cycling seriously. Anyone can cycle; however, to be adept at cycling for training purposes you should seek the advice of an experienced coach.

Cyclists usually develop great legs; but be careful if you want thin legs because cycling for more than a few hours a week can bulk up your muscle mass.

Benefits:

- Improves general fitness, and strengthens and tones muscles in legs.
- A non-impact activity (most of the time).
- A pleasurable outdoors activity, which can also be a means of transport.

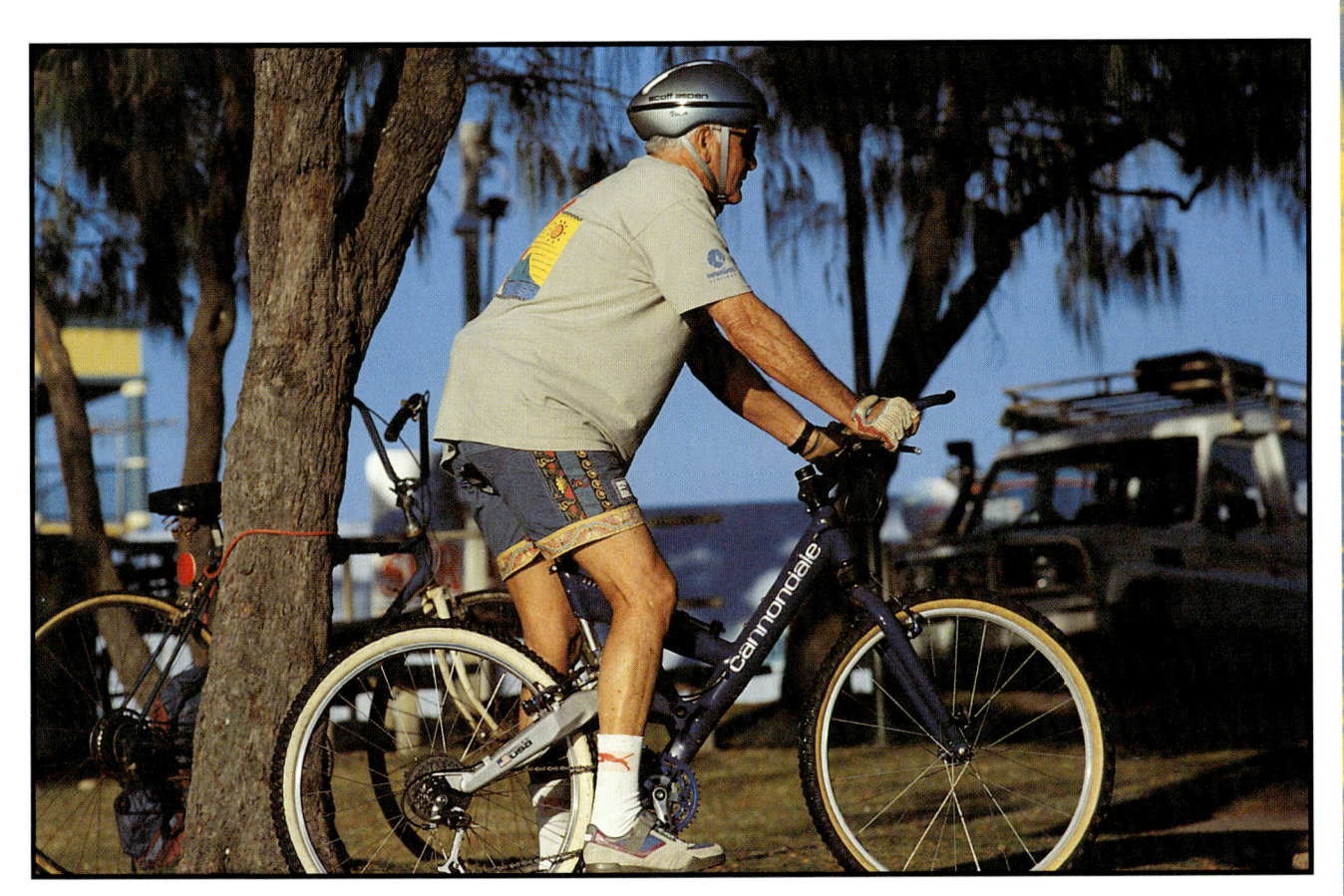

> *'Until you try, you don't know what you can't do.'*
> — Henry James

Cycling is a pleasurable, low-impact activity which is great for general fitness and strengthening leg muscles.

Smart Training

Aerobic and circuit classes

In recent years, the number of people participating in aerobic classes has been changing. A lot of people are now finding they get better results from weight training or activities other than just straight aerobic classes.

Aerobic classes can also be organised in a 'circuit' format, where the actual aerobics is mixed with other activities, such as weight training. Results can vary. People often set up their own circuit at home or at the local park, and it can all be very enjoyable even if the results may be slow. If this is what it takes to get you going, then go for it!

A sign that aerobics is decreasing in popularity is the trend for gyms to upgrade their cardiovascular and weight rooms at the expense of the aerobic floor. If you really enjoy aerobics, look into some of the new classes, such as Pump, that combine the best of both worlds, with aerobic activity *and* weight-training exercises.

Results possible:

Depending on who you listen to, the results can vary widely. Classes are great for first-time exercisers, for the unmotivated, for recovery training, for fun and social interaction, and for switching off from stress.

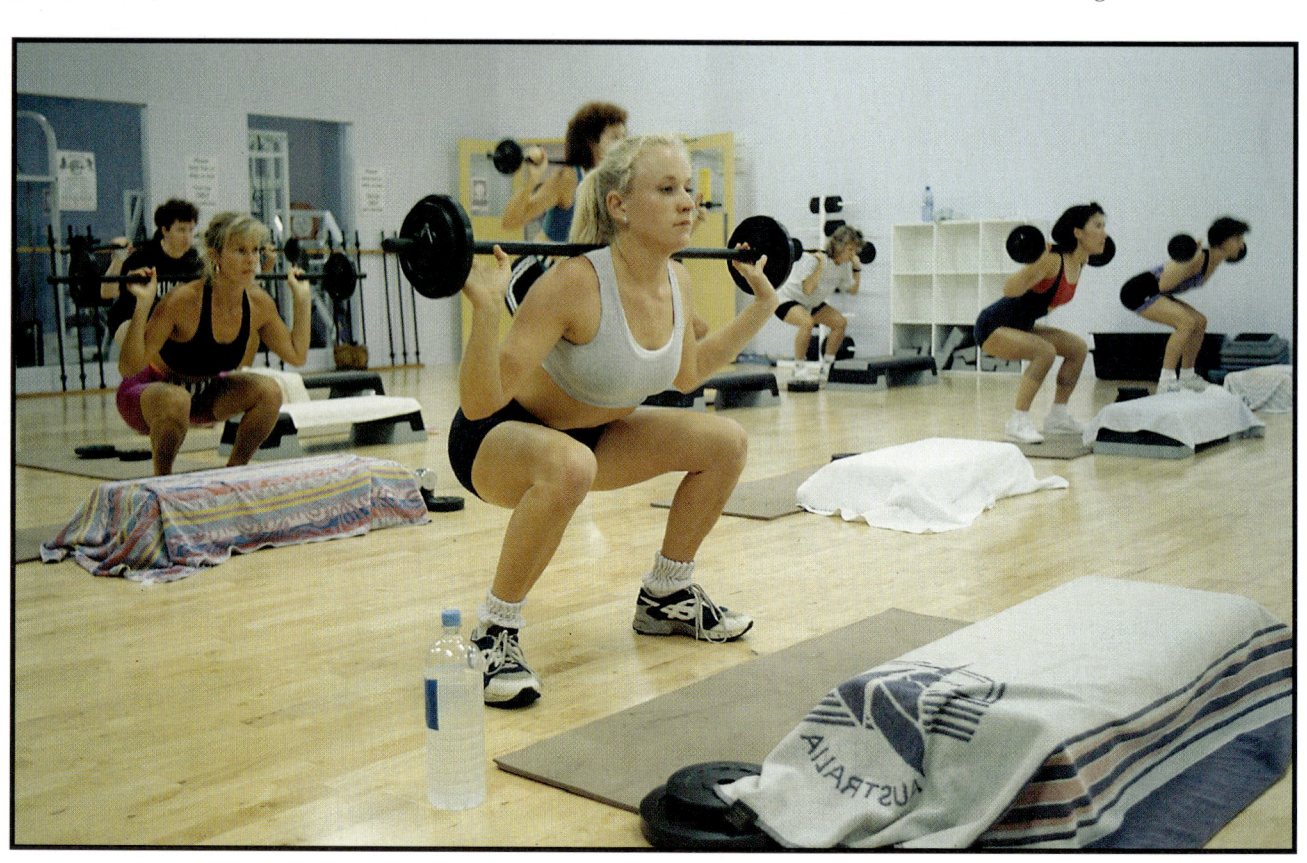

Pump classes are fantastic — weight training on the aerobics floor is a great way to train. Keep your movements controlled and always observe good technique.

The secret is to find a great instructor who'll make the time you spend with him or her worthwhile. Aerobics can improve your general fitness and result in fat loss and better muscle definition and shaping; but if you are a serious trainer or want results fast, then there are better options.

Some aerobic classes require very complicated movement patterns. Those who are more dance-oriented and have been doing aerobics for some time may have no problems, but people who are new to aerobic classes are often put off by the coordination required.

Another problem is that most classes don't sustain a training heart-rate level for long enough to be effective. Time is wasted on hip and thigh raises when it could be better spent on aerobic heart-rate training. To get better results, make sure you do ten minutes of weight training, including squats, immediately after your class. If you have access to Pump classes, these are a good option.

Circuit classes can help to promote general fitness and conditioning, as well as help with fat loss and muscular endurance. They can also improve your strength to a certain degree. Although there are better options for all of these, circuit classes can be tremendous fun and might provide just the kick to get you started.

Benefits:
- Aerobic classes help with fat loss, tone, shape and fitness.
- Circuit classes can help you to increase muscle strength and endurance, and improve muscle connective tissue strength.
- Properly performed aerobic classes can help you to use all your muscles, and improve and maintain your flexibility.
- Great social activity.
- Good for maintaining motivation.

Cross-training

Cross-training involves combining a range of different activities that use different muscles, different energy systems and different aspects of fitness in your training. It provides a balanced program if you include a variety of activities that exercise all your major muscle groups. One of the best things about cross-training is that you can attack training from different angles, giving you a better chance of success.

> 'If you really want to do something you'll find a way. If not, you'll find an excuse.'
> — Di Barr

Results possible:
Cross-training results can be varied depending on the combination of activities you put into your program. Boxing, running and weight training will give you different results to aerobics, swimming and netball.

Cross-training can comprise any number of activities in a combination that suits you. Try to select activities that complement each other, rather than repeating the same activities over and over again. This will help you to maintain your interest and motivation while training, and prevent you from suffering from overtraining or injuring the same muscles you are overusing.

Benefits:
- An interesting and varied way of training.
- Teaches you new skills.
- Involves many different types of training.
- A variety of results are possible.

Smart Training

Cross-training can be set up in a variety of ways — design your own session to suit your needs. The way you set it up depends on your goals:

If your goal is:

- **Muscle endurance** — circuit style on a time cycle with no rest in between.

- **Speed** — 4 sets of 6-8 reps for 5-6 exercises. Low volume, high intensity — long rest (45-60 secs between sets).

- **Strength** — 4 sets of 12-20 reps for 5 exercises. High volume — medium intensity — long rest (45-60 secs between sets).

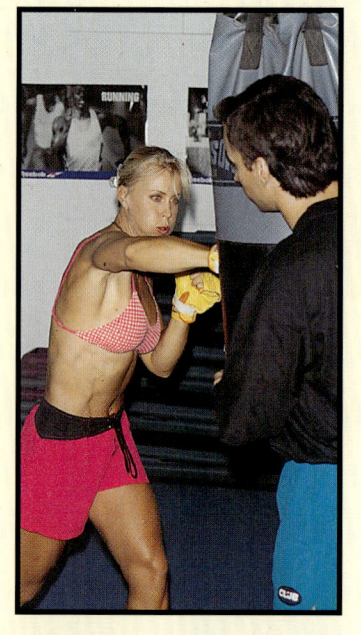

Boxercise/boxing training
Boxing will teach you new skills and work out your whole body. Take out your frustration and stress on a boxing bag!

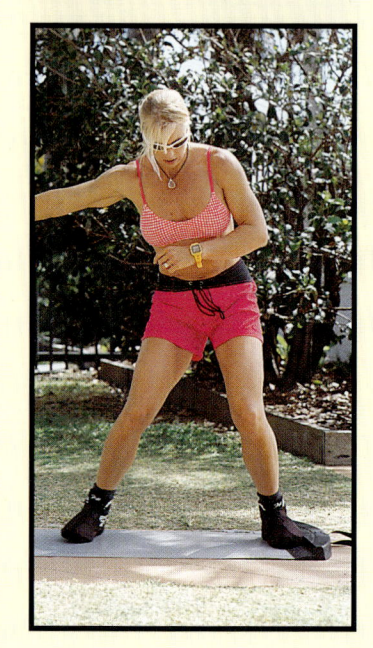

Slide Reebok
This is great for improving your balance and agility. It's low impact and it's easy to progress quickly — and you can do it anywhere with your own slide.
(Great for your legs and bottom.)

Smart Training

Five Great Cross-training Activities

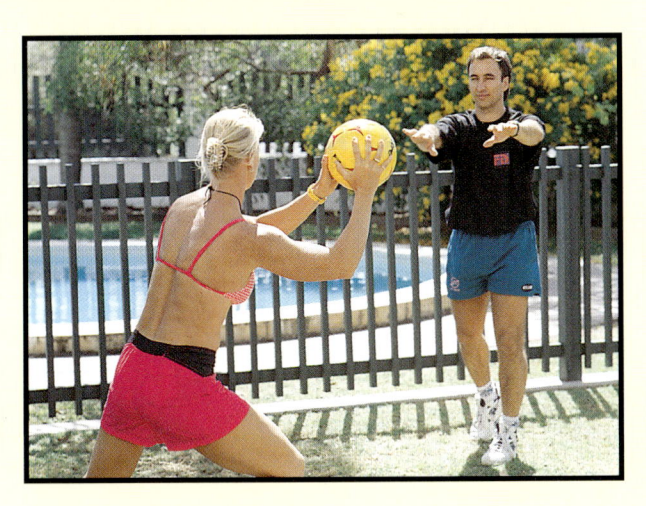

Agility drills
These drills will improve your agility and coordination, as well as your endurance and speed. They're good for all ages, but are especially good for helping children develop all-round skills.

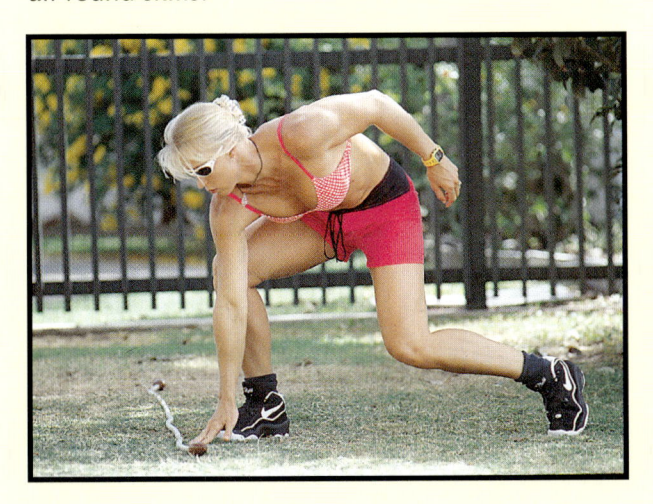

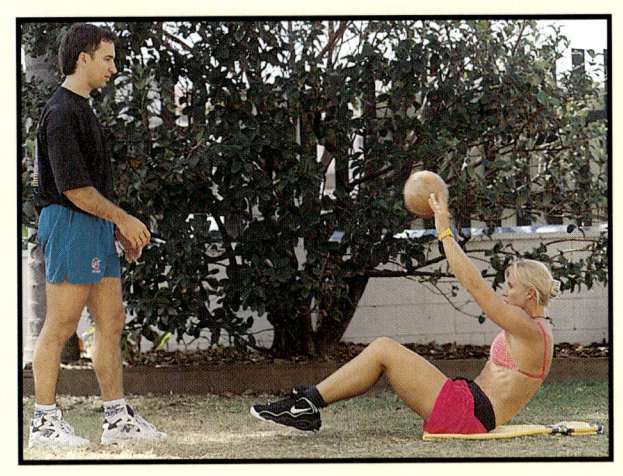

Medicine ball drills
These drills can be used for all parts of the body. An abdominal exercise has been illustrated in the photograph, but you could also include upper body throwing drills, overhead throwing drills — whatever suits your needs.

Interval or shuttle runs
These runs will improve your fitness quickly. They're great training for field and team sports as they involve movements very similar to those involved in most outdoor games. You don't need any equipment or a lot of space.

Smart Training

This is an Example of What I Include in My Sessions:

- Warm-up — 10 mins CV eg — exercise bike, treadmill, rowing ergo, stairmaster, walk/jog
- Stretch lightly for five minutes — using the five best stretches on pages 120–121
- 3 x 3 mins boxing (high and low on bag) — 1 min rest between
- 5 x 20 shuttle runs (easy/hard) continuous — 1 min rest between
- 5 x 1 min slide — 30 secs rest
- 3 x (30 sec fast skip + 1 min moderate skip) — 1 min rest in between
- 5 x 20 sit-ups with medicine ball — 30 secs rest
- 5 x 10-20 full or half push-ups — 1 minute rest in between
- 3 x 20 step-ups on each leg — 30 secs rest
- 5 x 10 squat jumps (reach your arms high) 1 min rest in between
- 3 x 20 burpees — 30 sec rest

Or

- (5 min bike / 5 min row ergo / 5 min treadmill / 5 min stairmaster) x 2 continuous eg 40 mins
- Finish off with a combination of the five best abdominal exercises on pages 212–213 plus five best stretches.

TOTAL workout time:
— warm-up 10-15 mins
— main set 40 mins
— abs and cool-down 10–15 mins

Sport

From backyard cricket and beach football to Olympic competition, sport in Australia is a great tradition. However, many people begin playing sport to get fit, when what they really should be doing is getting fit to play sport. How many times do we hear of middle-aged men heading off to the squash courts or a touch football field for the first time in years and collapsing after the first ten minutes because of their lack of fitness and the added stress of competition? The mind was willing, but the body was . . . simply unfit!

Sports range from the very physically demanding, such as football, triathlons and athletics, to the less demanding and more skill-oriented, such as golf, bowling, archery and pistol shooting. Select a sport that suits the level of exertion you want, as well as your skills and personality.

Results possible:

All kinds of things are possible here. If you take up touch football, fitness and agility can be developed quite well. If you take up archery, fitness isn't high on the list of benefits from this sport. If the sport you choose requires fitness, make sure you improve your fitness before you begin to play.

Smart Training

Benefits:
- Can be competitive and/or social.
- Can work on large muscle groups in all kinds of actions and can improve all components of fitness, from endurance to speed.

■ ■ ■

When deciding what you'd like to include in your training program, consider these three important points:
- enjoyment;
- suitability; and
- accessibility.

You need to select an activity that you'll enjoy. Then, you have to make sure it suits your fitness level, your skill level, and the level of your motivation. Finally, it must be accessible. If it's too far away, you'll use this as an excuse for not continuing your program. If you consider enjoyment, suitability and accessibility in your choices, you'll end up with a training program that will be much easier for you to maintain in the long term.

The Training Manual in the last section of this book will give you a range of training program options to consider.

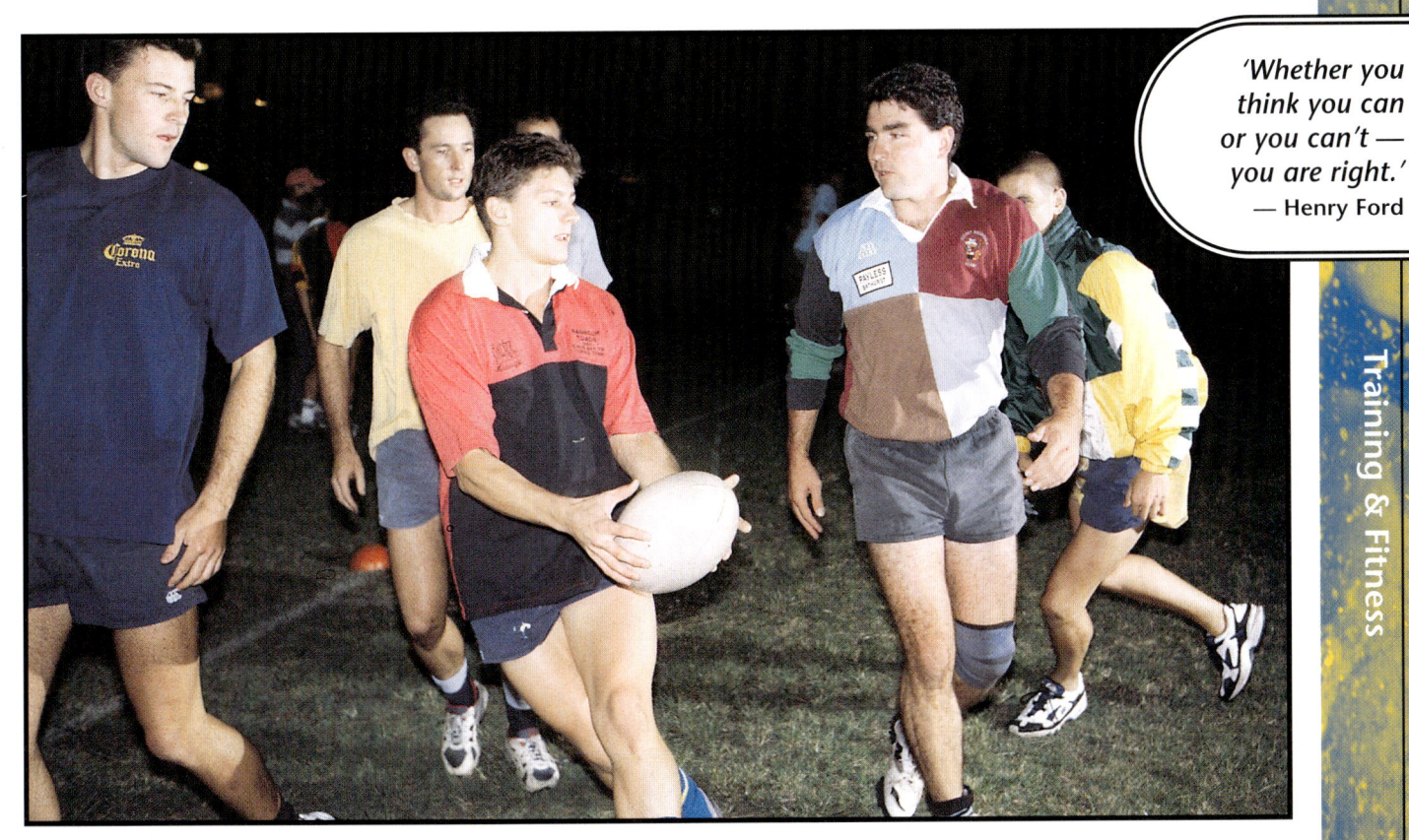

> 'Whether you think you can or you can't — you are right.'
> — Henry Ford

Being part of a team gives you an opportunity to develop good levels of fitness as well as being social and a lot of fun!

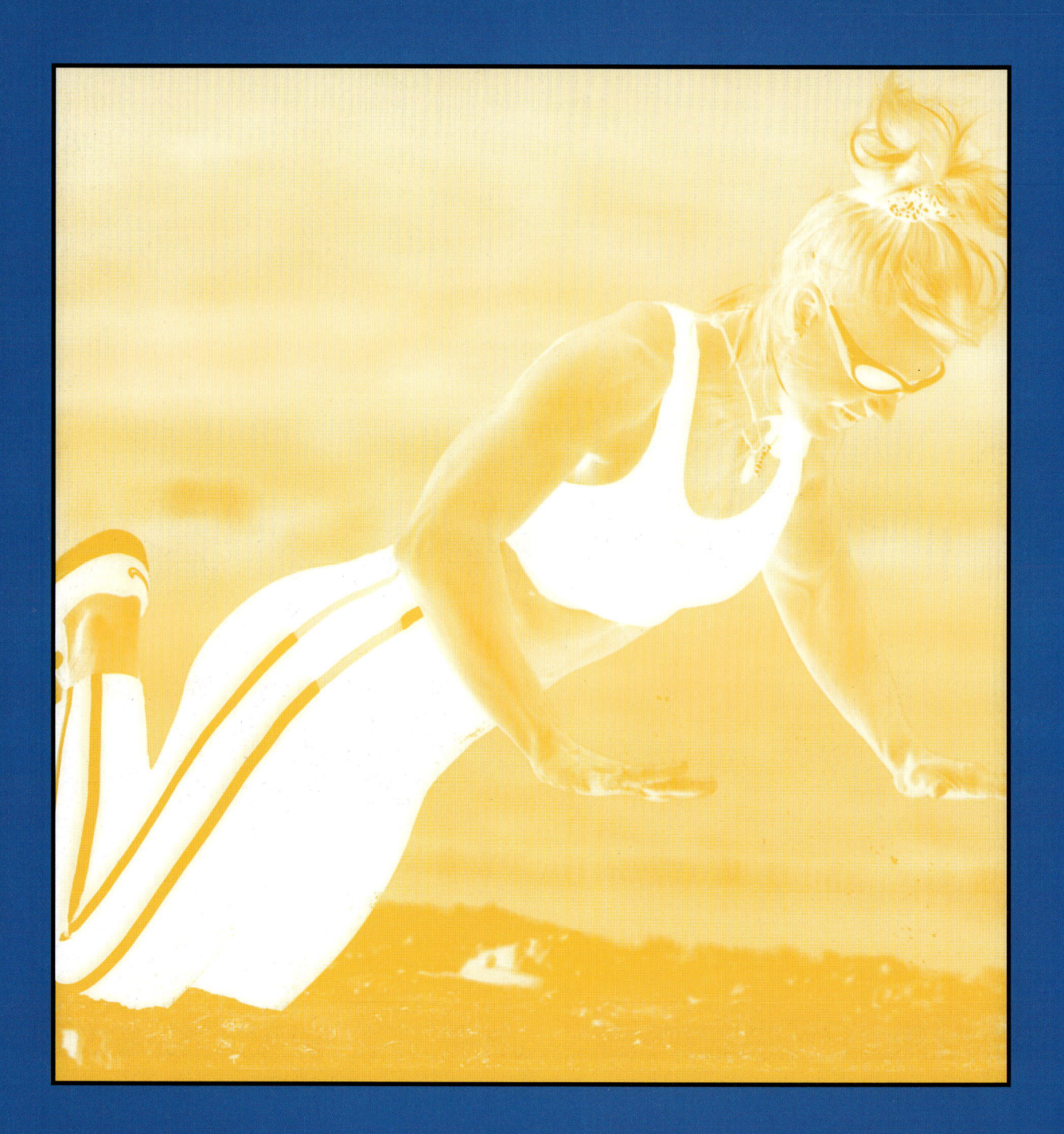

Training Manual

Introduction to Training Manual

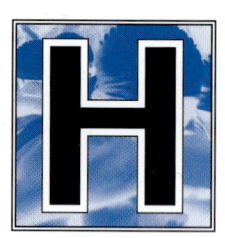

How to Use This Training Manual

There are several steps you should take in order to make the most of the programs in the Training Manual. Before commencing any of the programs you should get clearance from your doctor. Next you should make sure you have read all the chapters — so that you're familiar with the concepts involved (motivation, how your body works, the importance of diet, and the differences between exercise and training), and then write down your goals as outlined in Getting Started on page 13. Next, complete your personal fitness tests. Write down your scores and rate your fitness from the standards shown in Test Your Fitness starting on page 124. At this stage it's also beneficial to consult with a qualified nutritionist in order to establish your particular nutritional needs during training. You can then plan your normal weekly routine around your recommended sessions.

Take note of the recommendations for your posture on page 163, and then work through the training programs outlined in this manual. As you go, monitor your progress by occasionally re-testing your fitness. Don't forget also to monitor your diet — a return visit to your nutritionist at some stage would be beneficial. Consult your physio or trainer as to the specifics and progression of your program. Finally, write to us and tell us about your success story!

Goal-specific Training

Effective training combines a mixture of variables. Choosing exercises that are right for you will mean the difference between achieving the results and the success you want, and achieving nothing except the probability of injury and frustration. When putting together your training program, proper consideration needs to be given to your age, training history, current level of fitness and your specific goals.

Introduction to Training Manual

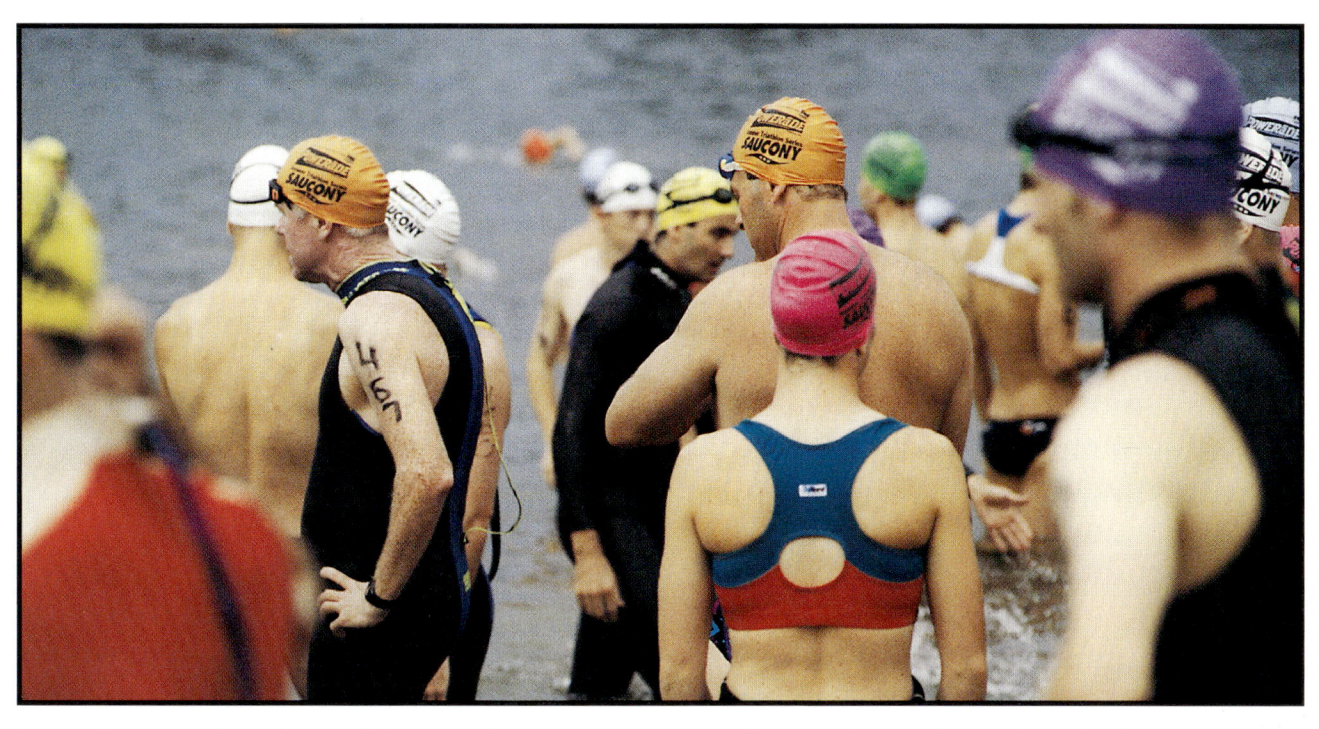

Improved posture and muscle control gives you a better opportunity to win when you take your place on the starting line.

The Importance of Posture and Control

Posture is something we should all be aware of. If you look around, there are more people with bad posture than good posture. Bad posture can include simple things such as a hunched back or uneven shoulders, or complex conditions such as pelvic imbalances or scoliosis (curvature of the spine). Some of these conditions can be fixed entirely, others can be stabilised, but unfortunately some will continue to give chronic discomfort.

Ideally, you need someone qualified in this area to give you an accurate assessment of your own condition. If you do have concerns about your posture, we recommend you see a physiotherapist who will give you a thorough examination and offer suggestions to suit your individual needs.

Posture and correct balance between muscles will benefit you greatly but only if you follow through with the advice from your physio or trainer. Stopping the exercises prematurely or doing them incorrectly will only harm your progress.

There are many general exercises which will assist in maintaining general stability for good posture. However, check beforehand that none of these exercises will aggravate your particular condition.

Poor posture and injuries often result from incorrect exercise technique. In general:

■ Try to avoid any exercises that use the shoulder or neck muscles or require you to lift above your shoulders or head — for example, the shoulder press

Get UP&GO! 163

Introduction to Training Manual

and the upright row. After you have learned how to keep your shoulder blades in a locked-down position, then you may add these types of exercises into your program.

■ Avoid using weights in exercises that are so heavy they cause your technique to change. Make sure you don't let your hips twist to one side or your knees collapse inwards during leg exercises. Similarly, don't allow your neck or shoulders to become too tight in upper body exercises.

■ Don't train under fatigued conditions where you are unable to assume the correct postural positions before you do each exercise.

■ Don't run if you have been diagnosed (by your physio) as having weak abdominals or poor hip stability. It's better to walk until you have overcome these problems.

General Guidelines for Improving Posture and Control

■ Select exercises appropriate to your level of ability. If your hips are weak, do a split squat instead of a full squat. Only do exercises you know you can do with control. If the exercise is too demanding, it may end up causing problems or reinforcing bad technique or poor posture.

■ Do only as many reps as you can control. Stop when you lose control and go on to the next exercise. Going past the number of reps where you lost control reinforces poor technique.

■ Keep the range of movement small and controlled. As control improves, increase the range of movement while steadily maintaining control.

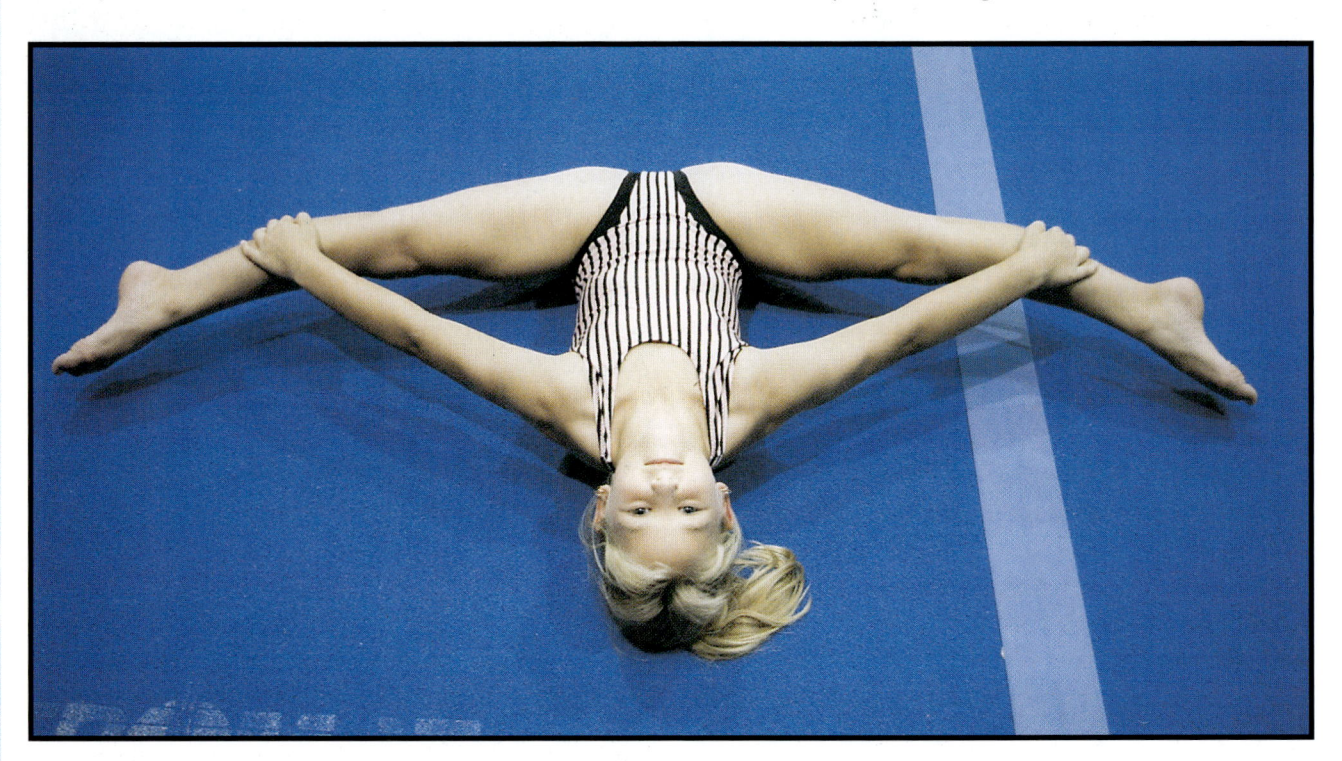

Maintaining flexibility from an early age can play a major role in good posture.

Get UP&GO!

■ Maintain good posture during all your exercises. Teach your body to hold a good position. Aim to be able to move your limbs yet hold your trunk in a controlled position throughout.

Are You Getting The Best Results?

When you train seriously for an extended period and don't get results, it's time to look at how you really train. There are some common mistakes people make when training:

It takes time to get results — People think they can get results overnight. They can't! If you are serious about changing your life, then be prepared to spend the time it takes to make it work. That's not to say that you won't see anything happening, but be prepared for the fact that it will take at least six months to make a *real* difference. While some people will start seeing and feeling the difference in four or five weeks, others may not notice any difference for up to three months. You just have to persevere because, even if you can't see it right away, believe me, it's happening for you! You must be patient.

I know nothing's happening! — If you feel you are not getting results after four weeks on a new program, and you feel like throwing it all in, then consider one of these three options:
1. The program doesn't suit you and you need to change it now. Get a program designed just for you — you may need a different program from your friend.
2. You are doing too much, so you should go into a rest cycle for at least a week to evaluate your training. If you do less your body has more of a chance to recover and you should get better results.
3. Your body is bored and you need to change your program more often so that your body has something to respond to.

Generally, most people have a combination of all three problems.

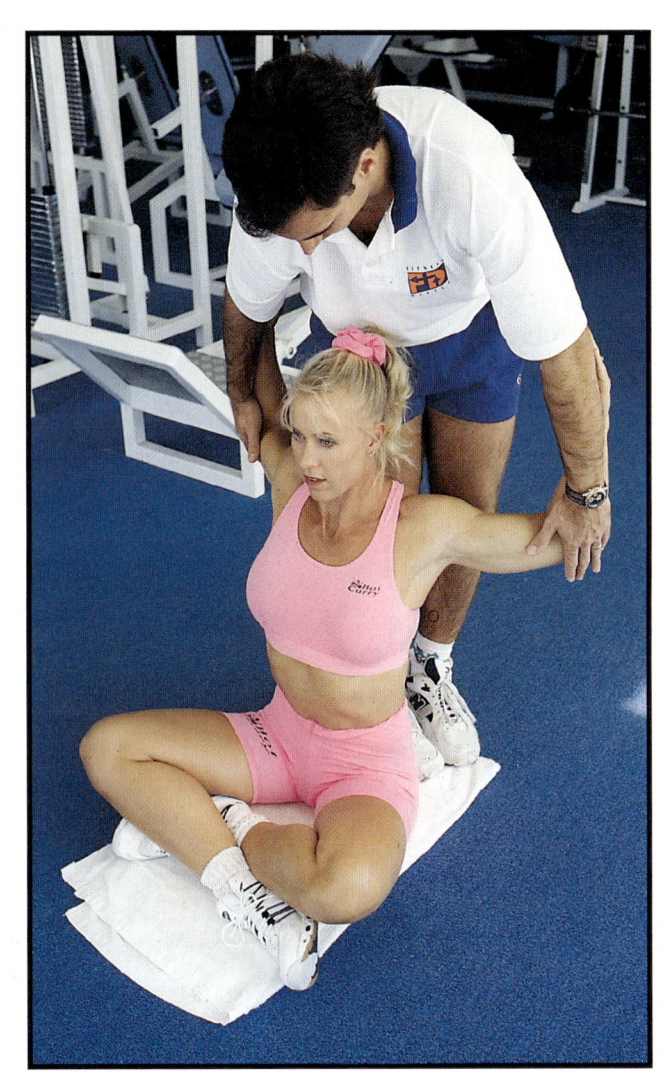

Holding your body in the correct posture is important in every facet of training, particularly stretching.

Introduction to Training Manual

Train less, rest more — A common mistake many people make is that, when they don't see results straight away, they think they have to do more work. This is wrong! The reason why most people fail to achieve results is that they are trying to do too much. Many people are pulling out of sport and training because of illness, injury, fatigue and boredom. You must rest.

You're training or playing sport for enjoyment, improvement and maintenance, not to feel tired and sick all the time. Train your body up to the point where you know you can't achieve much more and then have a period of rest appropriate to your exercise. When you start again after recovery, you'll perform better and achieve more.

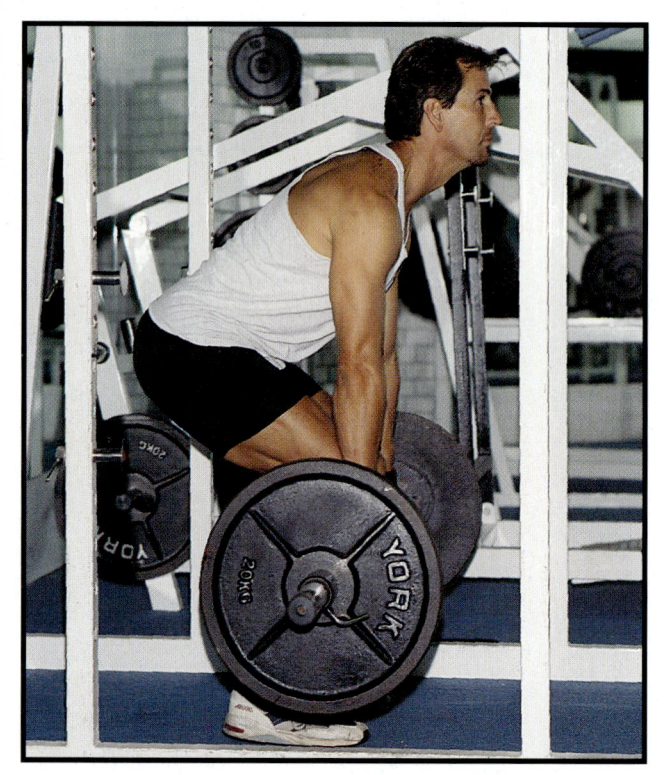

Progressing to heavy weights is possible if you train smart, train hard and rest regularly.

Train smarter and harder — You have a great program, you don't overtrain, you eat well and rest often. But it still doesn't work! In complete contrast to the problem just discussed above, the problem this time may be that you are just not training hard enough. Try to find your appropriate zone for training. It may help to exercise with someone a little more advanced than you. You will extend yourself and begin to see results.

One of the simplest things to teach people is how to train harder. If you use the correct muscles and do the right activity at a slightly harder level each week, then you are doing what we call 'progressive overload'. This leads to better results and, after rest, significantly improves your fitness, strength and shape, or whatever else you have trained for.

The smarter and harder you train, the less often you need to train.

Only do what you need to do — Only train as much as you need to, to achieve your goals. Just because the person next to you does 30 more crunches than you doesn't mean you have to try to emulate him or her.

Make your progressions regular and even, and only do what you set out to achieve for that session. Just because you can do 10 more chin-ups, ask yourself if it would be smart to do them now, or better to save them and do them tomorrow, when you'll have your last training session before your rest week. Progress training slowly and use your energy wisely.

Do what you need to do (and do it well) — The following programs will certainly give you a load of options and allow you to modify your training to see great results. Remember to tailor the programs to suit your lifestyle.

Introduction to Training Manual

The following programs have been divided into five goal-specific areas. Training for:
1. fat loss;
2. aerobic fitness;
3. increased muscle size;
4. muscle definition; and
5. shape.

The programs outlined in this section have been set up to help you get started and to suggest what you should do to progress in your training. All of the exercises included in the Training Manual are illustrated in the Appendix at the back of the book. Even if you are familiar with the exercises listed, you should still refer to the illustrations to ensure you use the correct technique.

Warming Up and Cooling Down

Warming up is necessary for injury prevention and, in some cases, enhancement of performance. Cooling down is also important, as it helps maintain flexibility and leads to faster recovery.

Your warm-up should always be specific to the kind of activities you are including in your training session. For example, you wouldn't warm-up the same way for a netball game as you would for a 5-kilometre run. Your warm-up should always be specific to the:
- energy systems you are going to use during training;
- joints and muscles that will be stressed during training; and
- timing and coordination of the movements you will include in your training.

Cooling down properly helps to prevent your blood pooling in the extremities, which can lead to fainting. It also helps in the removal of lactic acid, and increases your rate of recovery.

Stretching will make all the difference to the benefits of your training, and allow you to warm-up and cool down more effectively. Stretch for five minutes at the start of every session and again after each session. You must stretch as a warm-up and a cool-down. (Refer to 'Preparing to Train' on pages 120–121, for a guide to stretching.)

Delayed muscle soreness (DMS)

DMS is the stiffness that occurs after unaccustomed exercise. Eccentric activity (strain on the muscle as it is lengthening) is thought to promote this stiffness more than concentric activity (strain on the muscle as it is shortening). For example, in weight training this means that the lengthening phase is more likely to result in muscle soreness. In running, it is the landing (or absorbing phase) of each step that makes each muscle sore. DMS is thought to be caused by damage to the muscle-fibre membrane. Post-exercise stretching won't reduce DMS, but it *will* help to maintain your flexibility.

> 'Take rest; a field that has rested gives a beautiful crop.'
> — Ovid

Training for Fat Loss

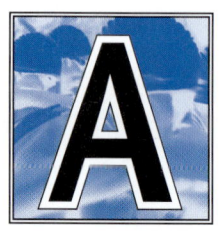

Achieving fat loss is as much a mental task as it is physical. No matter how hard you train or how much effort you put into changing your diet, to successfully lose body fat you have to *believe* that you can.

Before you begin training for fat loss, consider these essential points:

- You have to *feel good* about losing body fat. You might be carrying more body fat than you would like, but you still have to feel good about yourself while you are working on getting rid of the fat you don't want.
- Choose to lose body fat for the right reasons, such as health, fitness and lifestyle. Don't attempt to lose body fat just because you think it will make you more socially acceptable. Don't go on a fat-loss program for someone else's sake or you won't stick with it. It must be for you.
- It's important to have the support of your family and friends — without this it will be more difficult.
- You have to commit to achieving small goals on a weekly and monthly basis, with emphasis on your weekly goals. Try not to think of these goals as weight reduction; think of them as girth or body-fat reduction measures.
- Fat loss will not solve your relationship, family or financial problems, but improving your fitness will enable you to deal better with these types of stress.

Aerobic Training for Fat Loss

It's commonly believed that you need to perform three 20-minute aerobic training sessions a week to achieve fat loss. This is simply not enough. If you're untrained, it will take 10 of those 20 minutes for your aerobic system to kick in and start burning your fat reserves for energy. So, in 20 minutes you'll have achieved just over 10 minutes of effective fat burning.

To successfully lose fat, you must:

- train for at least 40 minutes at every session; and
- train three days a week as an absolute minimum and six days a week at the most; four to five sessions would be ideal.

Most people have heard that low-intensity exercise is best for burning fat, but the value of high-intensity exercise is that it increases your metabolic rate, which stays higher for longer after you finish exercising. For fat loss, a combination of high-intensity and low-intensity weight-bearing exercises are best — for example, walking, jogging and low-impact aerobic classes. An exercise can be high in intensity if it places a lot of stress on your body to complete it. In easy exercises such as walking, you'll have to stride out and pump your arms to increase the intensity.

When you first start training, begin with lower-intensity exercises. Your aim should be to slowly increase your intensity in at least one of your weekly training sessions. Monitoring the intensity you are training at is an important part of training for fat loss. Make sure you read the section on intensity in Smart Training and that you become proficient at taking your pulse before attempting any of the following programs. Training at the wrong intensity will alter your results significantly.

Training of any kind must include unloading (recovery) periods. For fat loss, you should take a minimum of one day off per week, and schedule every fourth or fifth week as an unloading week. On your rest day each week make sure you don't spend three hours doing the grocery shopping or place yourself in any situation that will cause you similar stress to that

Golden Rules of Training for Fat Loss

You must:
- Stretch to warm up and to cool down.
- Train for at least 40 minutes at every session — you have to do this for three days a week as a minimum, and six days as a maximum.
- Train at 60–80 per cent of your maximum heart rate.
- Include resistance training in your program.
- Rest at least one day a week.
- Unload every four to five weeks.

of your training. Rest means rest, so make this day as relaxing as possible. In your unloading week, reduce your training to a level that will allow your body to recuperate but still maintain everything you have worked so hard to achieve.

Aerobic Activities for Fat Loss

Walking/running

A session refers to a period of training on a per-week basis. Multiple sessions should also be completed per week. The minimum percentage refers to the intensity of your training — that is, the percentage of effort you should be training at. (Refer to the section on intensity in Smart Training to work out what your heart rate should be.) You shouldn't start a running program until you have achieved a minimum level of fitness and have cleared yourself from injuries or received medical clearance to run. To test your level of fitness, refer to the 12-minute run/walk test on page 131.

Training for Fat Loss

Fitness level	Walk or run	Surface	Weeks 1–2	Weeks 3–4	Week 5
Poor	Walk only	Flat and firm surface	2–3 x 30-minute sessions, minimum 60 per cent	3–4 x 30-minute sessions, minimum 60 per cent	2 x 30-minute sessions, minimum 60 per cent
Below-minimum	Walk only	Firm surface, occasionally trying small hills	2–3 x 30-minute sessions, minimum 65 per cent	2 x 35-minute sessions, minimum 65 per cent 2 x 40-minute sessions, minimum 60 per cent	3 x 30-minute sessions, minimum 60 per cent
Minimum	Walk only	Flat to small-to-medium hills with firm surface and occasionally soft grass or sand	2 x 40-minute sessions, minimum 70 per cent 2 x 45-minute sessions, minimum 65 per cent	2 x 40-minute sessions, minimum 70 per cent 1 x 60-minute session, minimum 65 per cent	1 x 30-minute session, minimum 65 per cent 1 x 60-minute session, minimum 60 per cent
Minimum	Walk and Run	Flat to small-to-medium hills with firm surface and occasionally soft grass or sand	2 x 40-minute sessions. Alternate between running and walking – walk for 2 minutes, run for 30 seconds 2 x 30-minute sessions. Alternate between running and walking – walk for 90 seconds, run for 30 seconds (For both, walk at a minimum of 60 per cent and run at a minimum of 70 per cent)	2 x 40-minute sessions. Alternate between running and walking – walk for 2 minutes, run for 30 seconds 2 x 30 minute sessions. Alternate between running and walking – walk for 90 seconds, run for 90 seconds (For both, walk at a minimum of 60 per cent and run at a minimum of 80 per cent)	1 x 60-minute walk at 60 to 70 per cent 1 x 30-minute session. Alternate between running and walking – walk for 10 minutes at 70 per cent, run at an easy pace for 5 minutes and repeat

Get UP&GO!

Training for Fat Loss

Fitness level	Walk or run	Surface	Weeks 1–2	Weeks 3–4	Week 5
Good	Walk only	Flat to hilly with firm surface or soft sand	2 x 40-minute sessions, minimum 75 per cent 2 x 50-minute sessions, minimum 70 per cent 1 x 60-minute session, minimum 65 per cent	3 x 50-minute sessions, minimum 75 per cent 2 x 60-minute sessions, minimum 70 per cent	2 x 40-minute sessions, minimum 65 per cent 1 x 60-minute session, minimum 60 per cent
Good	Walk and Run	Flat to hilly with firm surface or soft sand	2 x 40-minute sessions. Walk for 10 minutes (minimum 70 per cent), run for 20 minutes (minimum 70 per cent), run for 10 minutes (minimum 60 per cent) 2 x 40-minute sessions. Run for 20 minutes (minimum 60 per cent), then walk for 20 minutes (minimum 80 per cent)	2 x 40-minute sessions. Run for 20 minutes (minimum 70 per cent), walk for 10 minutes (minimum 60 per cent), run for 10 minutes (minimum 70 per cent) 2 x 60-minute sessions. Run 3 x 10 minutes, with 10-minute walk recovery after each 10-minute run.	2 x 60-minute sessions. Run for 20 minutes (at 80 per cent) and walk for 40 minutes at (60 per cent) 2 x 60-minute sessions, minimum 70 per cent Walk only
Excellent	Walk only	All manner of hills and sand surfaces	3 x 50-minute sessions, minimum 80 per cent 2 x 60-minute sessions, minimum 75 per cent	3 x 50-minute sessions, minimum 80 per cent 3 x 60-minute sessions, minimum 75 per cent	3 x 40-minute sessions, minimum 70 per cent

continued over page

Training for Fat Loss

Fitness level	Walk or run	Surface	Weeks 1–2	Weeks 3–4	Week 5
Excellent	Walk and Run	All manner of hills and sand surfaces	3 x 50-minute sessions. Run for 30 minutes (minimum 70 per cent), walk for 20 minutes (minimum 60 per cent) 2 x 50-minute sessions. Alternate between running and walking – walk for 3 minutes (minimum 70 per cent), run for 7 minutes (minimum 80 per cent)	2 x running sessions up to 50 minutes, at a very easy pace 2 x 60-minute sessions. Run for 30 minutes (minimum 70 per cent), run for a further 10 minutes (minimum 60 per cent), walk for 20 minutes (minimum 70 per cent) 1 x 30-minute run, minimum 80 per cent. 3 x 60-minute sessions	3 x 60-minute sessions, minimum 75 per cent. Alternate between walking for 5 minutes (minimum 60 per cent) and running for 5 minutes (minimum 70 per cent)

Swimming

How many metres can you swim in 12 minutes? Check the graph for your age on page 132 to determine your level.

Level   Intensity
Poor .... 60 per cent or below
Below-minimum............................... 60–65 per cent
Minimum .... 65–70 per cent
Good .... 70–75 per cent
Excellent.. 75–80 per cent

Kick with a board for all styles except backstroke. To do this backstroke kick, lie on your back with your arms extended above your head — keep them straight and together. Beginners may need a board held to the chest to start with.

Butterfly kick will sometimes be on your back — again, keep your arms extended, and you may need a board.

You will need to purchase the following swim gear: fins, kickboard, pull buoy, paddles, cap, goggles and a swimsuit.

Don't sit at the end of the pool and talk; keep your heart rate in the target zone.

After each set, take a minute's break, have a drink from your water bottle and breathe deeply. You may also like to stretch a little between sets.

It would be a good idea to photocopy the following swim programs, have them laminated, cut them up and arrange them in the order you're going to follow. Punch a hole through the corner, put a tie of some sort or a rubber band through the hole, and keep it with your swim things, waterproofed and ready to go!

Training for Fat Loss

Level – Poor

Swim twice a week until you get the 'feel' of swimming. It really doesn't take that long, maybe a couple of weeks, but it's worth persisting because of the great lifelong benefits you will get. Anyone, at any age, can learn to swim not only for enjoyment but also for health and fitness.

Every fifth week is an easier week. Remember to do this as it's necessary for recovery, and helps you to keep your motivation high while you improve. A major factor in sport drop-out is that many people who begin an exercise program try too hard and expect too much. Work into it easily — go with a friend or join a group. This is fun and motivating.

Do this five-week program as many times as you need to, so that you feel comfortable with your swimming. To get the most benefit out of sport and enjoy it, it helps to learn to get the basics right. Once you do, it will always be easier to get back into it after you have time off.

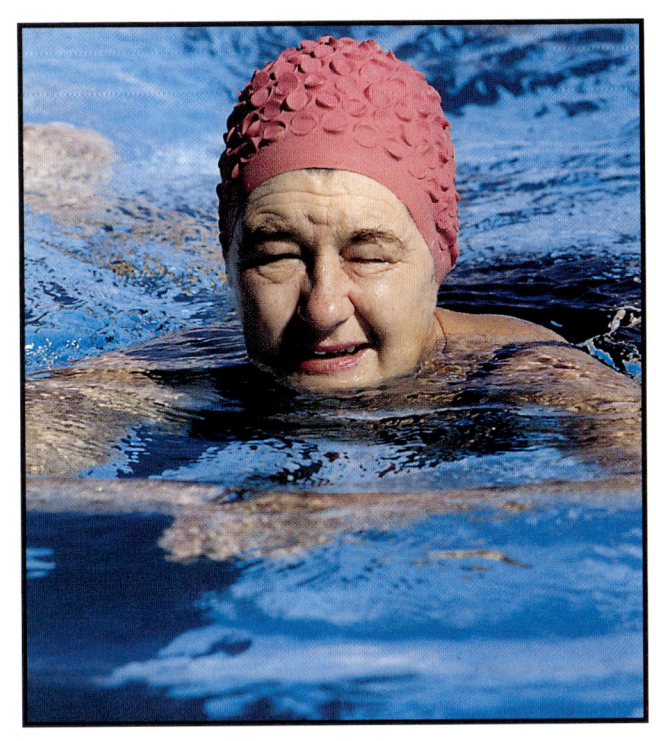

Swimming is great exercise for people of all ages.

- **Key:** FR — freestyle ■ BR — breaststroke ■ BK — backstroke ■ FLY — butterfly ■ H — Hard ■ M — Medium ■ E — Easy
- IM — individual medley (butterfly, backstroke, breaststroke, freestyle).
- Where there is no rest interval or intensity given, have your own rest and swim as you wish.

Session — Poor

Week 1–2 600 m–700 m	Week 3–4 900 m–1000 m	Week 5 800 m
4 x 25–50 m FR/BR/FR/BK	4 x 25–50 m FR/BK	4 x 50 m mixed
8 x 25 m FR 60 per cent 45 sec rest	12 x 25 m FR/BK 60 per cent 45 sec rest	6 x 50 m FR/BK 60 per cent 60 sec rest
8 x 25 m kick FR	6 x 50 m kick BR	8 x 25 m kick BK
2 x 50 m easy swim	4 x 50 m easy swim	4 x 25 m easy swim

Training for Fat Loss

Level – Below-minimum

Swim two to three times a week now, following these programs. After a while you'll understand how you should be training, and then if you want to substitute a set here and there, you may. For the third session repeat either of the first two sessions. Remember, once you have an understanding of what you need to do, how much you need to do, and how hard to do it, it's easy to write your own programs — just follow the guidelines in this book.

Session 1 — Below-minimum

Week 1–2 1.0 km	Week 3–4 1.2 km	Week 5 1.25 km
200 m mixed strokes	6 x 50 m mixed 45 sec rest	6 x 50 m mixed strokes
3 x 50 m + 6 x 25 m 65 per cent FR 45 sec rest	8 x 25 m + 4 x 50 m 65 per cent 45 sec rest	10 x 25 m + 4 x 50 m 60 per cent 45 sec rest
2 x 50 m BR + 2 x 50 m BK	2 x 50 m BR + 2 x 50 m BK	2 x 50 m BR + 2 x 50 m BK
4 x 50 m BK kick	4 x 50 m kick FR fast	4 x 50 m kick BR moderate
100 m easy	100 m easy	100 m easy

Session 2 — Below-minimum

Week 1–2 1.2 km	Week 3–4 1.4 km	Week 5 1.1 km
4 x 50 m FR/BK easy	4 x 50 m FR/BR easy	50 m + 100 m + 50 m FR easy
2 x 100 m non-stop FR 65 per cent	200 m non-stop FR 60 per cent	4 x 50 m kick FLY on back
6 x 50 m kick FR/BR 65 per cent 45 sec rest	(25 m kick + 75 m BR) x 3 65 per cent 45 sec rest	4 x 50 m FR 40 sec rest
4 x 50 m easy BR	4 x 50 m paddles FR	200 m BR kick moderate
2 x 100 m non-stop FR 60 per cent	2 x 100 m non-stop FR 65 per cent	100 m easy
2 x 50 m easy	(25 m easy + 25 m hard) x 4	4 x 50 m easy FR 30 sec rest
	100 m easy	

Level – Minimum

Remember to wear a cap and goggles — they'll help keep your hair from drying out and stop your eyes from stinging. If you sneeze after each swim, try wearing a nose clip. It took me 15 years to realise that a simple nose clip could stop my constant sneezing! Also, if you are prone to ear problems, buy some specially moulded ear plugs (from hearing aid specialists), or buy some ear putty. The ear putty is cheaper, but it gets dirty and you'll have to replace it every now and then.

Session 1 — Minimum

Week 1–2 1.5 km	Week 3–4 1.8 km	Week 5 1.5 km
(100 m FR/100 m BR/100 m BK) x 2	300 m mixed swim and kick	500 m swim non-stop
200 m non-stop FR 70 per cent	10 x 50 m (25 hard/25 easy)	500 m kick non-stop
2 x 50 m BR/BK easy	400 m kick non-stop 70 per cent	500 m pull non-stop
200 m non-stop FR 70 per cent	200 m paddles (25 hard/25 easy)	
3 x 100 m kick FR/BR/BK	200 m kick (50 hard/50 easy)	
100 m easy	200 m easy	

Session 2 — Minimum

Week 1–2 1.8 km	Week 3–4 2.0 km	Week 5 1.5 km
8 x 50 m FR 65 per cent 30 sec rest	(100 m swim + 100 m kick) x 3	10 x 50 m FR 20 sec rest
100 m BR easy	4 x 150 m FR 70 per cent 30 sec rest	400 m kick
6 x 50 m FR 65 per cent 20 sec rest	3 x 100 m BR 70 per cent 20 sec rest	6 x 50 m BR 20 sec rest
100 m BK easy	2 x 100 m BK 70 per cent 20 sec rest	200 m kick FLY on back
4 x 50 m FR 70 per cent 15 sec rest	4 x 50 m kick 70 per cent 20 sec rest	100 m BK easy
100 m BR easy	100 m easy	
2 x 50 m FR 70 per cent 10 sec rest		
3 x 100 m kick FR/BR/BK		
100 m BK		
100 m easy		

Training for Fat Loss

Level – Good

If you want to swim more than three times a week, you can choose another program from anywhere here, or you can try writing your own. Put together your favourite sets to make up a session. Remember to write it down and take it to the pool with you — that way you're more likely to do it.

Session 1 — Good

Week 1–2 2.0 km	Week 3–4 2.4 km	Week 5 2.0 km
4 x 100 m IM	300 m mixed strokes	400 m swim mixed strokes
3 x 200 m 70 per cent 30 sec rest	20 x 50 m FR 75 per cent 10 sec rest	400 m kick FR/BK
3 x 100 m 70 per cent 30 sec rest	100 m BK easy	400 m pull FR/BR
6 x 50 m 70 per cent 30 sec rest	3 x 200 m kick 75 per cent 20 sec rest	400 m kick BR/FLY
6 x 50 m kick (25 hard/25 easy)	6 x 50 m paddles (25 hard/25 easy)	400 m paddles FR/BK
100 m easy	100 m easy BR	

Session 2 — Good

Week 1–2 2.4 km	Week 3–4 2.6 km	Week 5 2.4 km
200 m swim + 200 m kick 200 m paddles + 200 m kick – every 3rd 50 m hard	(2 x 100 m FR + 2 x 100 m IM + 2 x 100 m kick + 2 x 100 m FR) x 2 75 per cent 20 sec rest	600 m FR breathe every 5
400 m 75 per cent 30 sec rest	200 m FLY kick on back	5 x 100 m BK/BR 65 per cent 20 sec rest
300 m 75 per cent 20 sec rest	2 x 200 m paddles 75 per cent	2 x 200 m kick FLY/BR
200 m 75 per cent 10 sec rest	8 x 50 m (25 hard/25 easy)	2 x 150 m FR/BK/BR
100 m 75 per cent		4 x 50 m IM order
8 x 50 m kick (H/M/E/M) x 2		100 m FLY kick
4 x 50 m BK/BR		300 m FR breathe every 5

Training for Fat Loss

Level – Excellent

Once again, if you want to swim more than twice a week, practise writing the third session yourself. The more you do it, the easier it becomes. When you start to feel really comfortable in the water, or if the session feels too easy, then you can increase the distance or reduce the rest time. Remember: for fat loss, stay within your target zone most of the time.

You can go harder for some sets, but make sure you don't overdo the intensity over a long period of time.

Remember to include paddles, pull buoys, fins, kickboards and stretch cords to give your swim session variety and 'overload'. Don't 'drag' on a swimmer in front of you. Lead the lane for clear water.

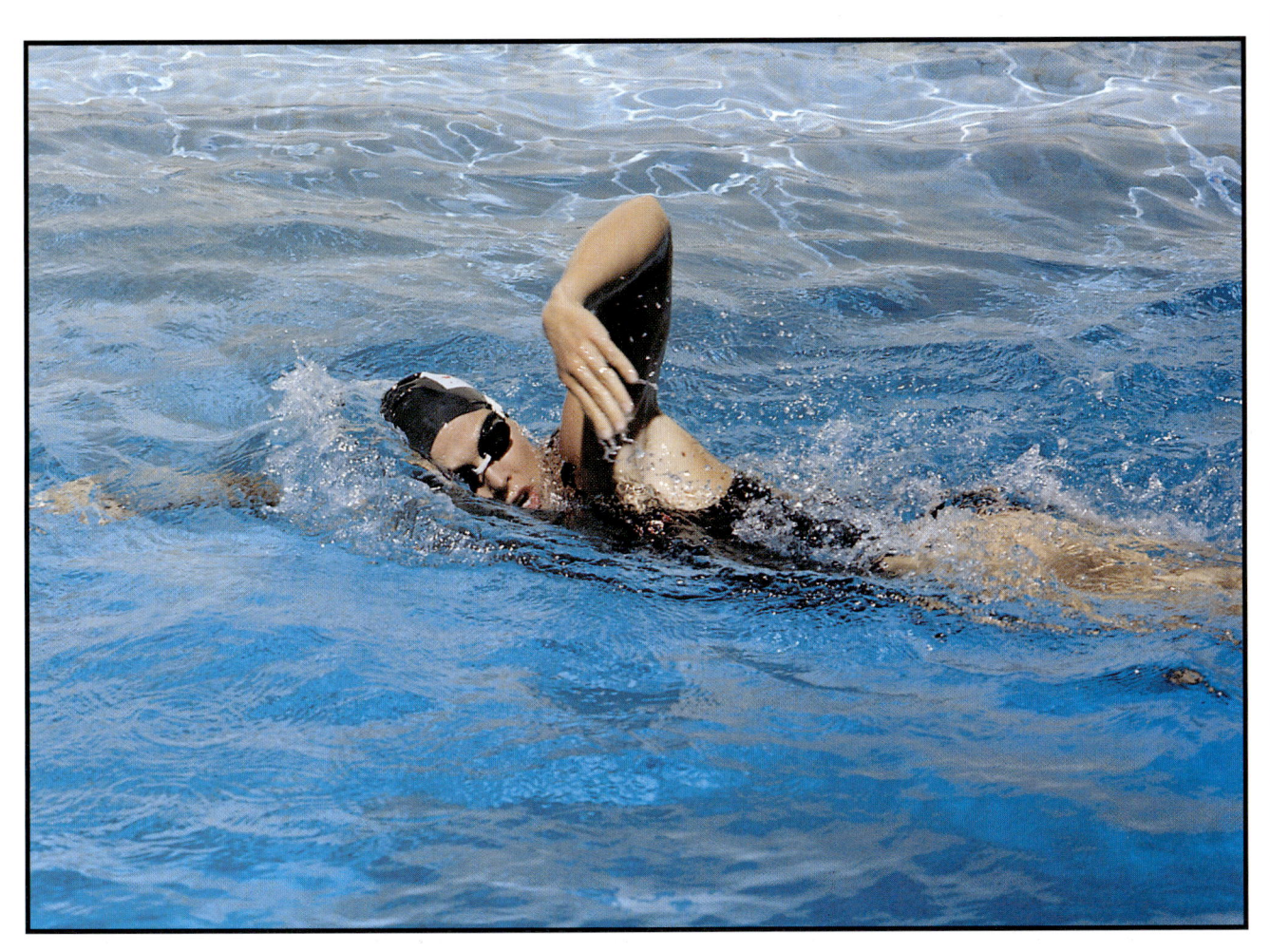

Learning the basics of swimming technique will enable you to swim efficiently and for longer periods.

Training for Fat Loss

Session 1 — Excellent

Week 1–2 3.0 km	Week 3–4 3.4 km	Week 5 2.6 km
(50 m FR + 100 m BR + 150 m BK + 200 m kick) x 2	300 m mixed strokes	300 m mixed strokes
5 x 200 m (50 m at 75 per cent/ 150 m easy)	16 x 50 m IM 80 per cent 15 sec rest	800 m FR/BK
3 x 200 m kick (100 m hard/ 100 m easy)	100 m easy	300 m kick FR
8 x 50 m mixed strokes 75 per cent 10 sec rest	4 x 200 m kick 1 of each stroke 75 per cent 30 sec rest	800 m FR/BK
	100 m easy	300 m kick BR
	400 m/200 m/100 m paddles and pull 75 per cent 20 sec rest	100 m easy
	10 x 50 m FR 75 per cent 10 sec rest	
	100 m easy	

Session 2 — Excellent

Week 1–2 3.2 km	Week 3–4 3.0 km	Week 5 2.5 km
4 x 100 m IM	(200 m FR/200 m IM/200 m kick/200 m pull) x 2	300 m mixed strokes
10 x 100 m 80 per cent 10 sec rest	8 x 25 m 100 per cent 45 sec rest	1000 m FR non-stop
200 m BK/BR	200 m easy	20 x 50 m alternate swim/kick no board 20 sec rest
12 x 50 m (25 hard/25 easy, 4 each of BK/BR/FR and some FLY if you can)	6 x 150 m FR/BK/FR 80 per cent 20 sec rest	4 x 50 m (hard/easy)
(100 m kick + 100 m swim) x 5 at 75 per cent	100 m easy	

Training for Fat Loss

Cardio equipment/cycling (indoor/outdoor)

Cardio equipment is that which is generally stationary, such as treadmills, rowers, stationary bikes and climbers. The session time allocated can be shared between different pieces of cardio equipment as long as the total target time is achieved.

Fitness level	Weeks 1–2	Weeks 3–4	Week 5
Poor	2–3 x 30-minute sessions, 60 per cent	3–4 x 30-minute sessions, 60 per cent	2 x 30-minute sessions, 60 per cent
Below-minimum	2–3 x 35-minute sessions, 65 per cent	2 x 35-minute sessions, 65 per cent 2 x 40-minute sessions, 60 per cent	3 x 30-minute sessions, 60 per cent
Minimum	2 x 40-minute sessions, 70 per cent 2 x 45-minute sessions, 65 per cent	2 x 40-minute sessions, 70 per cent 2 x 45-minute sessions, 65 per cent 1 x 60-minute session, 60 per cent	1 x 30-minute session, 65 per cent 1 x 60-minute session, 60 per cent
Good	2 x 40-minute sessions, 75 per cent 2 x 50-minute sessions, 70 per cent 1 x 60-minute session, 65 per cent	3 x 50-minute sessions, 75 per cent 2 x 60-minute sessions, 60 per cent	2 x 40-minute sessions, 65 per cent 1 x 60-minute session, 60 per cent
Excellent	3 x 50-minute sessions, 80 per cent 2 x 60-minute sessions, 75 per cent	3 x 50-minute sessions, 80 per cent 3 x 60-minute sessions, 75 per cent	3 x 40-minute sessions, 70 per cent

> 'A chain breaks at its weakest link, and so do we.'
> — Anonymous

Resistance Training for Fat Loss

The most effective programs for losing body fat include some form of resistance training. Resistance training increases your level of lean muscle mass, which in turn increases your resting metabolic rate. Resistance training needs to be performed at least twice a week and should include exercises for all the major muscle groups.

Your resistance program must make you train hard. If you are a beginner, this program needs to be only 20 minutes long, with perhaps three to four exercises per session. After a few months you can extend this to 40 minutes and six to eight exercises per session.

Incorporate your resistance training into your aerobic activity program. If your fitness level is between poor and below-minimum, you should do your resistance training on your easier days. All other levels of fitness should include resistance training on their shortest training days. For example, beginners would do the following: Monday: 60 minutes of aerobics; Tuesday: 30 minutes of gym; Wednesday: 60 minutes of aerobics, and so on.

The resistance program should involve major muscle groups (chest, legs, back) only. The bigger the muscles involved in each exercise the more energy you'll burn and the more lean muscle tissue you'll develop.

Avoid isolated exercises which only work one small muscle — that is, avoid exercises for specific sites on your body, such as side-lying leg raises, rear-leg lifts in a kneeling position — spot reduction doesn't work. Don't waste your time; go for the big exercises that use a lot of different muscles such as squats and deadlifts.

All training should be aimed at making you stronger over time. Keep the number of repetitions at between 6 and 15 only. To burn fat you don't have to do high repetitions. Going heavier with fewer reps is much more effective and good for variety.

Keep your rest between sets to 30–45 seconds and your intensity from medium to high.

It's best to do your resistance training before aerobic activity. Aerobic activity after weights will give you more opportunity to use your fat reserves for energy.

Do no resistance training in your unloading week.

Programs for Fat Loss

The following resistance training programs are varied to ensure you work your major muscle groups.

- A beginner is someone who has no previous gym experience.
- An intermediate trainer is someone who has had a small amount of gym experience, up to 6–12 months.
- An advanced trainer is someone who has had more than 12 months' experience.

Note: Reps refers to the number of times a load (the weight or resistance) is lifted. The first number refers to the number of sets you should do per session. For example: squats 3 x 8–12 reps = three sets of squats per session and you should lift your load between 8 and 12 times to complete a set. Your rest period refers to how many seconds you should rest between each set.

Training for Fat Loss

Resistance training programs for fat loss using small hand weights only.

Beginner (once per week)

Exercise	Weeks	Rest (in seconds)
Squats	3 x 8–12 reps	45
Split squats	2 x 6–10 reps	45
Wall push-ups	2 x 12–20 reps	30
Seated dips	2 x 12–20 reps	30
Alternate arm lifts	2 x 8–15 reps	30

Abdominals (Refer to the five abdominal exercises on pages 212–213 and choose exercises suited to your ability.)

Intermediate (2 times per week)

Exercise	Weeks	Rest (in seconds)
Squats	3 x 6–12 reps	45
Split squats	3 x 6–12 reps	45
Push-ups	3 x max. reps you can do	45
Bench dips	3 x max. reps you can do	45
Modified pull-ups	3 x max. reps you can do	45

Abdominals (Refer to the five abdominal exercises on pages 212–213 and choose exercises suited to your ability.)

Advanced (2–3 times per week)

Exercise	Weeks	Rest (in seconds)
Split squats	3 x 8–15 reps	45
Step-ups	3 x 6–10 reps	45
Squats	3 x 10–15 reps	45
Push-ups	3 x max. reps you can do	45
Bench dips	3 x max. reps you can do	45
Modified pull-ups	3 x max. reps you can do	45

Abdominals (Refer to the five abdominal exercises on pages 212–213 and choose exercises suited to your ability.)

Training for Fat Loss

Resistance training programs for fat loss requiring access to a fitness centre or home gym.

Beginner (once per week)

Exercise	Weeks	Rest (in seconds)
Squats	3 x 12–15 reps	45
Leg press	3 x 10–12 reps	45
Bench press	2 x 12–15 reps	45
Lat pull-downs	2 x 12–15 reps	45

Abdominals (Refer to the five abdominal exercises on pages 212–213 and choose exercises suited to your ability.)

Intermediate (2 times per week)

Exercise	Weeks	Rest (in seconds)
Lunges	3 x 8–10 reps	45
Leg press	3 x 10–15 reps	45
Leg curls	2 x 12–15 reps	45
Bench press	3 x 8–12 reps	45
Lat pull-downs	3 x 8–12 reps	45
Shoulder press	2 x 8–12 reps	45

Abdominals (Refer to the five abdominal exercises on pages 212–213 and choose exercises suited to your ability.)

Advanced (2–3 times per week)

Exercise	Weeks	Rest (in seconds)
Squats	3 x 6–10 reps	45
Split squats	3 x 10 reps	45
Dumbbell deadlifts	3 x 10 reps	45
Bench press	3 x 6–10 reps	45
Lat pull-downs	3 x 6–10 reps	45
Shoulder press	3 x 6–10 reps	45

Abdominals (Refer to the five abdominal exercises on pages 212–213 and choose exercises suited to your ability.)

Training for Aerobic Fitness

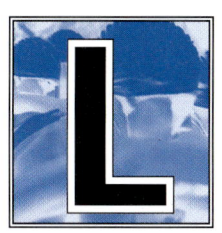

Like any other form of serious training, achieving aerobic fitness requires a long-term approach, although improvements in your fitness can be apparent quite quickly.

Training for high levels of aerobic fitness should only be considered after you've reduced your body-fat levels to the point at which you are happy to maintain them. Only then can you concentrate on increasing your aerobic fitness, mixing long and slow training methods with shorter, more intense training methods.

The decision to take on aerobic training might occur when you decide to become more active in sport; you might want to compete in some of the smaller triathlons that seem to be popping up all over Australia, or you might want to start coaching a junior sporting team.

Whatever the reason, you need to be aware that aerobic training requires a greater level of commitment, effort and intensity than other types of training.

When training for aerobic fitness, your intensity needs to be between 70 to 90 per cent of your maximum heart rate, and each session needs to last from 20 to 60 minutes. If you increase your percentage, make sure you decrease your session time. For example, train at 90 per cent for 20 minutes, 80 per cent for 30 minutes, or 70 per cent for 40 minutes. If you're going to compete in events longer than 60 minutes, your program will need to be slightly different, with some longer sessions included.

Due to the higher training intensity required for aerobic fitness, you'll need to rest more often each week than you would for most other types of training.

Training for Aerobic Fitness

> 'Nothing is so exhausting as indecision, and nothing is so futile.'
> — Bertrand Russell

You'll also need to train for a shorter block (number of weeks of training) before you have a recovery week. If you're just starting to improve your fitness, then you should only need to train three times a week, but advanced training systems for aerobic fitness can include as many as six to eight sessions a week. (Training this many times a week is for competing athletes, who might train for three weeks and then have the fourth week as unloading.)

The recommended rest cycle is to alternate your training days each week and recover every fourth week. In your unloading week you should only do two or three easy sessions for about 30 minutes, training at 60 per cent. During your weekly cycle you can include some lighter activities on your days off from fitness training, such as light walks, very easy runs, or a different sport other than the one you usually play.

Improving this component of fitness requires more control over your progression of training. If you slowly increase your training every week until your unloading week, you should start training on the first week back (week five) at the same intensity and volume you were training at in week two. In this way you get a stepped increment gradually over each four-week block.

After your initial training period — up to three months — you'll need to change the type of sessions you do. In the first three months, most of the training will revolve around increasing your *capacity* to train by slowly increasing the volume of work you do in each session each week. When you are able to train solidly for one hour, three to four times a week, it's time to increase the rate at which you train. You should then increase the intensity of your training in short bursts and in small amounts until you can gradually train harder for longer, or achieve a greater distance in the hour. Your diet may also need to be modified as your training goals and training methods change to achieve results.

This is called lactic tolerance training. The faster you become in training, the more likely you are to produce lactic acid (LA), so you need to teach your body how to cope with the feeling of high LA levels in your blood — this reduces your ability to sustain activity. Your body can cope with certain levels of LA, but when your speed increases to the point where you produce more LA than your body can cope with, you will feel tired and need to stop.

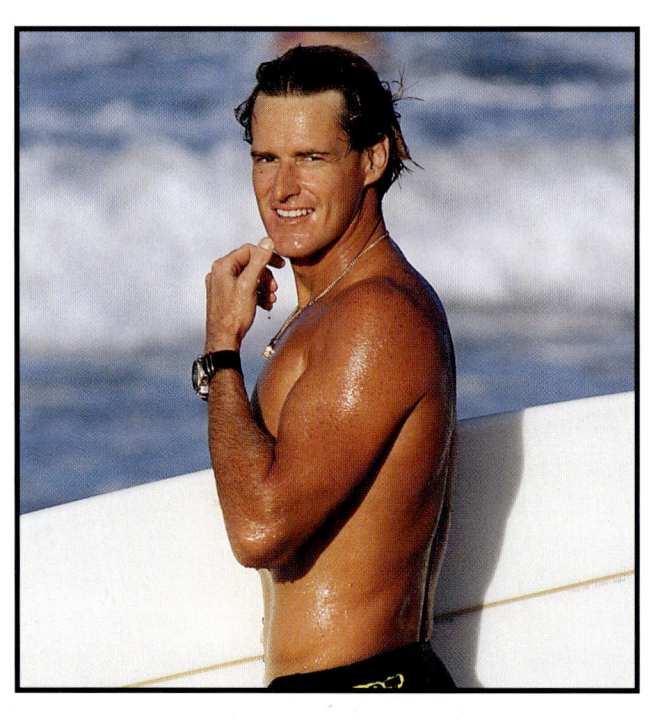

During unloading phases, choose an activity that is relaxing and enjoyable.

Programs for Aerobic Fitness

Walking/running/cardio equipment/cycling

Note: A session refers to a period of training. The percentage refers to the intensity of your training — that is, the percentage of effort you should be training at. Don't start training for aerobic fitness if your fitness level is below minimum. Ensure you are free from injury and have a medical check-up before undertaking the following programs. Each session can be made up of any combination of these activities as long as you achieve the total target time of training listed. Refer to page 145 to show you how to calculate your heart rate percentage.

Fitness level	Weeks 1–2	Weeks 3–4	Week 5
Minimum	2 x 60-minute sessions at 70 per cent, including 4 x 2 minutes at 90 per cent done at regular intervals 1 x 45-minute session at 80 per cent	1 x 60-minute session at 70 per cent 1 x 50-minute session at 80 per cent 1 x 30-minute session at 90 per cent	3 x 45-minute sessions at 60 per cent
Good	2 x 45-minute sessions at 70 per cent 1 x (3 x 10 minutes at 90 per cent, resting for 3–5 minutes between each 10-minute effort)	2 x 45-minute sessions at 80 per cent 1 x (3 x 10 minutes at 90 per cent 2–3 minutes rest) 1 x 60-minute session at 60 per cent	3 x 45-minute sessions at 60 per cent
Excellent	2 x 45-minute sessions at 80 per cent 1 x (2 x 10 minutes and 2 x 5 minutes, resting for 2–3 minutes between each effort) at 90 per cent	2 x 30-minute sessions at 90 per cent 1 x (2 x 25 minutes at 85 per cent, 2 x 5 minutes at 100 per cent) 1 x 40-minute session at 60–90 per cent	3 x 45-minute sessions at 60 per cent

Note: If a session requires you to do 45 minutes, you can break it down to 3 x 15 minutes, with small rests in between.

Swimming

Key:
UW — underwater swimming, usually breaststroke. Come up for a breath when you need to.
IM — individual medley (butterfly, backstroke, breaststroke, freestyle) continuous.
IM order — do 50s in the medley order but have a rest in between.
Breathe 3, 5, 7 — breathe every third or fifth or seventh arm cycle. Remember to blow out the bubbles — don't hold your breath.

Session 1 — Minimum

Week 1–2 1.6 km	Week 3 2.1 km	Week 4 1.5 km
3 x 100 m FR/BK/BR	6 x 50 m FR/BR	6 x 50 m FR/BR
4 x 50 m (25 m hard/25 m easy)	16 x 50 m 70 per cent 20 sec rest	500 m swim 60 per cent
8 x 50 m 90 per cent 1 min rest	3 x 100 m 70 per cent 20 sec rest	500 m kick 60 per cent
12 x 50 m 70 per cent 10 sec rest	6 x 50 m 70 per cent 20 sec rest	200 m pull 60 per cent
100 m easy	3 x 100 m kick 70 per cent 30 sec rest	
	100 m easy	

Session 2 — Minimum

Week 1–2 1.9 km	Week 3 2.0 km	Week 4 1.5 km
300 m mixed strokes	200 m swim FR easy	300 m mixed strokes
6 x 50 m (25 m hard/25 m easy)	200 m IM moderate	400 m FR/BR 60 per cent
4 x 100 m 90 per cent 90 sec rest	200 m kick 80 per cent	300 m kick 60 per cent
10 x 50 m kick 70 per cent 10 sec rest	200 m BR/BK easy	200 m BR/BK 60 per cent
100 m easy	16 x 50 m 80 per cent 20 sec rest	100 m FR 60 per cent
2 x 100 m kick FLY 80 per cent	4 x 50 m paddles	200 m easy
100 m easy	200 m easy	

Session 3 — Minimum

Week 1–2 1.9 km	Week 3 2.2 km	Week 4 1.5 km
200 m swim	4 x 100 m IM	6 x 50 m BR/BK
200 m kick	(4 x 50 m BR kick, 200 m FR, 4 x 50 m BR kick, 200 m FR, 4 x 50 m BK) 90 per cent 30 sec rest after each 200 m	(200 m + 100 m + 2 x 50 m) x 3, 60 per cent 30 sec rest (1 set FR/1 set BK/1 set BR)
200 m pull	(200 m FR, 4 x 50 m BR kick) 30 sec rest after each 50 m	
10 x 50 m FR/BR	4 x 50 m (25 m hard/25 m easy 1 of each stroke)	
10 x 50 m kick FLY/FR	200 m FR easy	
4 x 50 m (25 m hard/25 m easy)		
100 m easy		

Session 1 — Good

Week 1–2 2.5 m	Week 3 3.3 km	Week 4 2.1 km
4 x 50 m IM order easy	300 m mixed strokes	10 x 50 m 10 sec rest
4 x 100 m IM 70 per cent 20 sec rest	(400 m/200 m/100 m) x 2 FR 80 per cent 20 sec rest	(50 m FR/100 m BK/150 m BR/200 m IM) x 3, 60 per cent 30 sec rest
4 x 150 m FR/BK/FR 70 per cent 20 sec rest	(200 m BK/100 m kick no board/ 50 FLY) x 2, 80 per cent 20 sec rest	100 m easy
4 x 200 m IM 70 per cent 20 sec rest	8 x 50 m (25 m UW/25 m sprint)	
8 x 50 m kick 70 per cent 20 sec rest	16 x 25 m IM order own rest	
100 m easy	100 m easy	

Training for Aerobic Fitness

Session 2 — Good

Week 1–2 2.5 km	Week 3 3.0 km	Week 4 2.5 km
3 x 200 m swim/kick/pull 10 sec rest	20 x 50 m FR (every 5th FLY)	300 m easy
10 x 50 m 90 per cent 20 sec rest	(100 m kick/4 x 50 m pull/6 x 50 m FR) x 2 80 per cent 20 sec rest	(200 m/4 x 50 m/8 x 25 m) x 3, 1 set FR, 1 set kick, 1 set IM 60 per cent 20 sec rest
100 m easy BK	8 x 50 m (25 m UW/25 m sprint)	6 x 50 m pull FR/BR
10 x 50 m 90 per cent 40 sec rest	16 x 25 m IM order own rest	100 m easy
100 m easy BR		
10 x 50 m 90 per cent 60 sec rest		
200 m easy BK/BR		

Session 3 — Good

Week 1–2 3.0 km	Week 3 3.0 km	Week 4 2.4 km
100 m BR/200 m BK/300 m FR/400 m kick	(75 m easy/25 m hard) x 8	4 x 50 m FR 10 sec rest
5 x 200 m 1st 50 FLY/150 m FR 70 per cent 30 sec rest	5 x 100 m 90 per cent 30 sec rest	4 x 50 m BK 10 sec rest
200 m FLY kick on back	100 m easy BK	4 x 50 m BR 10 sec rest
200 m BR (50 m hard/50 m easy)	5 x 100 m 90 per cent 60 sec rest	4 x 50 m kick 10 sec rest
4 x 50 m (25 m UW/25 m sprint)	100 m easy BR	800 m non-stop FR 60 per cent
200 m BK (50 m hard/50 m easy)	5 x 100 m 90 per cent 90 sec rest	4 x 150 m kick FLY/BR 60 per cent
200 m mixed easy	500 m easy pull and paddles	200 m easy

Get UP&GO!

Training for Aerobic Fitness

Session 4 — Good

Week 4	3.0 km
1000 m swim	
1000 m kick	
1000 m pull	
All at 60 per cent, concentrate on swimming well	

Session 1 — Excellent

Week 1–2 3.0 km	Week 3 2.8 km	Week 4 2.5km
3 x 100 m IM	4 x 100 m IM	300 m mixed strokes
6 x 50 m kick (25 m hard/25 m easy)	8 x 25 m FLY/FR	10 x 50 m FR/BK 60 per cent
200 m easy	20 x 50 m (25 m at 90 per cent/ 25 m easy)	10 x 50 m IM 60 per cent
600 m/400 m/200 m/100 m FR 80 per cent	10 x 50 m kick (15 m at 90 per cent/ 35 m easy)	5 x 100 m kick 30 sec rest 60 per cent 20 sec rest
3 x 300 m pull/kick/swim 80 per cent 20 sec rest	4 x 25 m dive 1 of each stroke 100 per cent	5 x 100 m pull FR/BR 60 per cent
	400 m pull 80 per cent	200 m easy
	200 m easy	

Get UP&GO!

Training for Aerobic Fitness

Session 2 — Excellent

Week 1–2 3.8 km	Week 3 3.1 km	Week 4 2.5 km
200 m FR/BK 300 m kick/swim	10 x 50 m FR/BK 8 x 25 m IM order	3 x 100 m IM 3 x 100 m FR
3 x 200 m FR 80 per cent 20 sec rest	25 m dive + 25 m easy 50 m dive + 50 m easy 8 times, 90 per cent, own rest	3 x 100 m IM
6 x 100 m FR 80 per cent 20 sec rest	400 m pull breathe 3, 5, 7	3 x 100 m BR
12 x 50 m FR 80 per cent 20 sec rest	12 x 50 m alternate hard/easy 15 sec rest	500 m kick
2 x 200 m/4 x 100 m/8 x 50 m kick 80 per cent 20 sec rest	200 m easy	8 x 100 m pull and paddles
300 m mixed strokes easy		

Session 3 — Excellent

Week 1–2 2.6 km	Week 3 3.0 km	Week 4 2.5 km
4 x 100 m IM	200 m mixed strokes	10 x 50 m mixed strokes
4 x 25 m dive fast	2 x 200 m IM	2 x 200 m IM 60 per cent 30 sec rest
2 x 200 m FR/BK 4 x 100 m FLY/FR 16 x 25 m FR/FLY 90 per cent, 1 min rest in between	4 x 25 m dive fast	400 m pull 60 per cent 30 sec rest
400 m easy	2 x 400 m FR 85 per cent 2 min rest	2 x 200 m kick 30 sec rest
2 x 100 m FR 100 per cent own rest	2 x 200 m kick 60 per cent 30 sec rest	400 m pull 60 per cent 30 sec rest
100 m easy BK	400 m pull 60 per cent 30 sec rest	8 x 50 m FR 30 sec rest
2 x 50 m FR 100 per cent own rest	100 m easy	
100 m easy	4 x 25 m FR fast	
	300 m FR/BK easy	
	4 x 50 m pull breathe every 6	

Session 4 — Excellent

Week 1–2 3.0 km	Week 3 3.0 km
400 m mixed strokes	500 m mixed strokes
800 m FR/600 m kick/400 m pull/200 m BK. Once every 100 m, sprint for 15–20 m at 90 per cent then swim easy for the rest at 60 per cent	400 m FR/300 m kick/200 m pull/100 m BK 60 per cent 20 sec rest
12 x 50 m IM order 80 per cent	16 x 50 m (15 m easy/20 m hard/15 m easy) 20 sec rest 6 x 100 m kick (25 m hard/75 m easy for 3, 75 m hard 25 m easy for 3) 15 sec rest
	100 m easy

Golden Rules of Training for Aerobic Fitness

You must:
- Maintain a training heart rate of 70–90 per cent of your maximum heart rate for a minimum of 20 minutes each session, but up to 60 minutes depending on intensity.
- Complete at least three sessions a week.
- Rest one out of every four weeks and complete two or three 30-minute sessions of low intensity (60 per cent) training during your unloading week.
- Follow a high-energy eating plan.
- Progress your fitness program in small but regular amounts each week up to your unloading week.

Resistance Training for Aerobic Fitness

You should also incorporate some resistance training in your program. Refer to 'Resistance Training for Fat Loss' (on page 180). Resistance training is best done on the shortest training days, regardless of your level of fitness. It will assist in strengthening your muscles, which will increase your body's endurance. This all helps to increase the efficiency of our aerobic system. Programs which include major muscle groups only, are best for aerobic fitness. Reps of 12–30 can be used, but 6–15 will still work the best with rest periods of 30–60 seconds.

Training for Increased Muscle Size

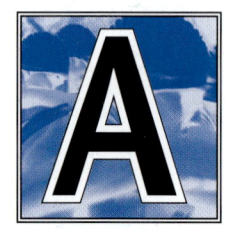

Any sort of training to increase your muscle size requires a very careful assessment of your eating plan. Your body needs a lot of energy just to maintain its current muscle mass, so if you want to increase your muscle mass, you need to eat more of the correct food to cope with the extra training.

Before attempting any of the following programs, you should have already completed a general strength program (such as fat loss, aerobic fitness, improved posture and control, or muscle definition) to condition your body to training. A general strength program allows your muscles, ligaments and tendons to strengthen before you start training them at the intensity needed to gain muscle.

The programs which follow are aimed at those who wish to get bigger all over. Later in this Training Manual there are specific guidelines for those who want to concentrate on specific shaping goals. However, regardless of whether you want to be a body builder or just wish to increase the width of your shoulders, the same principles apply.

Principles of Training for Increased Muscle Size

When training for increased muscle size, strength and size go together in a 50:50 ratio. You can't be muscular without being strong, and vice versa. Many female athletes or parents of female athletes don't

Training for Increased Muscle Size

want to lose their 'feminine look', but if you want to be a strong athlete you have to develop powerful muscles.

The two most important factors in training for increased muscle size are:

The tension placed on a muscle — that is, the intensity of the weight you are lifting. It has to be medium to high all the time. To maintain the intensity it's important not to swing the weights up and down, as this results in lost muscle tension. Keep a smooth steady action through the full movement.

The duration of the training stimulus — that is, the longer the set takes the more the stimulus is transferred. Between 40 and 70 seconds for each set can be used as a guideline (three seconds up and three seconds down per rep), so keep your movements slow. Everyone has different potential to increase their amount of muscle. Women will always find it very difficult to put on muscle mass, so they need to be patient. Young men will find it the easiest during their late teens when their body is developing naturally.

If you are taller, thinner or leaner than average, you'll need to be very careful about just how much of this sort of training you do. It's very easy to do too much and burn off your extra energy in some other activity instead of saving it for building your body. If you are naturally heavy with muscles, or 'chunky', you'll find it easier to increase or maintain muscle mass than most others.

If you want to build up but have a job that requires heavy physical work, you'll need to eat enough to carry out your physical job as well as the extra you'll need to fuel your body in training. Most people fail to put on muscle mass because they train too much and/or eat too little. Simple if you think about it, isn't it?

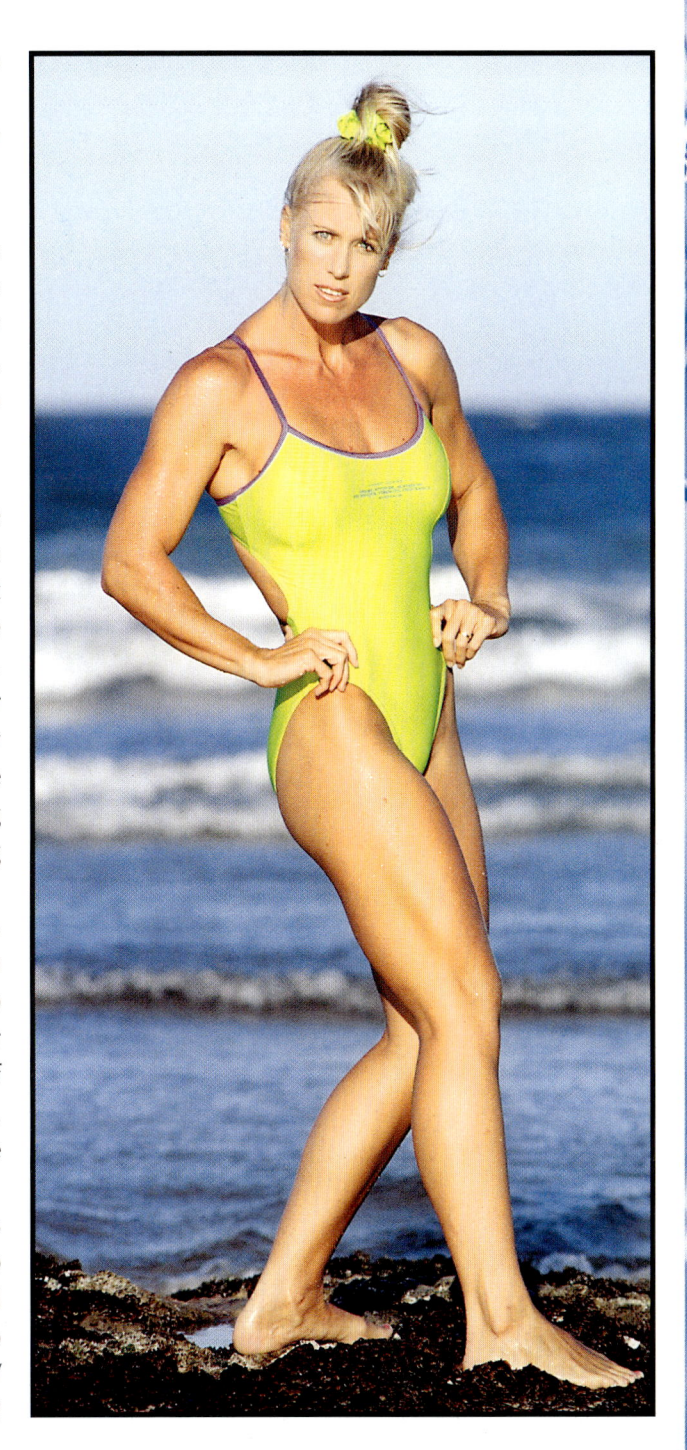

Training for Increased Muscle Size

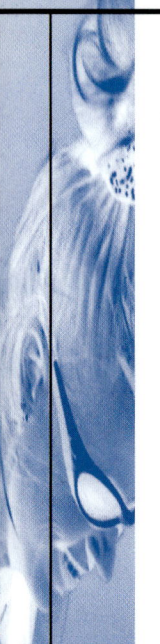

Eat more and train less! You need to find out how much training you can do without weight loss and how much rest you need to allow for full recovery.

Increases in muscle mass occur slowly. You might find that you put on 2 kilograms and then lose 1 kilogram — this isn't unusual. Things in your life can change and cause extra stress, or business and/or social commitments may make it hard for you to maintain your normal eating pattern. All these factors will influence your rate of muscle growth.

Weight training will always be the best way to achieve a balanced approach to muscle gain. Free weights are better than pin weight machines (stacks of weights in which a pin is inserted at the desired level). Hydraulic machines (operated on a cylinder of oil or air, much like a car shock absorber) aren't nearly as beneficial due to the lack of an eccentric contraction (as the muscle is not under stress while lengthening). Body-weight exercises are good initially, but at some time you'll need to do some resistance training in the form of weights to make the best gains.

Some sports and other activities will develop muscles in certain areas of your body, due to the sheer repetition of work performed by these muscles, but this won't be balanced development and it won't increase the size of *all* your body's muscles. For example, kayakers who mainly use their upper body and torso need to incorporate strength programs for their legs and hips. For all-over gain you need to have a program that works all the major muscles in your body.

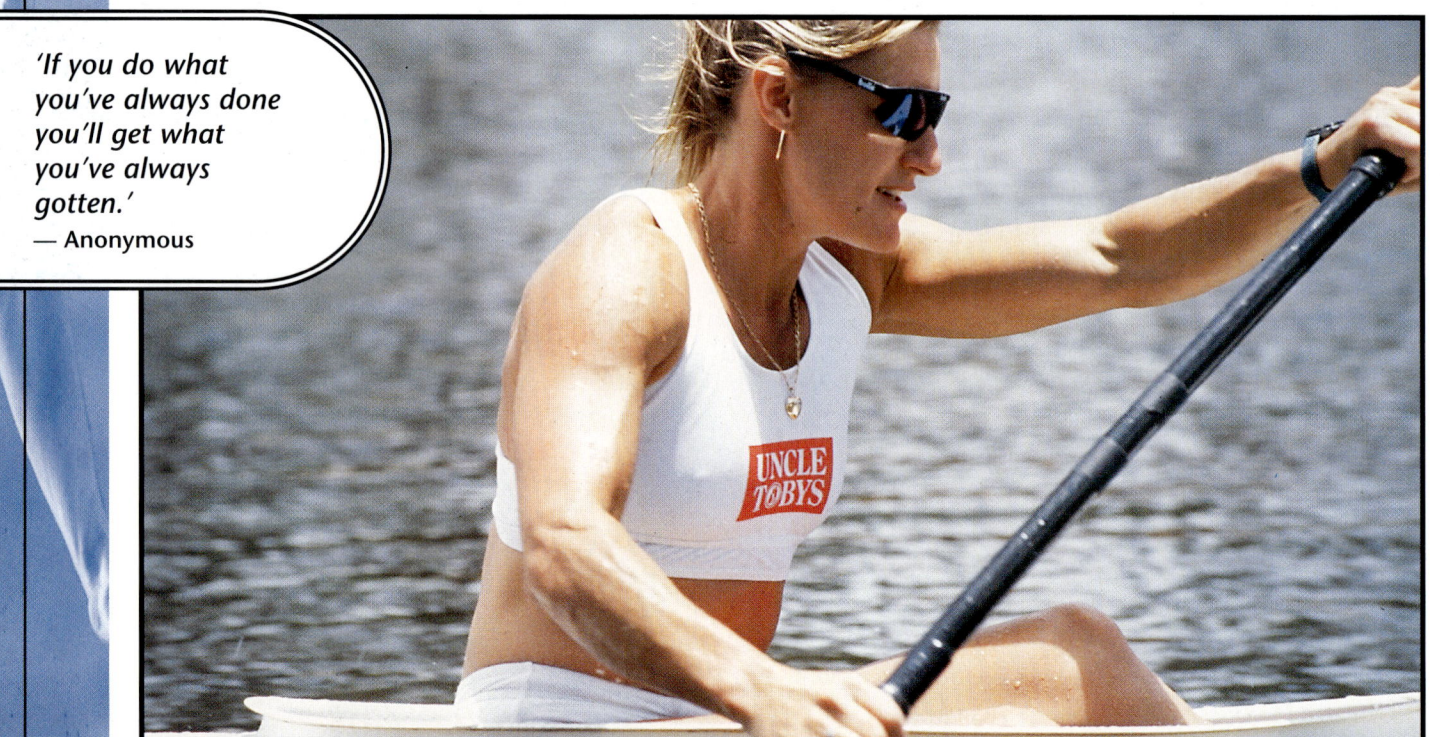

> 'If you do what you've always done you'll get what you've always gotten.'
> — Anonymous

Some sports develop muscle size in specific areas. Kayakers develop muscle size predominantly in the upper body.

Training for Increased Muscle Size

General Guidelines for Training for Increased Muscle Size

- Complete three to five strength sessions (gym programs) a week.
- Train each muscle group only once or twice a week. The more you train them, the less time they have to recover and grow.
- Keep the number of repetitions between 8 and 15 for most of the time, but occasionally vary the number of repetitions — sometimes choosing to train between 1 and 6 and sometimes including sets of higher reps, between 15 and 20.
- A high total number of reps in your workout is preferable. Try to complete around 300 reps per workout. This may equal 30 sets of 10, 20 sets of 15, etc.
- Complete between 6 and 10 sets per muscle group, decreasing the number of reps as you increase the number of sets. For example, if you do 6 sets, you'll do 10–12 reps; and if you do 10 sets, you'll do 6–10 reps. Put simply, the more reps you do, the fewer sets you need to do; or, the fewer reps you do, the more sets you need to complete.
- A significant factor is how much weight you lift in total tonnes each workout. The more you can lift in the time allowed, the better. Weight x reps x sets = load. High training volume requires greater recovery considerations after the workout.
- Keep your rest between sets to between 45 and 90 seconds. The fewer reps you complete, the longer you should rest.
- Avoid high-intensity and long sessions of regular aerobic activity, such as team sports or cardio training, as they will reduce your ability to gain muscle.
- Make each session last for only 60–75 minutes. The longer the session, the less effective the training. Some people will train for two hours on their weight program. If you are training this way, you might like to consider how 'well' you are training.
- Aim at increasing the weight on each exercise each session of each week, regardless of how many reps you do, but still aim to stay around the number of reps shown in the program. The increase may only be half a kilogram each week. Always make the increase in weight small and regular to allow your body time to adjust to each increment. It's amazing how much you can improve when you increase the weights slowly.
- Aim to follow the order of exercises as outlined in the programs. Exercises are given in a specific order for best results, so try to stay with them.
- Weigh yourself and measure your girths before you start. Weeks 6 and 12 will be the best times to gauge results.

Golden Rules of Training for Increased Muscle Size

- Complete three to five strength sessions a week.
- Train each muscle group only once or twice each week.
- Ensure that you do *rest* on your rest days to allow time for recovery and muscle growth, and have one week off every six weeks.
- Make each session last for only 60–75 minutes.
- Eat smart, and enough of the right foods (see 'Food for an Active Lifestyle' on page 91).
- Don't compromise technique for more reps. This leads to injury.

Programs for Increased Muscle Size

The following programs provide options for three different levels of training: beginner, intermediate and advanced:

A beginner is someone who has trained for up to six months on general fitness and conditioning, and now wants to change their muscle size. If you are a beginner, you should train hard but you shouldn't work to 'failure' (when you can't do another rep due to complete fatigue) until after you have been training for 12 months.

An intermediate trainer is someone who may have been training for 12 months and doing a general program for weight gain. You should approach 'failure' with most sets with the help of a spotter.

An advanced trainer is someone who has trained for more than 12 months and is more committed to gaining muscle mass. You can train at all intensities, but will need much more variety in your training to get continued results.

The following programs span a six-week period. Aim to be training your hardest in weeks 4–5. Build up to these. Rest at least two days a week for recovery and muscle growth, and have one week off every six weeks to let your whole body rest. Technique is always more important than the amount of weight you lift in weeks 1–3. In the other weeks you can concentrate more on weight, knowing your technique has improved. You should repeat this section again to make up a 12-week program. Essentially, the programs outlined adhere to the following structure:

Weeks 1–3: General strength-type exercises aimed at increasing the weight lifted in each set of each exercise of each week. More reps and shorter rests are standard.

Weeks 4–5: Maximal strength week with fewer reps, more rest periods between sets, and a greater weight improvement on each exercise.

Week 6: Unloading (or recovery) week. No gym at all this week, but you can walk or swim at a very low intensity. Rest is the main option, aerobic activity is okay. The less you do the better. Don't worry about losing condition or size, your muscles need time to repair. Rest is necessary if they are to grow.

Beginner level

Program: Weeks 1–5 (Week 6 is a rest week).
Four gym sessions per week.
Follow this training program over a 12-week period, referring to the preferred training sequence below.
Day 1 = Program 1
Day 2 = Program 2
Day 3 = Rest
Day 4 = Program 1
Day 5 = Program 2
Day 6 and 7 = Rest

Program 1

Note: The first number refers to the number of sets you should do per session, while the second number refers to the number of reps you should include in each set. For example: 3 x 12 means you need to do three sets of the exercise in question, lifting your load 12 times in each set. Your rest period refers to how many seconds you should rest between each set.

Training for Increased Muscle Size

Program 1 — Beginner Level

Exercise	Weeks 1–3	Rest (in seconds)	Weeks 4–5	Rest (in seconds)
Bench press	3 x 12	60	3 x 10	60
Pec deck	3 x 15	60	3 x 12	60
Push-ups	2 x 8–12	60	2 x 12–20	60
Dumbbell shoulder press	3 x 12	60	3 x 10	60
Upright rows	3 x 15	60	3 x 12	60
Lat raises	2 x 10	60	2 x 8	60
Tricep extensions	2 x 12	60	2 x 10	60
Bench dips	2 x 12	60	2 x 15	60

Abdominals (Refer to the five abdominal exercises on pages 212–213 and choose exercises suited to your ability.)

Program 2 — Beginner Level

Exercise	Weeks 1–3	Rest (in seconds)	Weeks 4–5	Rest (in seconds)
Incline leg press	3 x 12	60	3 x 10	60
Squats	3 x 10	60	3 x 8	60
Leg curls	2 x 15	60	2 x 12	60
Lat pull-downs	3 x 12	60	3 x 10	60
Single arm rows	3 x 10	60	3 x 8	60
Prone raises	2 x 15	60	2 x 12	60
Dumbbell curls	2 x 12	60	2 x 10	60
Calf raises	2 x 15	60	2 x 12	60

Abdominals (Refer to the five abdominal exercises on pages 212–213 and choose exercises suited to your ability.)

Training for Increased Muscle Size

Intermediate level

Program: Weeks 1–5 (Week 6 is a rest week).
Four gym sessions per week.
Follow this training program over a six-week period, referring to this preferred training sequence. You can start the program on any day, whatever suits your schedule.

Day 1 = Program 1
Day 2 = Program 2
Day 3 = Rest
Day 4 = Program 3
Day 5 = Rest
Day 6 = Rest
Day 7 = Rest

Day 8 = Program 2
Day 9 = Rest
Day 10 = Program 3
Day 11 = Rest
Day 12 = Program 1
Day 13 = Program 2
Day 14 = Rest

Program 1 — Intermediate Level

Exercise	Weeks 1–3	Rest (in seconds)	Weeks 4–5	Rest (in seconds)
Dumbbell press	4 x 12	60	4 x 8	90
Dips	3 x max.	60	3 x max.	90
Push-ups	2 x max.	60	2 x max.	90
Upright rows	4 x 12	60	4 x 8	90
Forward raises	3 x 12	60	3 x 8	90
Lat raises	2 x 10	60	2 x 8	90
Overhead tricep extensions	3 x 12	60	3 x 10	90
Lying tricep extensions	2 x 15	60	2 x 10	90

Abdominals (Refer to the five abdominal exercises on pages 212–213 and choose exercises suited to your ability.)

Program 2 — Intermediate Level

Exercise	Weeks 1–3	Rest (in seconds)	Weeks 4–5	Rest (in seconds)
Squats	4 x 12	60	4 x 8	90
Leg extensions	3 x 10	60	4 x 8	90
Leg curls	2 x 15	60	4 x 12	90
Lat pull-downs	4 x 12	60	6 x 8	90
Seated rows	3 x 10	60	3 x 8	90
Bent-over raises	3 x 15	60	3 x 12	90
Bicep curls	3 x 12	60	3 x 10	90
Calf raises	2 x 15	60	2 x 12	60

Abdominals (Refer to the five abdominal exercises on pages 212–213 and choose exercises suited to your ability.)

Program 3 — Intermediate Level

Exercise	Weeks 1–3	Rest (in seconds)	Weeks 4–5	Rest (in seconds)
Incline dumbbell press	6 x 8	90	6 x 6	120
Lunges	6 x 6 on each leg	90	6 x 4 on each leg	120
Chin-ups	6 x 8	90	6 x 6	120

Abdominals (Refer to the five abdominal exercises on pages 212–213 and choose exercises suited to your ability.)

Do one lot of each set of reps, increasing the weight each time.

Advanced level

Program: Weeks 1–5, Week 6 Rest.
Four gym sessions per week.
Follow this program for the first six weeks, referring to the training sequence outlined.

Day 1 = Program 1
Day 2 = Program 2
Day 3 = Rest
Day 4 = Program 3
Day 5 = Rest
Day 6 = Program 1
Day 7 = Rest
Day 8 = Program 2
Day 9 = Rest
Day 10 = Program 3
Day 11 = Rest
Day 12 = Program 1
Day 13 = Program 2
Day 14 = Rest

Program 1 — Advanced Level

Exercise	Weeks 1–3	Rest (in seconds)	Weeks 4–5	Rest (in seconds)
Leg extensions	2 x 12	60	3 x 8	90
Leg curls	2 x 12	60	3 x 8	90
Deadlifts	12/10/8	120	10/8/6	120
Squats	12/6/10/6/8	120	10/4/8/4/6	120
Calf raises	3 x 12	60	3 x 15	90
Back extensions	3 x 15	60	3 x 8	90

Abdominals (Refer to the five abdominal exercises on pages 212–213 and choose exercises suited to your ability.)

The lower the reps, the heavier the weight. Always maintain good control and technique.

Training for Increased Muscle Size

Program 2 — Advanced Level

Exercise	Weeks 1–3	Rest (in seconds)	Weeks 4–5	Rest (in seconds)
Chin-ups	3 x max.	120	3 x max.	120
Lat pull-downs	12/10/8	90	10/8/6	90
Seated rows	12/10/8	60	3 x 8	90
Single arm rows	3 x 12	120	8/6/6	120
Prone raises	2 x 15	60	2 x 20	90
Preacher curls	12/10/8	60	10/8/6	90
Bicep curls	3 x 12	60	3 x 10	90

Abdominals (Refer to the five abdominal exercises on pages 212–213 and choose exercises suited to your ability.)

The lower the reps, the heavier the weight. Always maintain good control and technique.

Program 3 — Advanced Level

Exercise	Weeks 1–3	Rest (in seconds)	Weeks 4–5	Rest (in seconds)
Incline bench press	12/10/8	90	10/8/6	90
Wide grip dips	3 x max.	120	3 x max.	120
Dumbbell press	3 x 12	60	3 x 8	90
Dumbbell pullovers	10/8/8	120	8/6/6	120
Dumbbell flyes	2 x 15	60	2 x 20	90
Close grip dips	12/10/8	60	10/8/6	90
Lying tricep pullovers	3 x 12	60	3 x 10	90

Abdominals (Refer to the five abdominal exercises on pages 212–213 and choose exercises suited to your ability.)

The lower the reps, the heavier the weight. Always maintain good control and technique.

Training for Increased Muscle Size

After you have finished the first six weeks of the advanced level program, follow this program for the remaining six weeks of your schedule, referring to the training sequence outlined.

Program: Weeks 7–11, Week 12 Rest. Three gym sessions per week.

Weeks 7, 9 and 11
Day 1 = Program 1
Day 2 = Rest
Day 3 = Program 2
Day 4 = Rest
Day 5 = Program 1
Day 6 = Rest
Day 7 = Rest

Weeks 8 and 10
Day 1 = Program 2
Day 2 = Rest
Day 3 = Program 1
Day 4 = Rest
Day 5 = Program 2
Day 6 = Rest
Day 7 = Rest

Program 1

Exercise	Weeks 7–9	Rest (in seconds)	Weeks 10–11	Rest (in seconds)
Squats	6 x 8	120	6 x 6	120
Lunges	4 x 12 each leg	60	4 x 8 on each leg	60
Lat pull-downs	6 x 8	120	6 x 6	120
Bent-over rows	4 x 8	60	4 x 6	60
Calf raises	4 x 15	60	4 x 12	60
Dumbbell curls	4 x 8	60	4 x 6	60

Abdominals (Refer to the five abdominal exercises on pages 212–213 and choose exercises suited to your ability.)

Program 2

Exercise	Weeks 1–3	Rest (in seconds)	Weeks 4–5	Rest (in seconds)
Bench press	6 x 8	120	6 x 6	120
Dumbbell press	4 x 6	120	4 x 4	120
Upright rows	6 x 8	120	6 x 6	120
Lat raises	4 x 8	60	4 x 6	60
Dips	4 x max.	120	4 x max.	120

Abdominals (Refer to the five abdominal exercises on pages 212–213 and choose exercises suited to your ability.)

Training for Muscle Definition

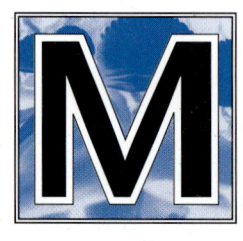

Muscle definition is the correct term for what some people call 'tone'. If you have good muscle definition, it means you can see the shape of your muscles, and you have low body-fat levels. Tone actually refers to the degree of tension in your muscles when they are at rest. The stronger a muscle the better the tone and, if you have a low level of body fat, the more obvious a muscle will be.

Training for muscle definition is the most common training goal that people choose. It involves a combination of training for lower body fat, strength and fitness.

When training for muscle definition, your first goal should always be fat loss. You need to get your body fat down to a level you're happy with and be able to maintain this level, to do this you need to eat well. Your next goal should be to improve your fitness.

You'll need to include two to three aerobic activity sessions, as well as two resistance training sessions, per week. To achieve *great* definition, you'll need to train just that little bit harder. Each aerobic session should be different, with some being longer and lower in intensity and others being shorter but harder in intensity. Aerobic training activities at higher intensities, such as running, sprinting, sports-based activities and triathlon training, are good activities to try.

Resistance-training sessions should be varied. The first phase of training should be aimed at general strength and establishing good technique. The next phase should be more muscle endurance-

Training for Muscle Definition

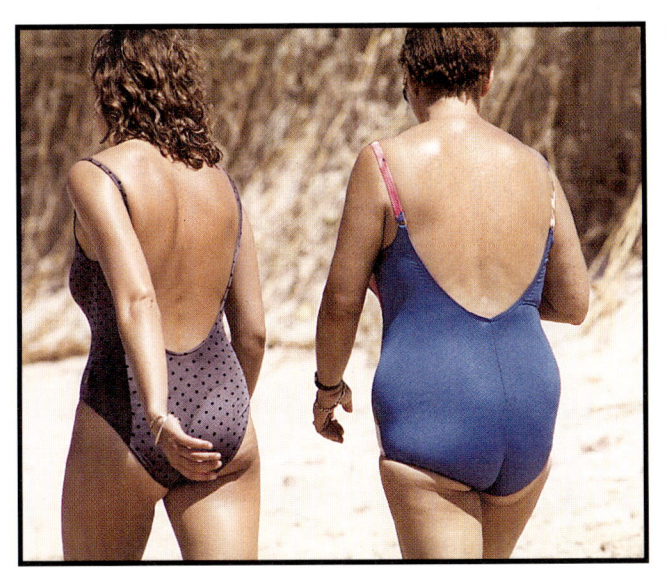

Reducing body fat is the key to increasing muscle definition.

have access to weight-training equipment or to buy some basic equipment (such as dumbbells or a skipping rope).

You should rest for one week every five weeks, with the rest week having no gym work but low-intensity aerobic sessions of 30–45 minutes. Cross-training will certainly be the most enjoyable and effective for definition. (See 'Cross-training' on page 155.)

Once you have achieved a low body-fat level and a good level of fitness, then you can start working on those areas that need special attention. (See 'Training for Shape', on page 207 of this Training Manual.)

based, with the aim of doing higher reps and working at medium-to-high intensities. The aim of the resistance training is to increase the demand on your fat reserves through having higher levels of muscle mass. Initially, this can be done with very little equipment, but you may need to join a gym to

Aerobic Activity Programs for Muscle Definition

The following programs assumes that you have at least a minimum level of fitness. Refer to 'Training for Fat Loss', on page 168 of this Training Manual, for suggested aerobic activities to include in your program. These activities can be mixed within the session if you wish.

Golden Rules of Training for Muscle Definition

- Complete a combination of two to three aerobic activity sessions and two resistance training sessions a week.
- Each aerobic session should be different, with some being longer and lower in intensity and others being shorter but harder in intensity.
- Each gym session should be based around a strength program with the aim to increase the strength and shape of muscles rather than the endurance ability of the muscle.
- Rest one week every five weeks with the rest week having no gym but easy aerobic sessions of 30 minutes at lower intensities.
- Follow a low-fat, high-energy eating plan (see 'Food for an Active Lifestyle' on page 91).

Get UP&GO!

Training for Muscle Definition

Aerobic Activity Programs for Muscle Definition

Fitness level	Weeks 1–4	Weeks 5	Week 6-9	Week 10
Minimum	2 x 50–60-minute sessions at 70 per cent 1 x (3 x 10 minutes at 80 per cent)	2 x 60-minute sessions at 60 per cent	2 x (3 x 15 minutes at 90 per cent) 2 x (45 minutes at 80 per cent)	2 x 60 minute sessions at 60 per cent
Good	2 x 60-minute sessions at 70 per cent 1 session of (5 minutes at 90 per cent and 5 minutes at 70 per cent) x 4	2 x 60-minute sessions at 70 per cent	2 x (4 x 10 minutes at 90 per cent) 2 x 45-minute sessions at 80 per cent	2 x 60-minute sessions at 70 per cent
Excellent	2 x 60-minute session at 80 per cent 1 x 60-minute session, alternate between 7 minutes at 90 per cent and 3 minutes at 60 per cent	2 x 60-minute sessions at 80 per cent	2 x 45-minute sessions at 80 per cent 2 x 60-minute sessions at your maximum effort	2 x 70-minute sessions at 80 per cent

Guidelines for Resistance Training for Muscle Definition

■ This program is done in two lots of five week blocks. Note that the reps, sets and rest periods change from weeks one to four and weeks six to nine.

■ Make sure you change your exercises after the ten week period is completed, if you want to use the same system again. Your body gets used to the same exercises and can become lazy if you don't challenge it.

■ Make your resistance training sessions short, only 20–30 minutes in the first five weeks and 30–40 minutes in the second five weeks. It's best to do your resistance training after the aerobic activity in the first five-week period, and before the aerobic activity in the second five-week period.

■ At the end of each five week period, spend one week in recovery. Do no resistance training in these weeks and drop off the higher-intensity aerobic training, doing only low-intensity training like that used for fat loss.

■ Also refer to the general resistance training guidelines as outlined on page 148.

Training for Muscle Definition

Programs (for home without any equipment)

Beginner (2 times per week)

Exercise	Weeks 1–4	Rest (in seconds)	Weeks 6–9	Rest (in seconds)
Squats	3 x 8–12	45	3 x 12–20	30
Step-ups	2 x 6–10	45	2 x 10–15	30
Push-ups	2 x max.	45	2 x max.	30
Bench dips	4 x 6–10	45	2 x 10–15	30
Bent-over raises	2 x 8–12	45	2 x 12–20	30

Abdominals (Refer to the five abdominal exercises on pages 212–213 and choose exercises suited to your ability.)

Intermediate (2 times per week)

Exercise	Weeks 1–4	Rest (in seconds)	Weeks 6–9	Rest (in seconds)
Lunges	3 x 8–10 on each leg	45	3 x 12–15 on each leg	30
Squats	3 x 10–15	45	3 x 15–20	30
Push-ups	3 x max.	45	3 x max.	30
Bench dips	2 x 12–15	45	2 x 15–20	30
Modified pull-ups	3 x 4–8	45	3 x 8–12	30
Bent-over raises	2 x 12–15	45	2 x 15–20	30

Abdominals (Refer to the five abdominal exercises on pages 212–213 and choose exercises suited to your ability.)

Advanced (2–3 times per week)

Exercise	Weeks 1–4	Rest (in seconds)	Weeks 6–9	Rest (in seconds)
Squats	3 x 15	45	3 x 20	30
Lunges	3 x 12 on each leg	45	3 x 15 on each leg	30
Step-ups	3 x 12 on each leg	45	3 x 15 on each leg	30
Push-ups	3 x max.	45	3 x max.	30
Bench dips	2 x max.	45	2 x max.	30
Modified pull-ups	3 x max.	45	3 x max.	30
Bent-over raises	2 x 15	45	2 x 20	30

Abdominals (Refer to the five abdominal exercises on pages 212–213 and choose exercises suited to your ability.)

Training for Muscle Definition

Programs (with equipment)

Beginner (2 times per week)

Exercise	Weeks 1–4	Rest (in seconds)	Weeks 6–9	Rest (in seconds)
Squats	3 x 8–12	45	3 x 12–20	30
Leg curls	2 x 6–10 on each leg	45	2 x 10–15 on each leg	30
Bench press	2 x 8–12	45	2 x 15–20	30
Bench dips	2 x 6–10	45	2 x 10–15	30
Lat pull-downs	2 x 8–12	45	2 x 12–20	30

Abdominals (Refer to the five abdominal exercises on pages 212–213 and choose exercises suited to your ability.)

Intermediate (2 times per week)

Exercise	Weeks 1–4	Rest (in seconds)	Weeks 6–9	Rest (in seconds)
Lunges	3 x 8–10 on each leg	45	3 x 12–20 on each leg	30
Squats	3 x 10–15	45	2 x 15–20	30
Bench press	3 x 8–12	45	3 x 12–20	30
Bench dips	2 x 12–15	45	2 x 15–20	30
Lat pull-downs	3 x 6–12	45	3 x 12–15	30
Bent-over raises	2 x 12–15	45	2 x 15–20	30

Abdominals (Refer to the five abdominal exercises on pages 212–213 and choose exercises suited to your ability.)

Advanced (2–3 times per week)

Exercise	Weeks 1–4	Rest (in seconds)	Weeks 6–9	Rest (in seconds)
Squats	3 x 15	45	3 x 20	30
Lunges	3 x 12 on each leg	45	3 x 15 on each leg	30
Step-ups	3 x 12 on each leg	45	3 x 15 on each leg	30
Bench press	3 x 6–10	45	3 x 10–15	30
Bench dips	2 x max.	45	2 x max.	30
Lat pull-downs	3 x 6–10	45	3 x 10–15	30
Bent-over raises	2 x 15	45	2 x 20	30

Abdominals (Refer to the five abdominal exercises on pages 212–213 and choose exercises suited to your ability.)

Training for Shape

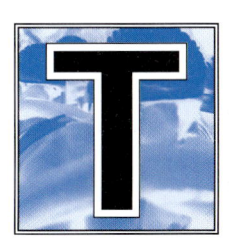

This is a goal you might like to pursue after you have achieved great fitness, low body fat and, possibly, enhanced muscle definition. As you trained towards these goals, you will have noticed a change in your shape. And now, as you look at yourself in the mirror, you might feel that there are some areas where you would like to see other small differences — wider-looking shoulders, a smaller waist, thinner thighs, bigger arms, etc.

Training for shape is a very individual thing — you have to look at what you have to work with and what you want to change. If your goals now include building muscle in a few areas, you'll need to look at changing your diet to include more energy foods to help you with this. If you have been on a fat-loss diet, this won't build you up, but more muscle definition will be gained. Your eating plans will need to change to suit different goals.

Start in the area of most need. If you need to lose fat, then you should train for this goal first. If you need to improve fitness, then start there. Prepare your body to do the work. Assess your needs for shape reduction or shape increase, and start there. Always start on your priority first and work towards one main goal at a time. Training for too many different goals at the same time reduces your chance of achieving them.

Once you've achieved suitable fat levels, you can work towards shape modification. This might mean you need to reduce your fat levels further if you want great thighs, or it may mean a change in training — for example, a combination of weight training and aerobic activity for muscle definition. At this time you'll generally need to include at least two strength sessions a week, aimed at either making certain muscles bigger or giving them better tone, as well as aerobic sessions aimed at maintaining fitness and further reducing body fat.

Training for Shape

> ## Golden Rules of Training for Shape
>
> - Start in the area of most need.
> - Once you've achieved suitable fat levels, work towards modification of your shape.
> - Alternate your weight and aerobic training in cycles.
> - Remember to include unloading weeks in your training program.
> - Be prepared to take enough time to get to the shape that best suits your body. Plan a program that will get you there over a period of at least 12 months, as quick-fix programs don't give lasting results.
> - Follow a low-fat, high-energy eating plan (see 'Food for an Active Lifestyle' on page 91).

Because weight training and aerobic training don't give the best results when done together, you'll need to alternate the different types of training you choose. For example:

For fat loss — include three weeks of an activity you need to do most, such as aerobic training, with one session a week of strength training. After the three-week block, you might do only two sessions of low-intensity aerobic activity and three sessions of weights for two weeks before having an unloading week.

For muscle size — train for four to five weeks, including two to three sessions of weights and one or two 30-minute sessions of low-intensity aerobic activity each week. After this, you should go into a one-week recovery plan of very easy activity of a different kind, such as swimming, and then start again.

Be prepared to take a long time to get to the shape that best suits your body. Plan a program that will get you there over a period of at least 12 months. Each time you set a new program and achieve your small goals, it means your program must become more specific to the areas on which you still wish to work. But it must still include training to maintain all those results you worked so hard to achieve early in your training.

Specific Shaping Goals

The following information provides you with a starting point to achieve specific shaping goals. All the suggested exercises have been illustrated in the Appendix.

Wider-looking shoulders

To achieve the look of having wider shoulders you need to make your shoulders slightly bigger and your waist and hips smaller. Everything is gauged on the rest of the body and what you compare it to. If you have small hips and a small bottom, then your shoulders will automatically look bigger.

Shoulders are made up of many muscle groups and you need to train all of these to achieve the wider look. Training should focus on improving the size of your chest, back and arms in general, but mostly on the muscles known as Deltoids which give shape to the top of your shoulders and width to your shape.

Be careful in exercising the muscles high on your shoulders near your neck (Trapezius) too much, as this can give you a rounded shape and cause imbalances in your back.

You should include some of the following exercises in your training program: upright rows, dumbbell shoulder presses, forward raises, lat raises and bent-over raises.

V-shaped back

A V-shaped back is made more pronounced by having broad shoulders and a narrow waist. Training for these changes in your body will further exaggerate the shape of your back. The 'V' shape is due to the shape of your 'Lat' muscle (Latissimus Dorsi), which flares out from under your shoulder and trims down into your lower back.

Some people have a greater potential to achieve this look than others, due to the shape of their ribs and the length of their back. Shorter people tend to be able to achieve this look more easily, as there is less room to spread the muscle over and it grows thicker with less training.

You should include some of the following exercises in your training program: lat pull-downs (with a wide grip), chin-ups, seated rows (with a wide grip), and single arm rows (with your elbow out to the side).

Note: The wider grip places more emphasis on the lats doing the work instead of your biceps. However, you should still train with your normal grip as well, as this will eventually make you stronger and enable you to lift more.

Great-looking legs

If the amount of body fat in your legs is low, you'll have great legs. Thin legs don't mean low body fat — you can have thin legs but high body fat, with very little lean muscle mass to give them shape. You need to reduce your body fat first and then aim to increase the muscles in your legs through training. Any form of high-intensity aerobic training will change the shape of your legs. Running and high-intensity walking

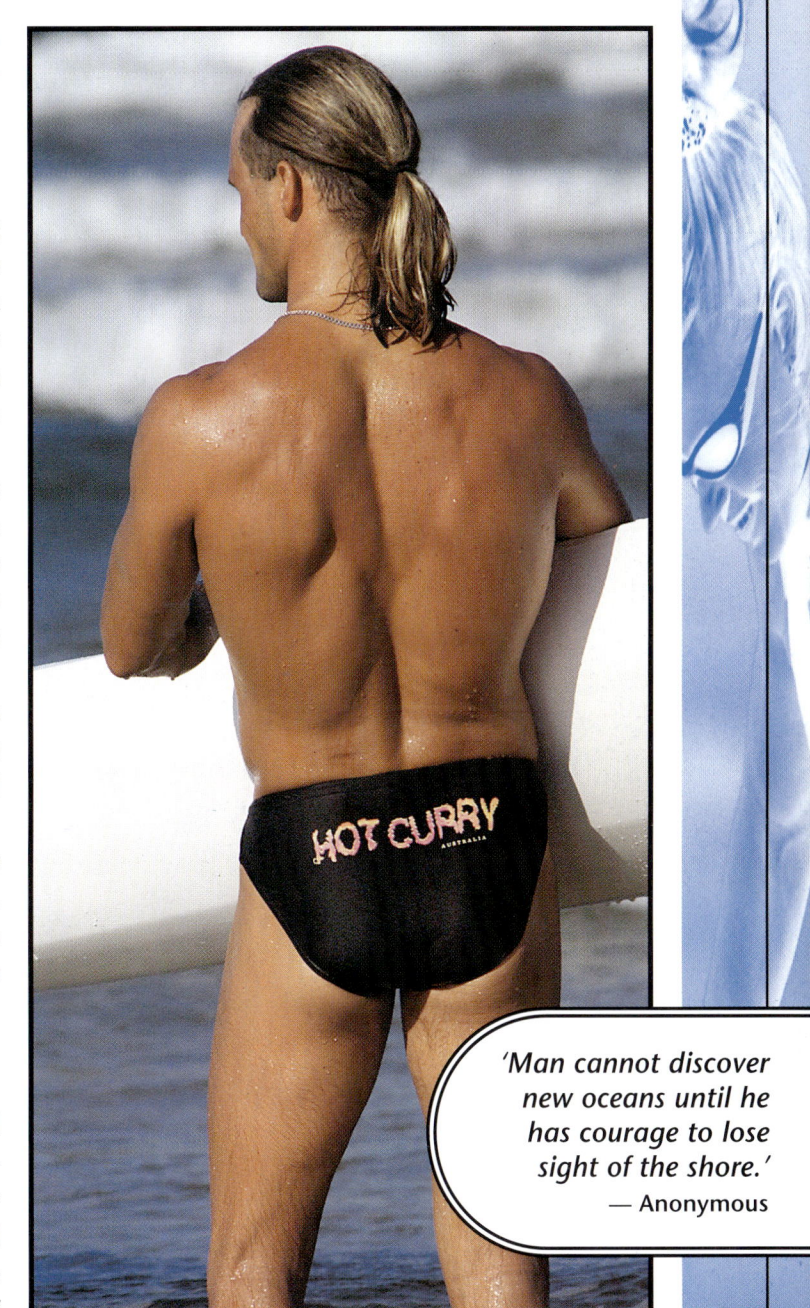

The classic V-shaped back. Some sports, like surf lifesaving, promote specific shape development.

> 'Man cannot discover new oceans until he has courage to lose sight of the shore.'
> — Anonymous

Training for Shape

(up hills or stairs, for example) gives the best results, so get into those exercises for a start.

Once you have reduced your body fat you can begin to train to increase muscle mass in your legs — some form of resistance training will work best. You should include some of the following exercises in your training program when training your legs, or after your aerobic activity: squats, lunges, split squats, step-ups and bent-leg deadlifts.

Note: Exercises such as leg extensions and leg curls are isolated exercises that don't train the whole leg. Use big muscle group exercises that make every muscle in your legs active.

Great-looking arms

Great-looking arms come from having enough muscle to give them some shape. Your shoulders also affect the appearance of your arms, so having shape in your shoulders will help your arms look better, too.

Arm exercises should always be done after all major exercises, and you'll get as much benefit for your arms as for all muscle groups by training for a good back, chest and shoulders.

Try to include exercises with a lot of the arm muscles involved, such as standing bicep curls, standing dumbbell curls, seated incline dumbbell curls, tricep extensions and overhead tricep extensions.

Other exercises done in a slightly modified way will place more emphasis on your arms, for example:

Biceps — Close-grip lat pull-downs and seated rows.

Triceps — Close-grip bench presses and push-ups, as well as close-grip dips.

Continue to train your whole body, with a little more emphasis on these areas, but don't overdo it.

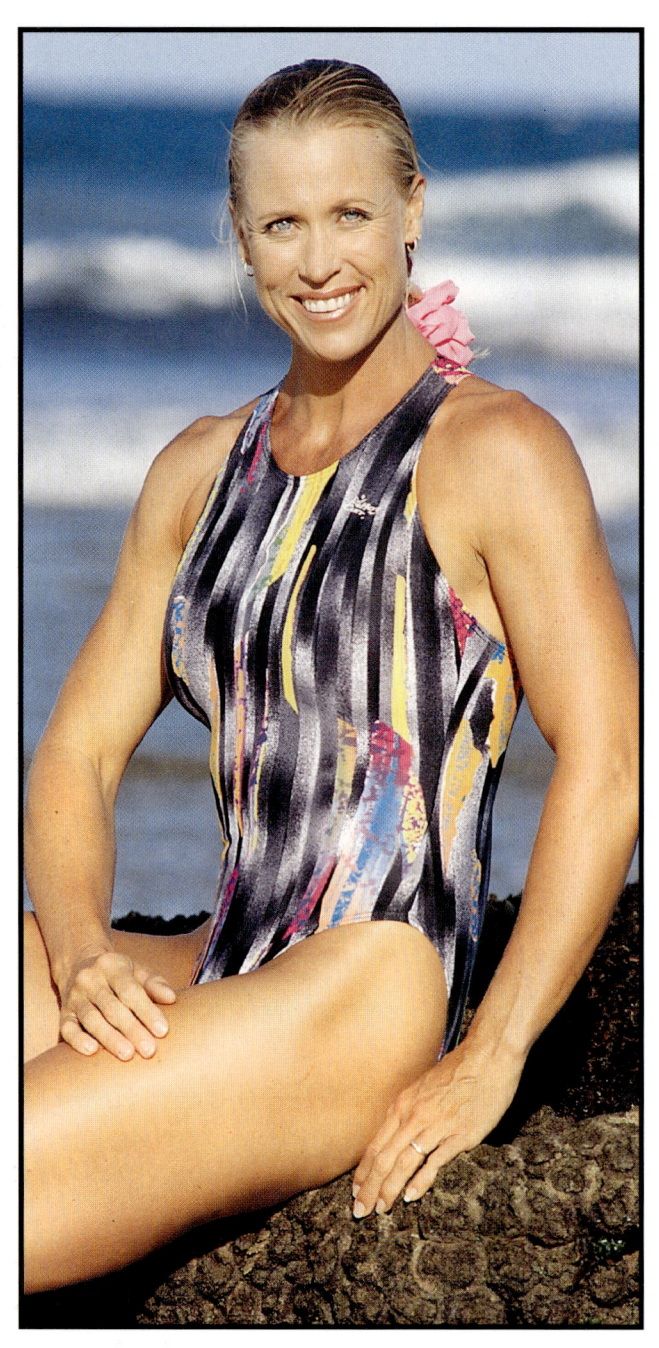

Training for shape should be incorporated into your training programs for sport.

Great-looking abdominals

Great abdominals are the envy of all. Again, the secret is to have low body fat. It's easy to have great abs, but if you can't see them for the body fat, then who will know? Always do your abdominal exercises last. They act as your trunk stabilisers and you need them to hold you steady when you squat or do any other trunk-supported exercises.

On pages 212–213 are the five best abdominal exercises to get you started. Do them in the order set down. If you can't do one, go back to the previous one and work on that until you can move on to the next.

It's commonly thought that you should never do full sit-ups, especially with your feet locked or held down. I've gained tremendous benefit from full sit-ups, and so have a lot of other people I train with, but only after we've been able to perfect the initial exercises described above. Once you have achieved good abdominal strength and stability, the full sit-ups are much easier and of greater benefit.

Tight, toned bottom

Imagine having a bottom that sat out nicely without hanging down or having any floppy bits. Sure, there are a few specific exercises you can do to improve your bottom muscles, but if you use them well in all other exercises you won't need specific exercises for them.

I had to learn how to use my bottom muscles properly because I used to be very dependent on my big thigh muscles and it took some time to make adjustments to this. After I learned how to make use of such big muscles, my strength in all leg exercises doubled and my kicking in the pool changed significantly.

Whenever you do leg exercises that include the bottom — such as squats, lunges, leg presses, step-ups — you have to squeeze your bottom consciously to make it work. It may have forgotten how, so you may need to spend some time practising this before results will start to show. Exercises such as leg lifts or side leg raises are great to learn postural control, but they are a waste of time for improving your bottom shape.

On pages 214–215 are some of the best bottom exercises to get you started.

It should feel a bit like an elevator ride, as your bottom muscles will lift you up without you having to rely purely on your big quad muscles. Once they are tired and you can't get them to squeeze any more, stop and try again in the next session.

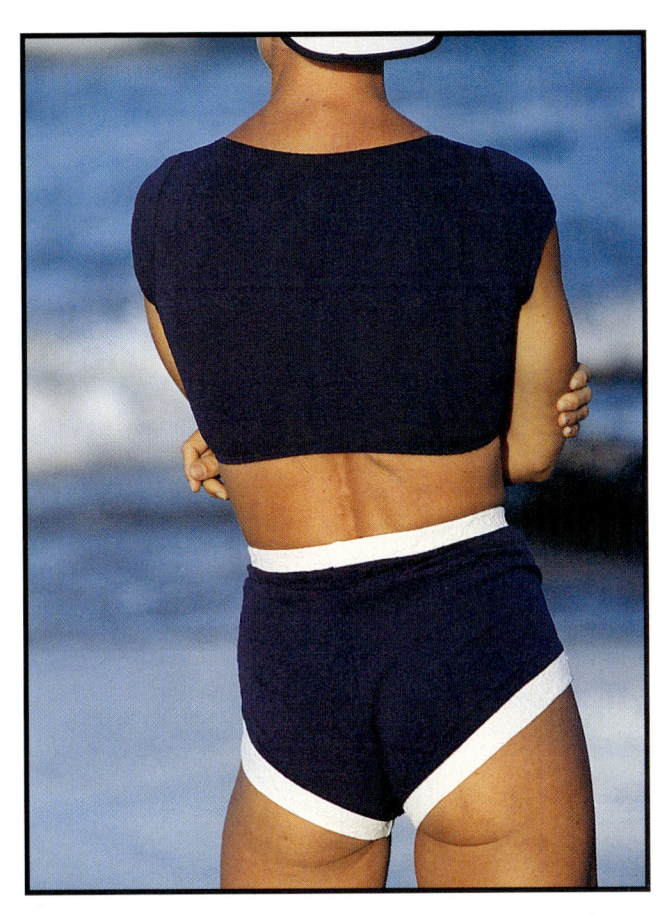

Great shape takes a lot of work and time. The results are well worth the effort.

Training for Shape

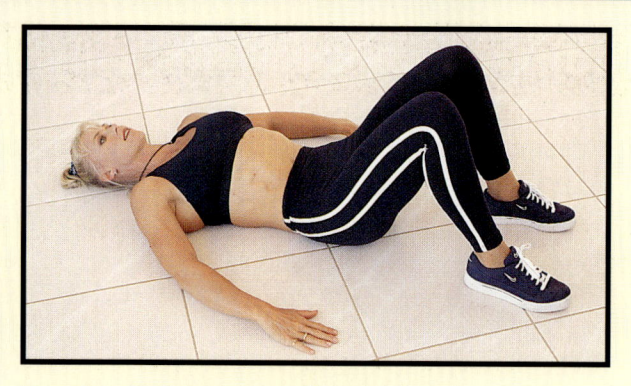

Exercise 1: Contract and hold (above)
This abdominal exercise is the first step in all weight-training exercises. Holding your lower abdominals contracted, breathe out and suck your tummy down and hold for three to five seconds and then try to breathe in without losing the tightness you feel in your lower abdominal area. You should be able to feel your upper abdominal area and it should be relaxed. You should not be trying to squeeze anything tight. Simply sucking down will bring tension into your lower abdominal region either side of centre. Once you have the hang of this exercise you can practise all the time so that you become conscious of holding your lower abdominals in.
- Beginner: 4 x 5 sec hold
- Intermediate: 3 x 30 sec hold
- Advanced: 3 x 1 min hold

Exercise 2: Bent-leg fallout (below)
From this position try to keep your contraction as in Exercise 1, and roll one leg out to the side. Stop when you feel like you have lost your contraction or you feel your hips move. Go back to the top and start again.
- Beginner: 2 x 8 each side
- Intermediate: 2 x 15 each side
- Advanced: 2 x 20 each side

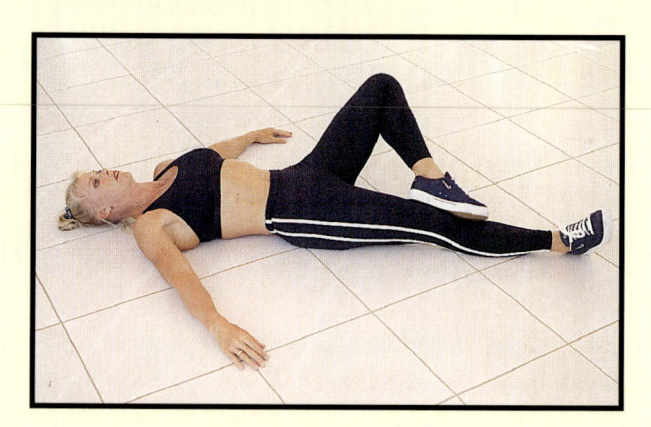

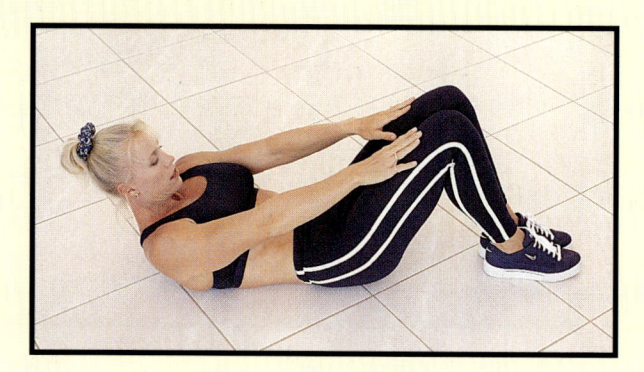

Exercise 3: Crunch and hold (left)
Contract your lower abs as in Exercise 1, and roll into a crunch and hold for five seconds. The aim here is to make sure that you maintain the lower abdominal feeling, then bring in the crunch position and hold there. You should not get too high with your crunch.
- Beginner: 2 x 10
- Intermediate: 3 x 12
- Advanced: 3 x 15

Training for Shape

Five of the Best Abdominal Exercises

Note: these abdominal exercises are slow, precise and controlled. A conscientious decision to regularly complete these simple exercises will help maintain a flat and strong stomach.

Exercise 4: Roll down (below)

From a seated position, suck in and hold your lower abs and roll down to the floor keeping your back in a curved position. Aim to touch your lower back to the floor before you touch your shoulder blades to the floor. Start with your arms outstretched and, as you get better, bring your arms into your chest and then behind your head. Your feet should stay on the floor at all times. If you fall backwards, try to move your heels away from your bottom until you can go all the way down slowly and with full control.

- Beginner: 2 x 6 heels away from bottom
- Intermediate: 2 x 12 heels closer to bottom
- Advanced: 2 x 15 heels almost touching bottom

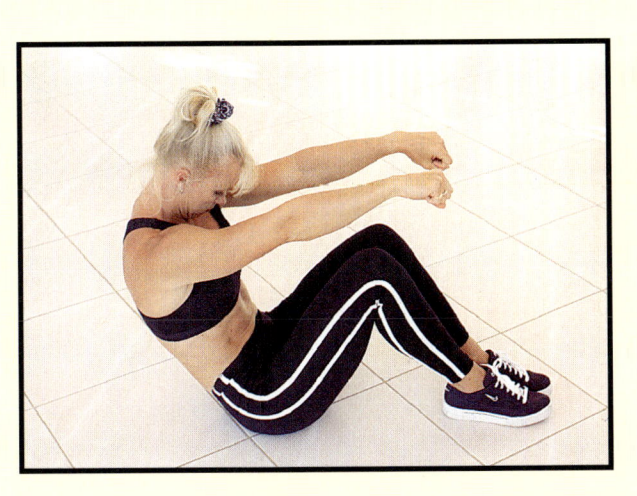

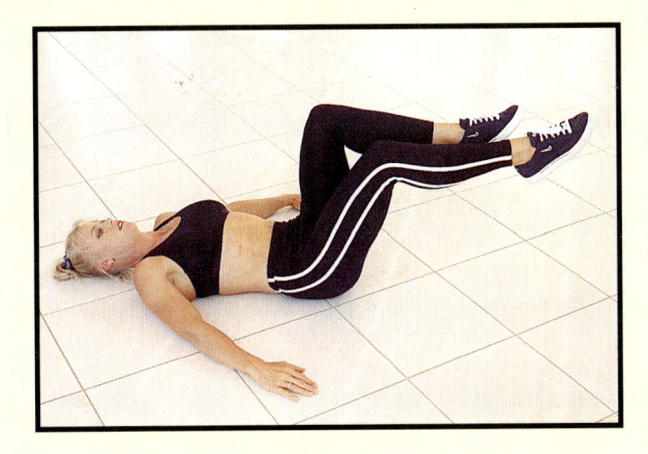

Exercise 5: Alternate leg lifts (above)

Maintain the abdominal feeling as in Exercise 1, and slowly lower one leg to the floor without losing the abdominal contraction and without your hips rolling slightly to one side, then lower the second leg to the floor. As you improve, progress to holding the first leg in the air and moving the second leg down and back up to meet it, without losing control and keeping the abs tight.

- Beginner: 2 x 6 each leg, start with both feet on the floor
- Intermediate: 2 x 12 each leg, start with both feet in the air
- Advanced: 3 x 12 each leg, start with both feet in the air

Training for Shape

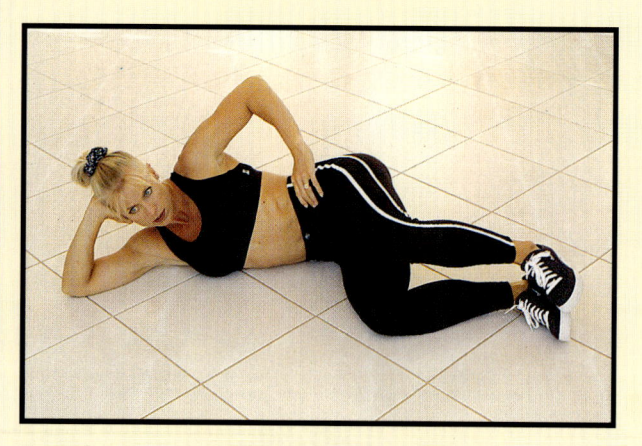

Exercise 1: External hip rotation
With your knees bent, heels together and abs held tight, slowly try to lift the top leg keeping your heels together, hips still and abs tight, so the bent knee is raised off the leg on the floor. Stop lifting the knee when you feel a change in any of these positions. The height isn't important, but the control is. Slowly lower your leg to your starting position and repeat.
- Beginner: 2 x 6 each leg
- Intermediate: 2 x 20 each leg
- Advanced: 2 x 40 each leg

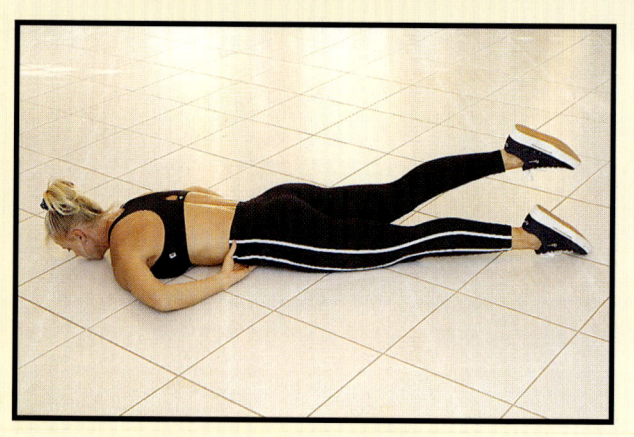

Exercise 2: Prone hip extension
Lie face down with your abs and glutes held tightly. Place your hands under your hip bones to give you an idea of how much your hips are moving. Slowly lift one leg. Having your hands under your hips will let you know when to stop as you'll feel your hips either pushing into your hands or lifting away from them. Your leg should only be lifted about 2–5 centimetres off the ground. Control is the most important part of this exercise. Slowly lower to the ground and repeat.
- Beginner: 2 x 6 each leg
- Intermediate: 2 x 12 each leg
- Advanced: 2 x 20 each leg

Five of the Best Bottom Exercises

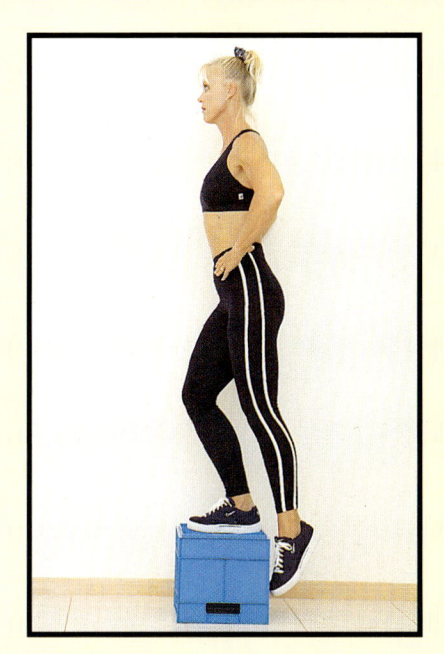

Exercise 3: Step-ups

Place your right foot on the box and move your weight onto this leg. Take your weight off your left leg and lean forwards over the box using your right leg only to lift you off the floor. Keep your hips steady and facing forwards. Slowly lower your leg and repeat.
- Beginner: 2 x 10 each leg
- Intermediate: 3 x 15 each leg
- Advanced: 3 x 20 each leg

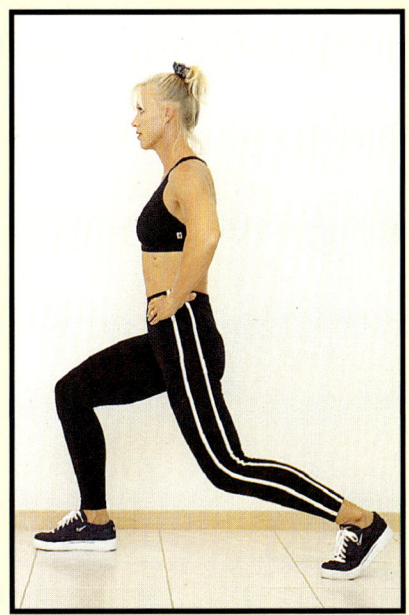

Exercise 4: Lunges

Step forward onto your right foot, upper body slightly leaning forward keeping the knee above the toes. Keep the weight on the right leg. Slowly lower your body weight until your left knee touches the floor (or as low as you can go). Keep your head up and body upright. Pause, squeeze your bottom, push with your foot and push your body weight back to the start position.
- Beginner: 2 x 6 each leg
- Intermediate: 2 x 12 each leg
- Advanced: 3 x 15 each leg

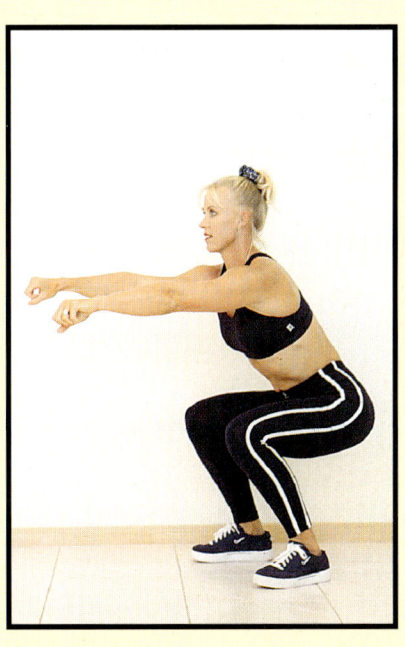

Exercise 5: Squats

Feet shoulder-width apart, arms extended, face forward. Poke your hips out backwards, bend your knees over your toes, and back flat, lean slightly forward. Lower your bottom towards the ground, pause, squeeze your bottom tight, and hold for 3–5 seconds. Use this squeeze to help lift you back to the top position.
- Beginner: 2 x 12
- Intermediate: 3 x 15
- Advanced: 3 x 20

Appendix

Index of Exercises

Alternate Arm Lift	218
Back Extensions	218
Bench Dips	219
Bent-leg Deadlift	219
Bent-over Raises	220
Bent-over Row	220
Bench Press	221
Bicep Curls	221
Seated Calf Raises	222
Chin-ups	222
Dips	223
Dumbbell Curls	223
Dumbbell Deadlift	224
Dumbbell Chest Press	224
Dumbbell Pull-over	225
Dumbbell Flyes	225
Dumbbell Shoulder Press	226
Forward Raise	226
Incline Bench Press	227
Incline Dumbbell Press	227
Incline Leg Press	228
Lateral Pull-down	228
Lateral Raises	229
Leg Curls	229
Leg Extensions	230
Lunge	230
Modified Pull-up	231
Pec Deck	231
Preacher Curl	232
Prone Raises	232
Push-ups	233
Modified Push-ups	233
Seated Dips	234
Seated Row	234
Shoulder Press	235
Single Arm Row	235
Split Squat	236
Squat	236
Step-ups	237
Tricep Press-down	237
Overhead Tricep Extension	238
Lying Tricep Extension	238
Wall Push-ups	239
Upright Row	239

Alternate Arm Lift

- Neck relaxed
- Shoulder blades held together and down
- Elbows level with shoulders
- Lift left arm off floor, then lower

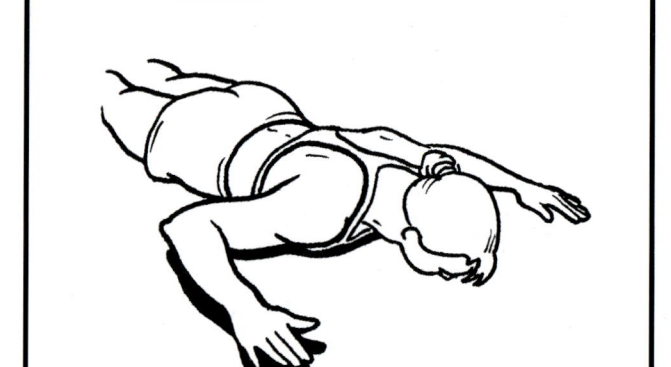

- Lift right arm off floor, then lower
- Keep shoulder blades held together
- Keep muscles in neck relaxed
- Keep abs tight

Back Extensions

- Arms crossed on chest
- Back rounded
- Abs tight

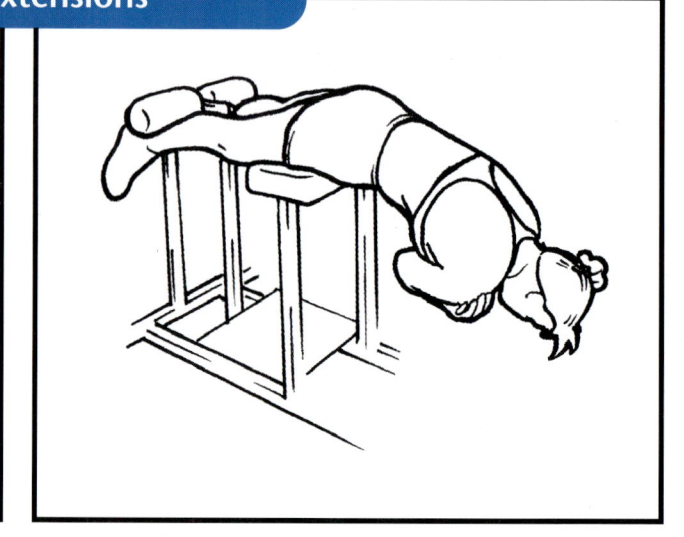

- Squeeze bottom and hamstrings
- Raise upper body
- Maintain rounded back

Appendix

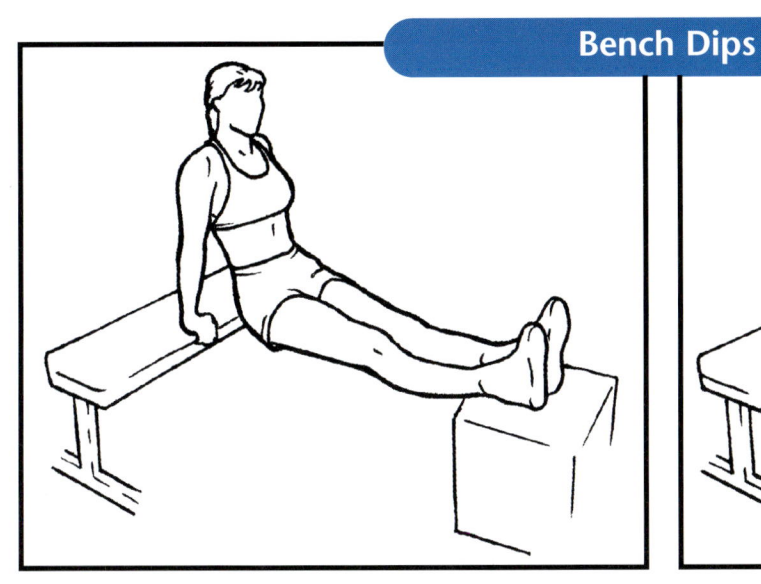

Bench Dips

- Feet straight
- Fingers over side of bench
- Upper body straight

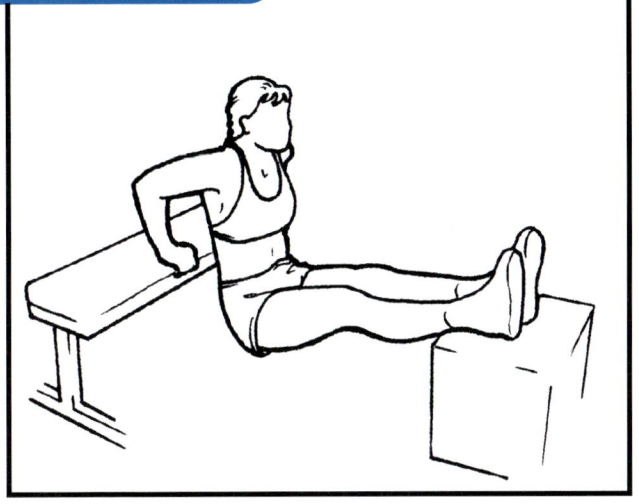

- Bend from elbows
- Shoulders and elbows even at bottom position

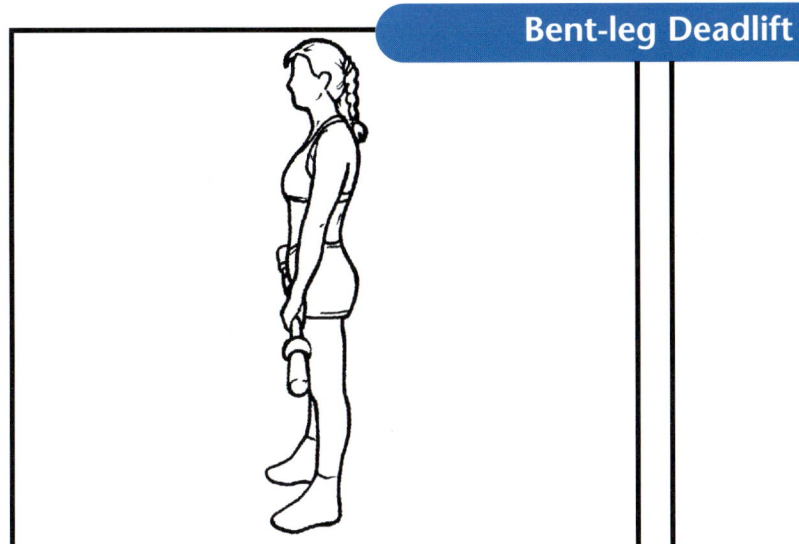

Bent-leg Deadlift

- Feet shoulder-width apart
- Elbows point sideways
- Abs tight

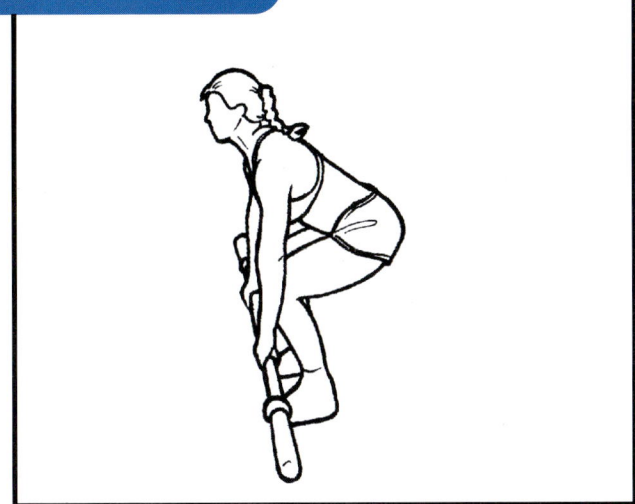

- Bend at hips first
- Back flat
- Shoulders forward of bar
- Squeeze bottom to push up

Get UP&GO!

Appendix

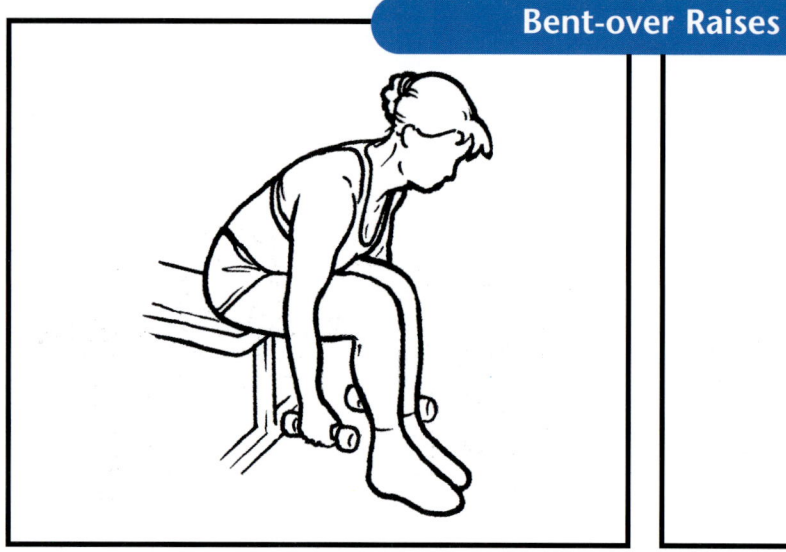

Bent-over Raises

- Shoulders held together and down
- Elbows slightly bent

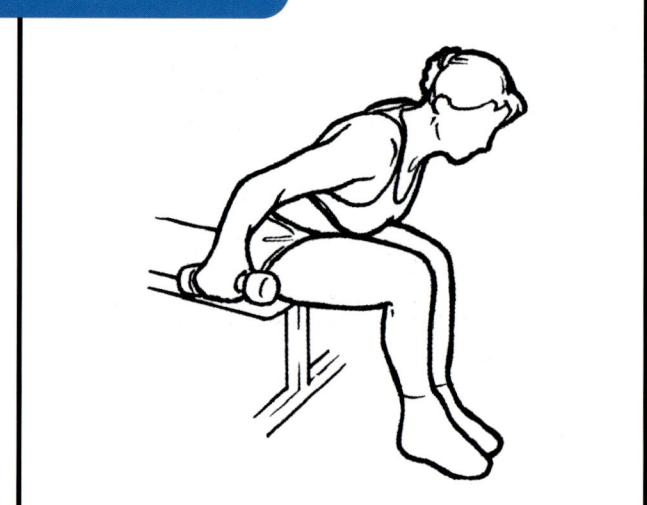

- Lift arms sideways
- Keep shoulders down as you lift
- Back stays slightly curved

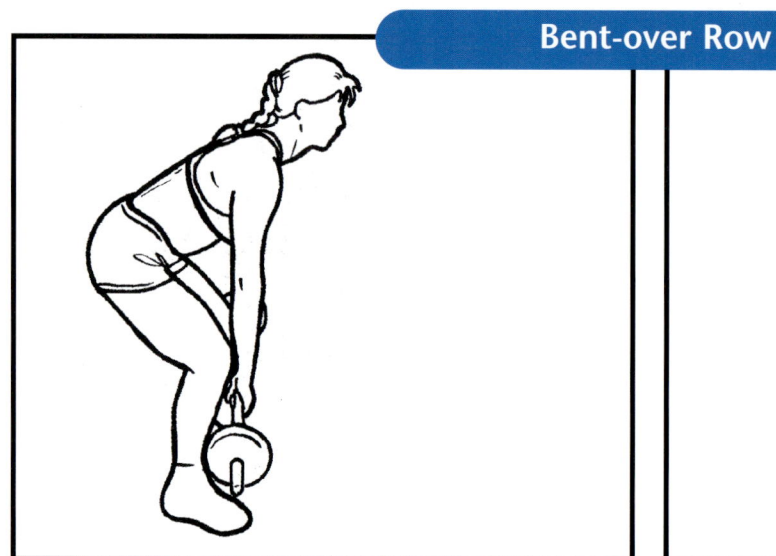

Bent-over Row

- Back flat, hips bent 90°, knees soft
- Shoulder blades together and down

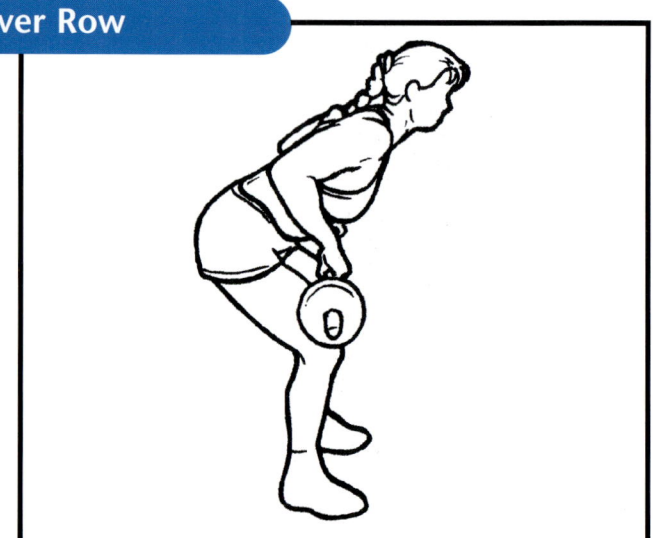

- Pull bar to bottom of ribs
- Stop when elbows get just past back

Bench Press

- Back flat, abs tight, feet flat

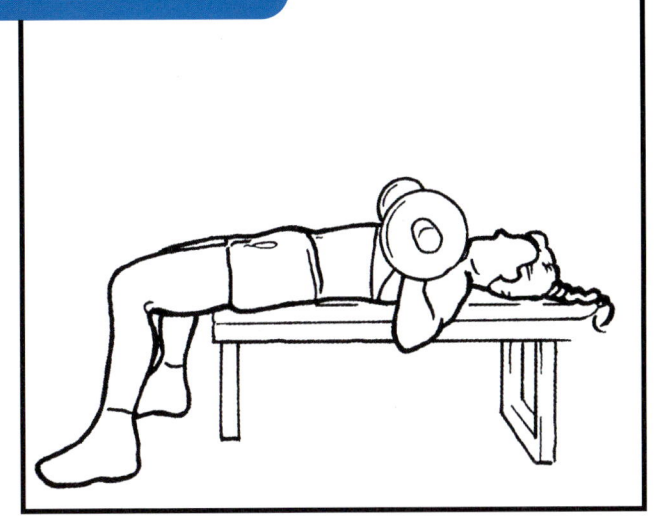

- Lower bar to mid chest
- Elbows stay under bar
- Push bar back to starting position

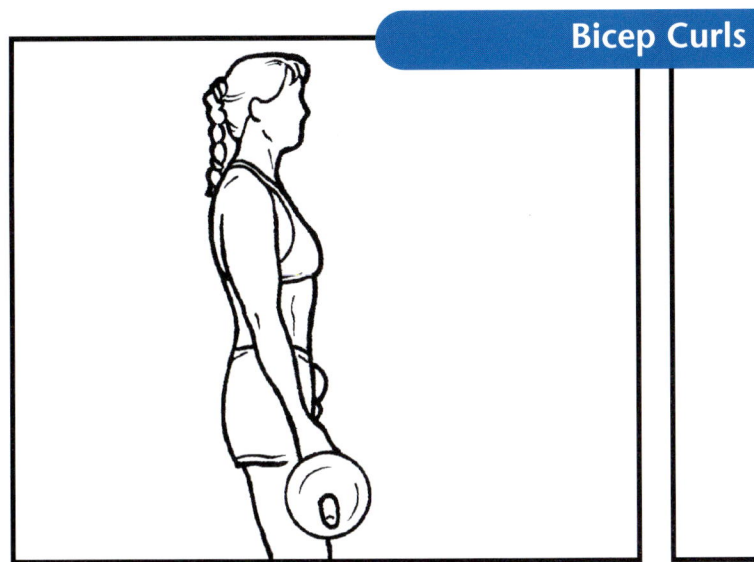

Bicep Curls

- Stand tall, abs tight, shoulders back
- Hands shoulder-width apart

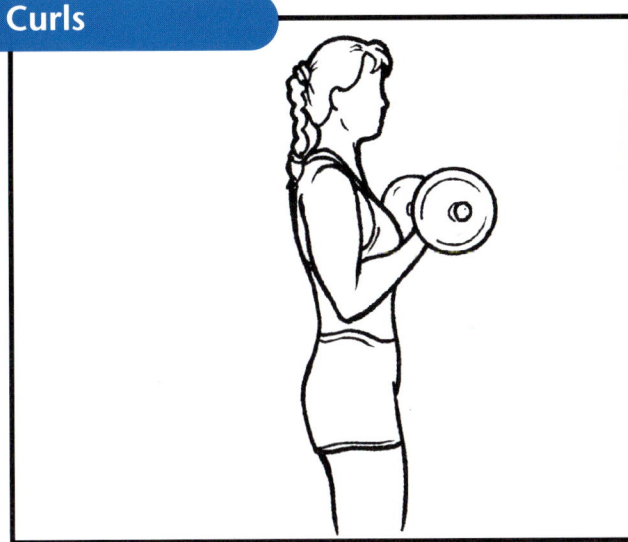

- Keep elbows by side
- Bend arms at elbows
- Lift bar to chest

Appendix

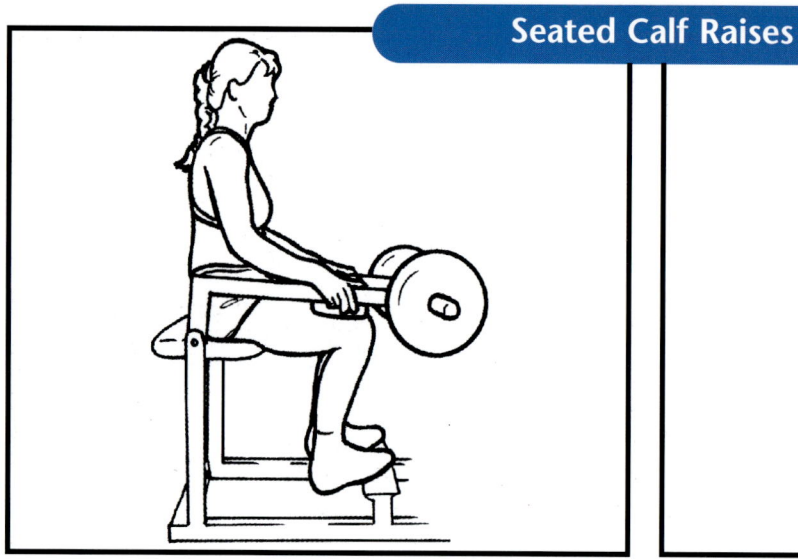

Seated Calf Raises

- Ball of foot on platform
- Knees above ankles
- Heels as low as possible

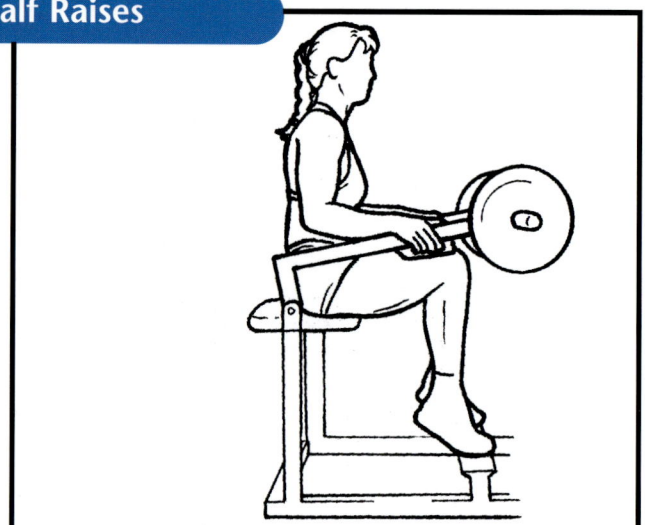

- Lift feet onto tiptoes
- Knees over toes

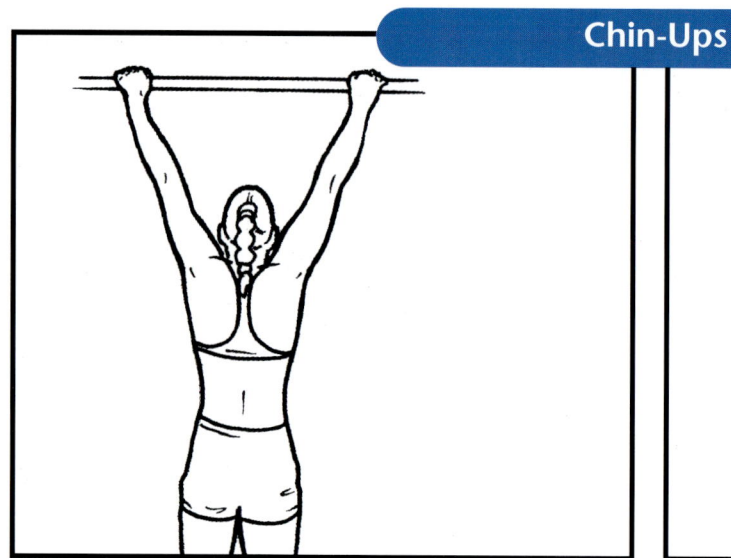

Chin-Ups

- Legs crossed
- Back flat
- Pull shoulder blades down and together

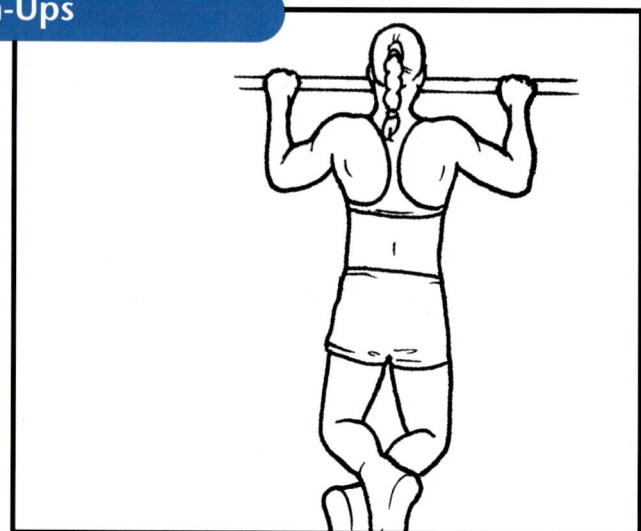

- Shoulder blades stay down
- Pull chin towards bar
- Keep elbows under bar
- Body remains vertical

Get UP&GO!

Appendix

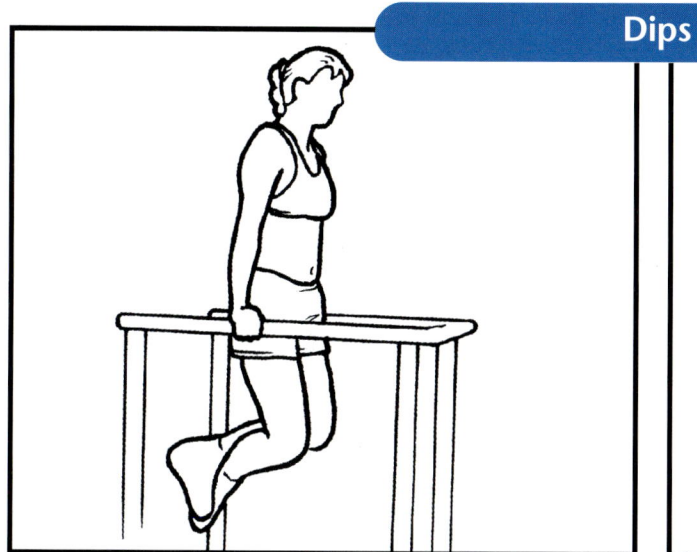

Dips

- Abs tight, legs crossed

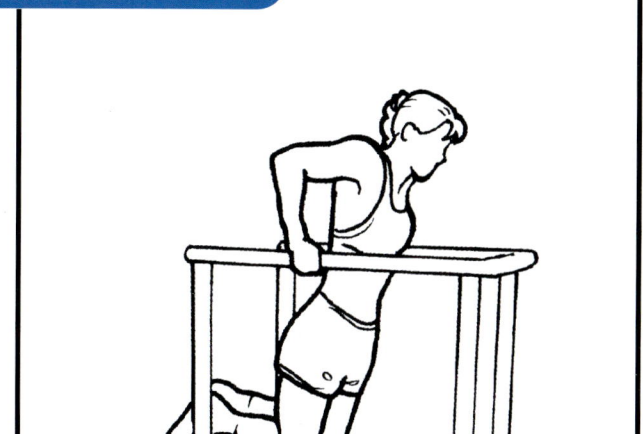

- Lower body, elbows and shoulders even at the bottom position
- Body leaning slightly forward

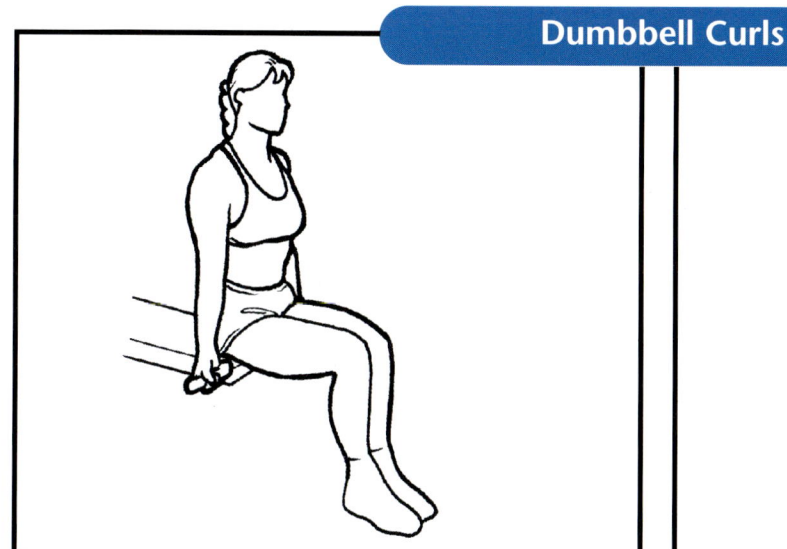

Dumbbell Curls

- Seated, elbows by side
- Body upright

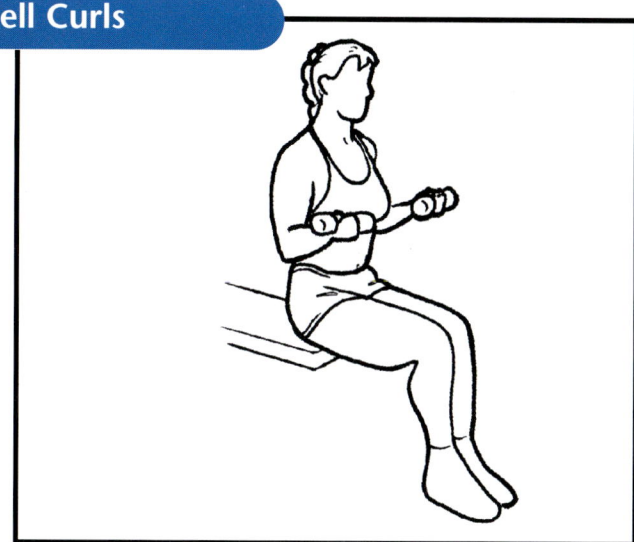

- Keep elbows still
- Bend elbows lifting dumbbells to chest

Appendix

Dumbbell Deadlift

- Abs tight, dumbbells by side

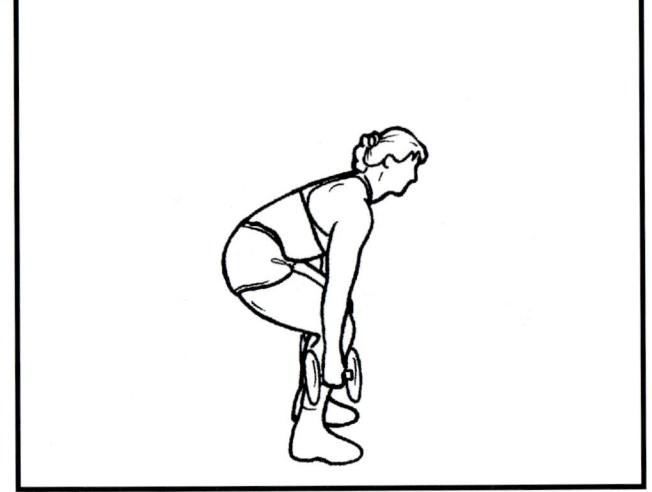

- Bend at hips first, bottom out, back flat
- Dumbbells slide down outside of each leg
- Shoulders over knees
- Squeeze bottom to return to top

Dumbbell Chest Press

- Back flat, feet flat
- Dumbbells together

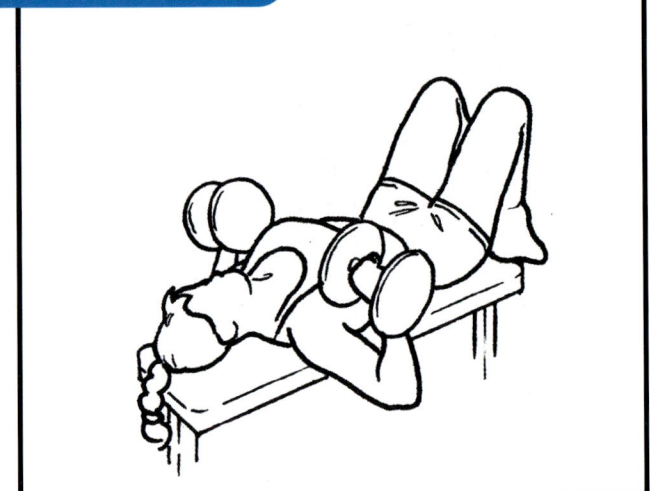

- Lower dumbbells to each shoulder
- Elbows stay under dumbbell
- Push back to starting position

Appendix

Dumbbell Pull-over

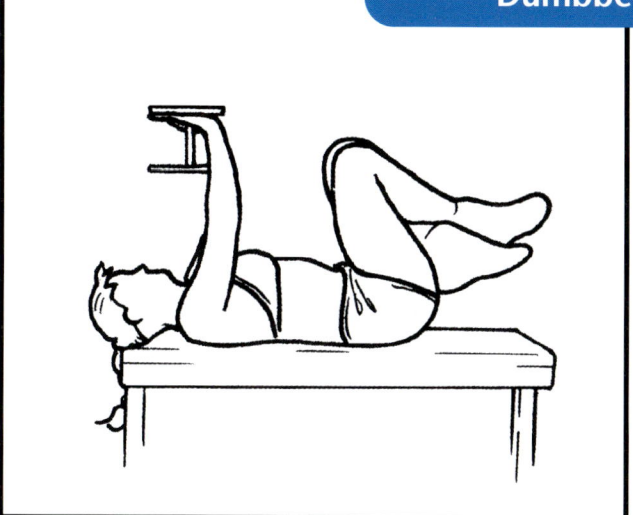

- Back flat, feet up
- Palms face up under dumbbell
- Elbows point to knees
- Elbows stay slightly bent

- Lower dumbbell over head
- Elbows held slightly bent
- Back remains flat

Dumbbell Flyes

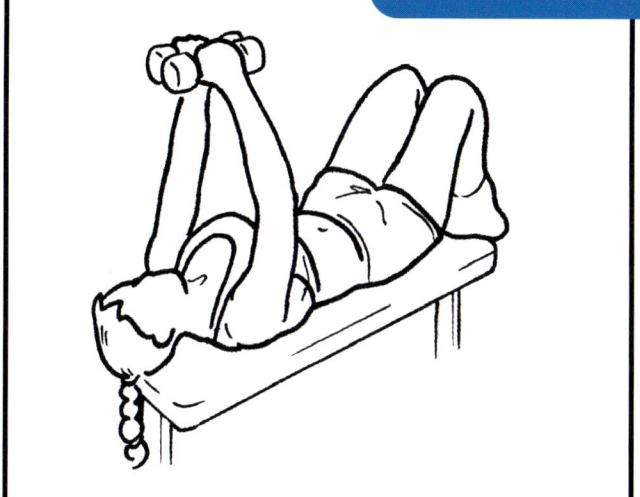

- Back flat, feet flat
- Elbows facing out to side
- Dumbbells held together

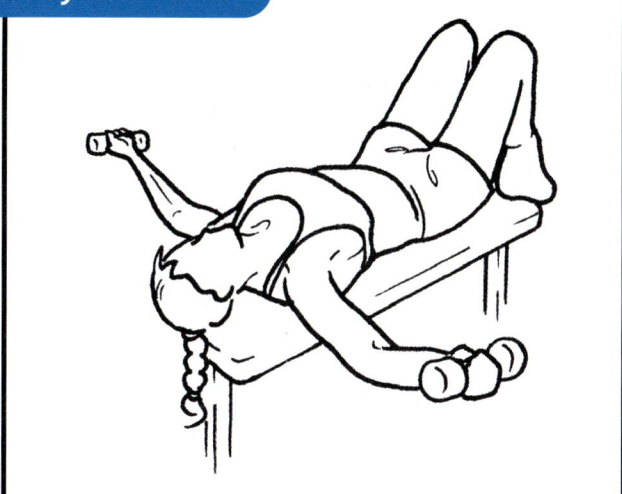

- Keep elbows slightly bent
- Lower dumbbells to side
- Back stays flat

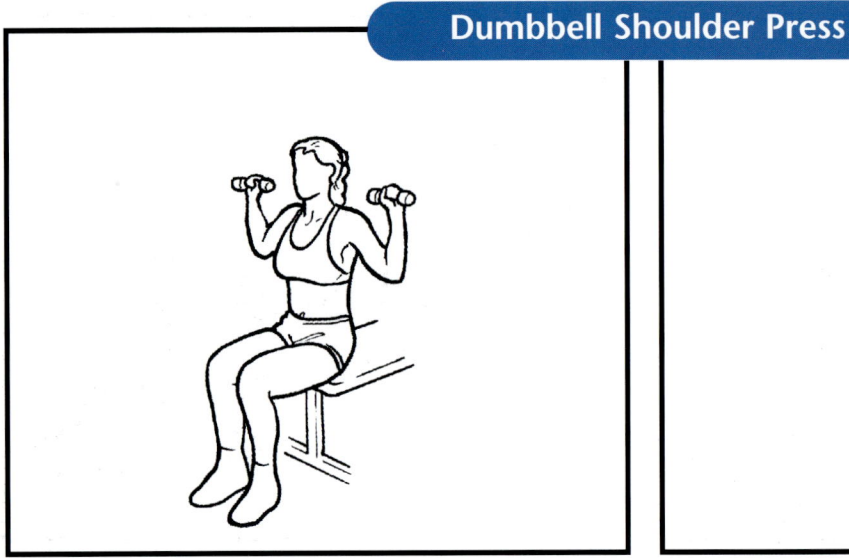

Appendix

Dumbbell Shoulder Press

- Sitting upright abs tight, back flat
- Dumbbells held level with shoulders

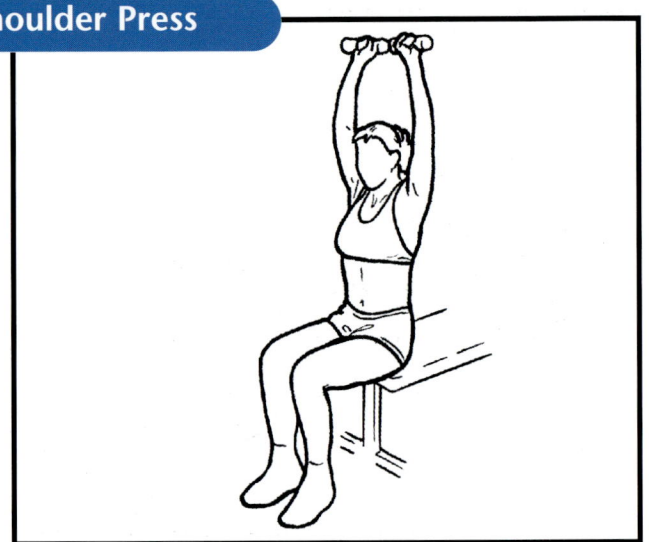

- Push dumbbells overhead and together
- Keep dumbbells in line with shoulders when lowering

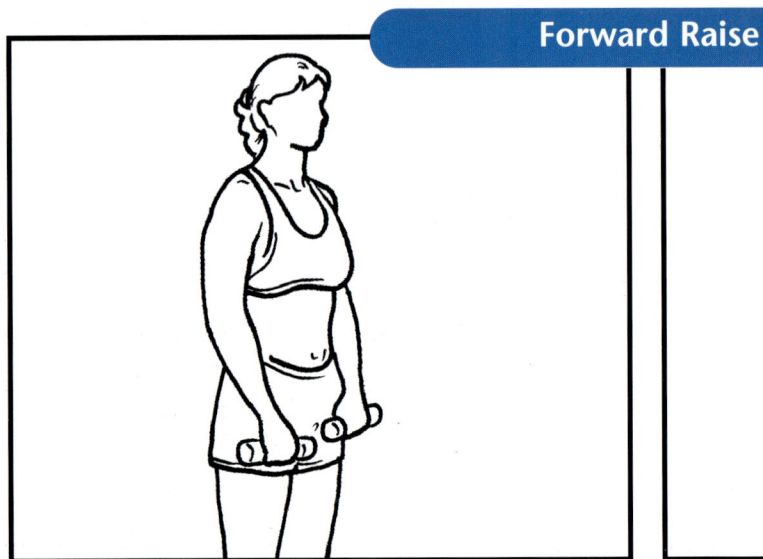

Forward Raise

- Stand tall, abs tight
- Dumbbells held on thighs, arms straight

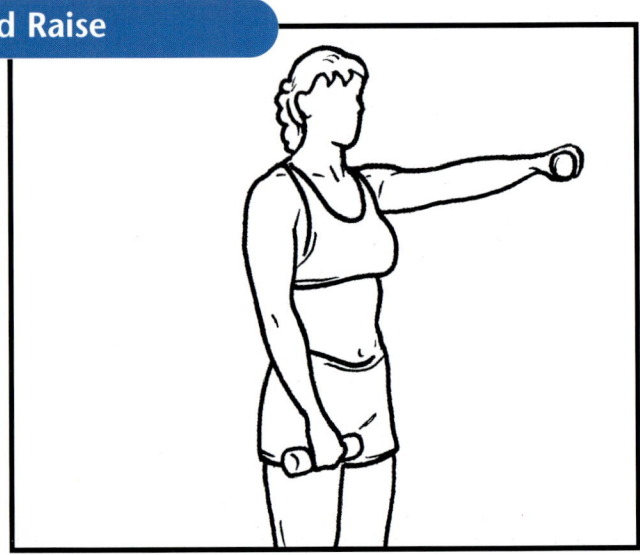

- Alternately lift one arm
- Keep shoulders together and down

Appendix

Incline Bench Press

- Back flat, abs tight, feet up

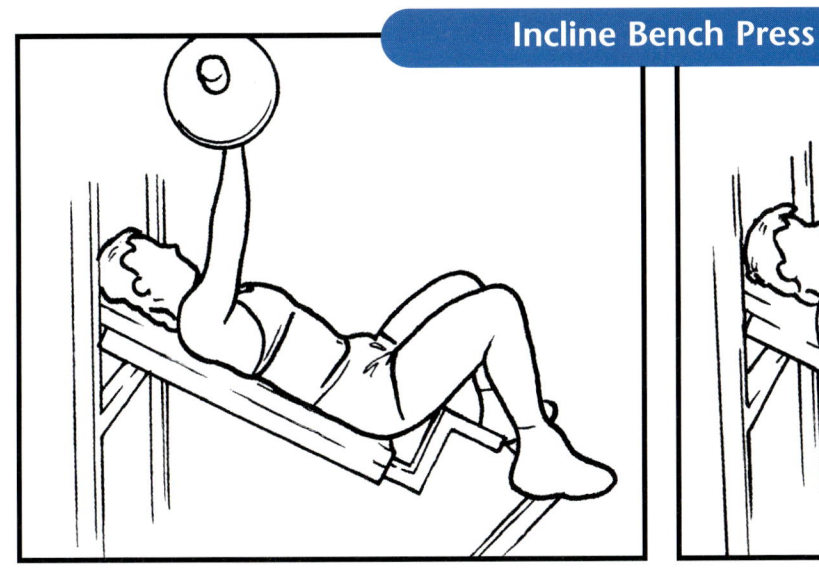

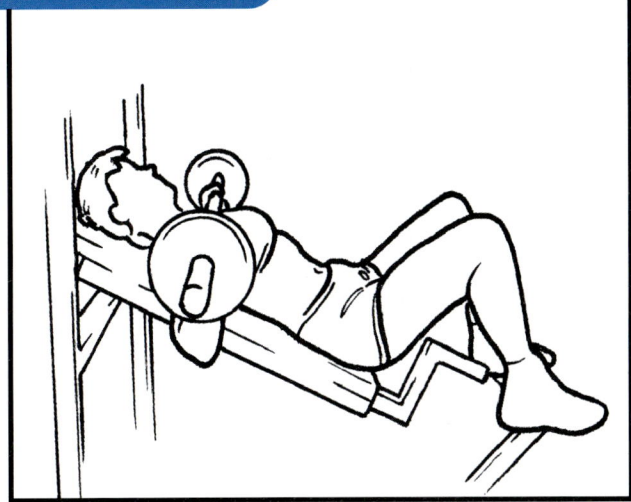

- Lower bar to upper chest
- Elbows stay under bar
- Push back to starting position

Incline Dumbbell Press

- Back flat, abs tight, feet flat
- Dumbbells together

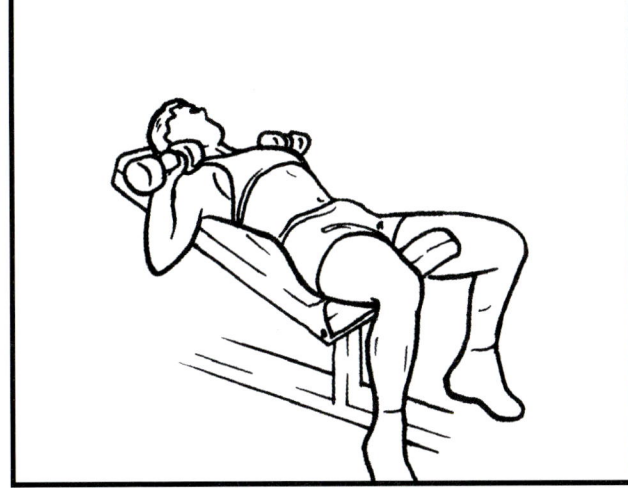

- Lower dumbbells to shoulders
- Elbows stay under dumbbells

Get UP&GO!

Appendix

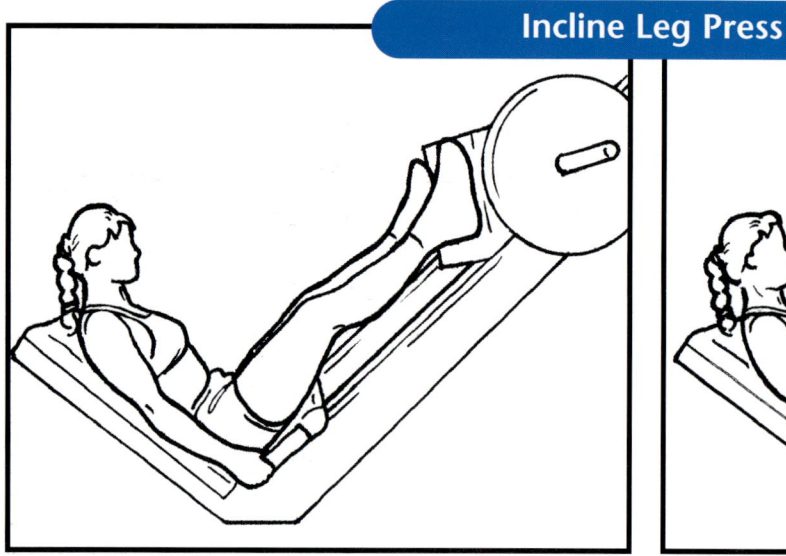

Incline Leg Press

- Bottom tight in seat
- Back flat
- Feet shoulder-width apart
- Toes high on plate

- Lower knees to 90°
- Push with heels and squeeze bottom tight
- Bottom stays tight in seat

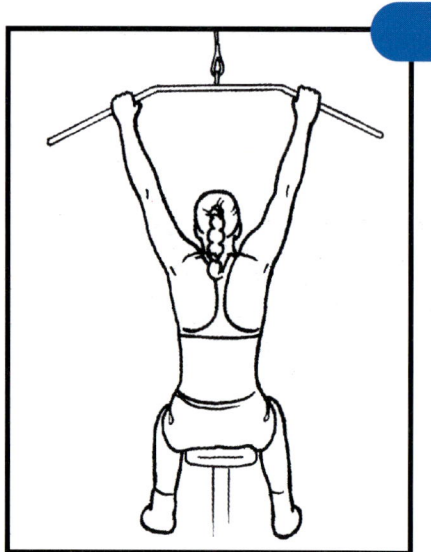

Lateral Pull-down

- Back flat, abs tight
- Hands outside shoulder-width

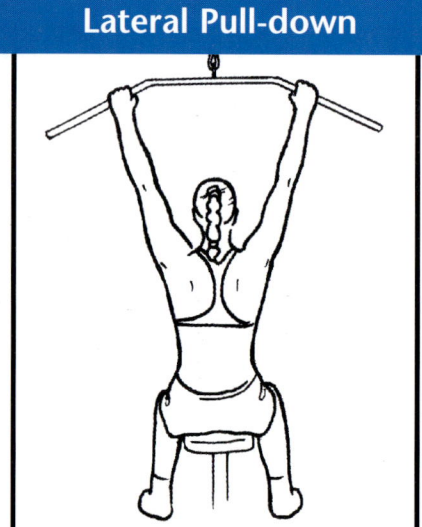

- Pull shoulder blades down and hold together
- Keep elbows straight

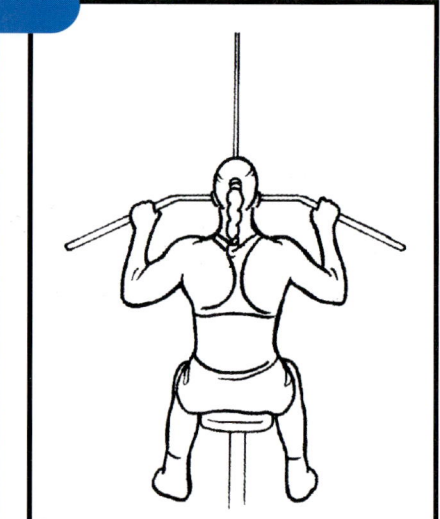

- Pull bar to nose level
- Keep back flat, shoulder blades down

Appendix

Lateral Raises

- Stand tall, abs tight
- Shoulders down and relaxed
- Arms slightly bent by side

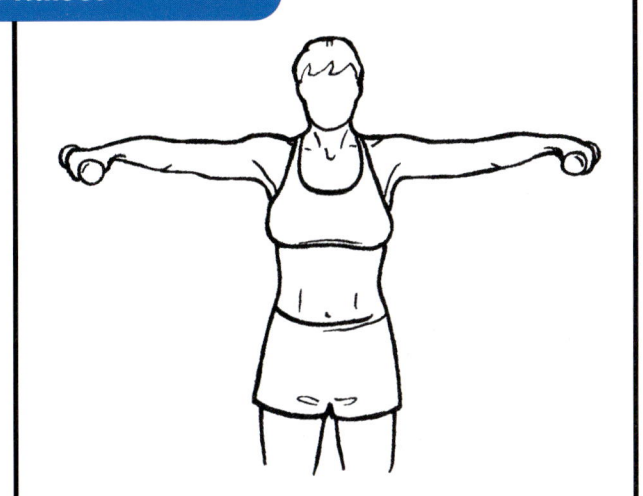

- Lift arms out to side
- Keep elbows slightly bent
- Keep palms face down

Leg Curls

- Bottom and abs tight
- Keep feet and ankles relaxed

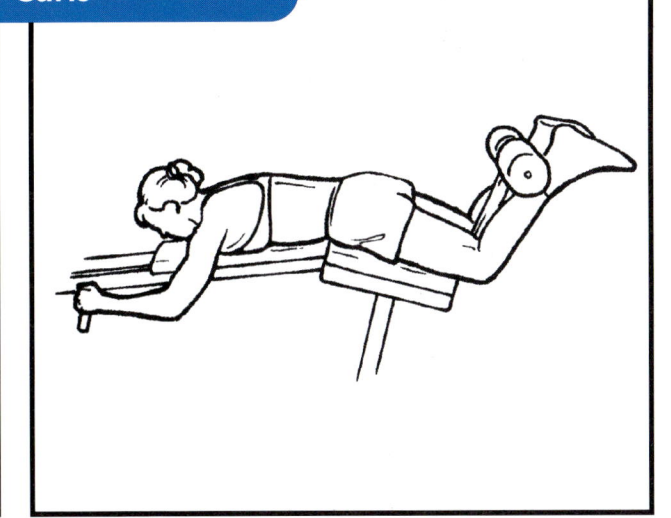

- Lift feet towards bottom
- Stop when abs or bottom relax or lift

Appendix

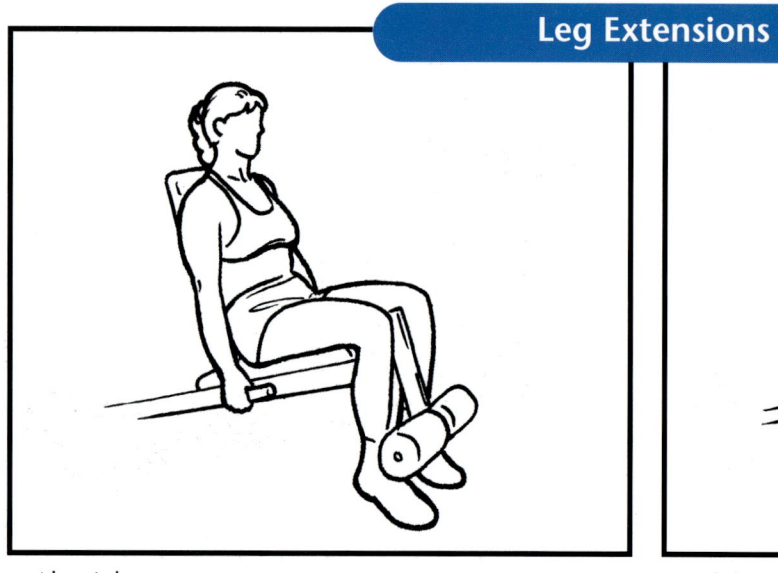

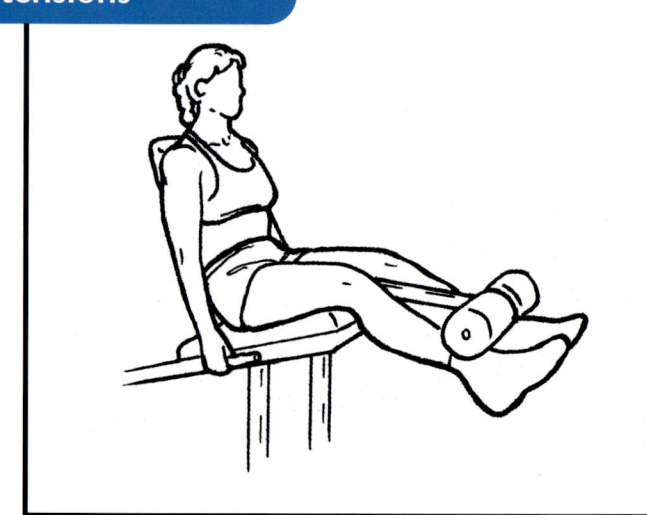

Leg Extensions

- Abs tight
- Bottom firm in seat

- Lift legs
- Keep toes relaxed

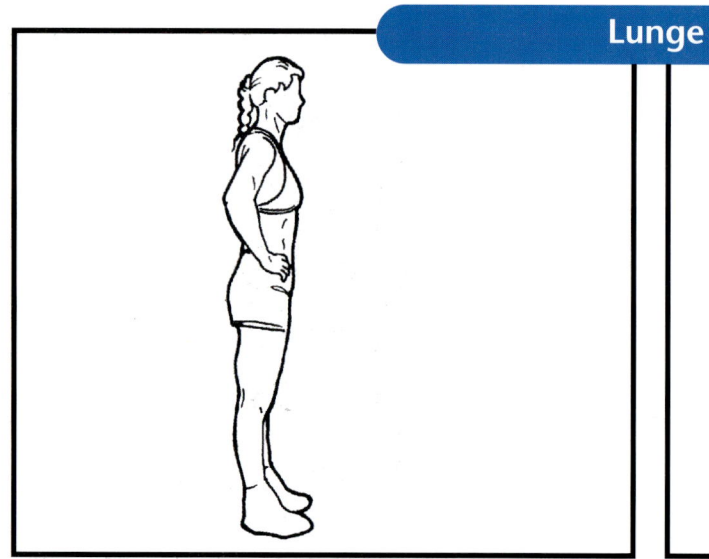

Lunge

- Abs tight

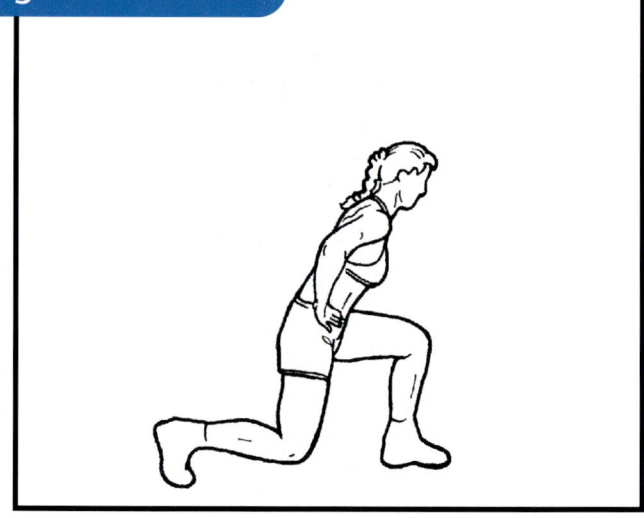

- Step forward with a slight upper body lean
- Weight onto front foot
- Squeeze bottom to push back to starting position

Appendix

Modified Pull-up

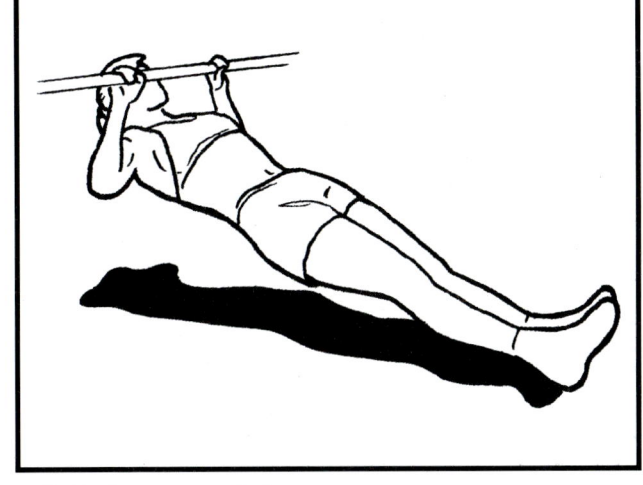

- Lie flat, hanging onto bar
- Keep body tight and rigid, heels on ground

- Pull chest towards bar
- Keep shoulders together and back
- Lower to the floor

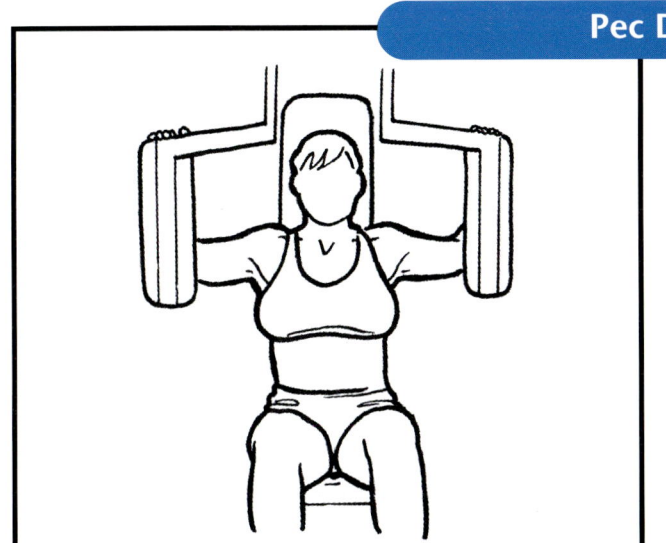

Pec Deck

- Back flat against seat
- Elbows at shoulder level
- Hands relaxed

- Push with elbows, not hands
- Bring pads to middle of body
- Keep shoulders together and back
- Hold abs tight throughout

Get UP&GO!

Appendix

Prone Raises

- Pull shoulder blades together and down
- Elbows slightly bent
- Neck relaxed

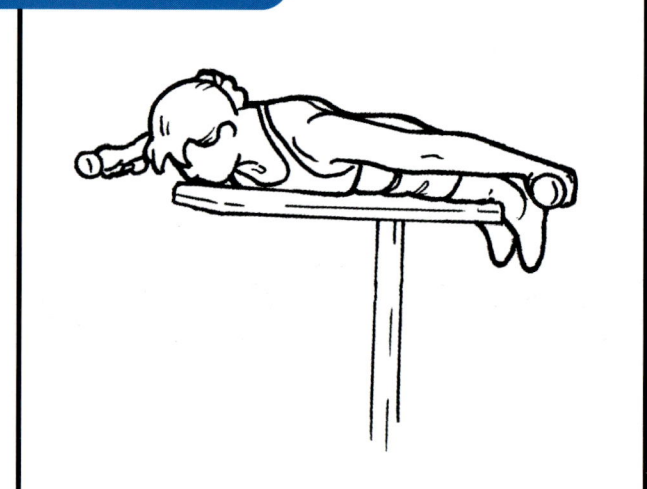

- Lift arms to side
- Keep muscles in upper neck relaxed
- Palms remain face down
- Stop if muscles in neck get tight

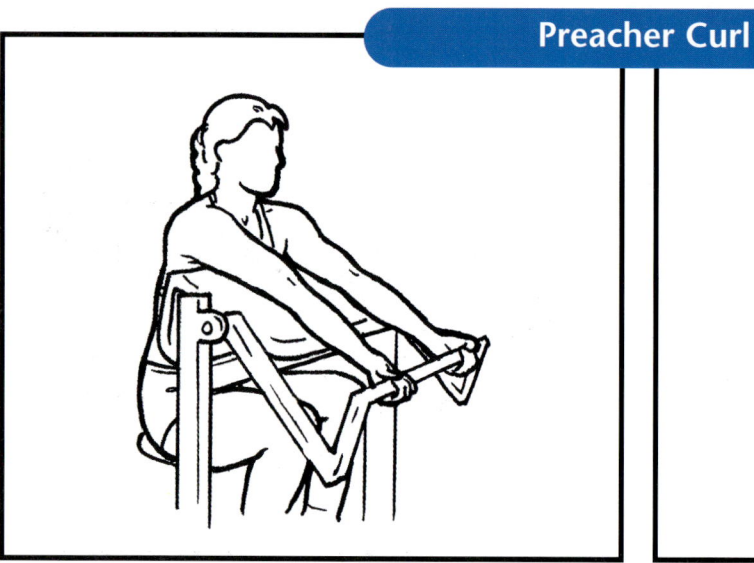

Preacher Curl

- Armpits firmly against pad
- Palms face up

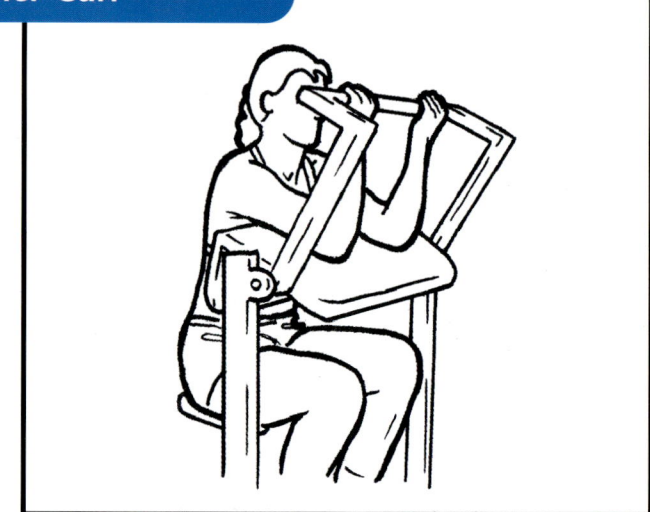

- Lift back to forehead, keeping wrists straight
- Keep elbows firmly on bench

Appendix

Push-ups

- Body flat on floor
- Palms face down level with shoulders
- Abs tight, body rigid
- Toes together

- Keep body tight
- Push to straight arms
- Toes straight on floor
- Lower to starting position

Modified Push-ups

- Body flat on floor
- Legs bent, and crossed
- Abs tight

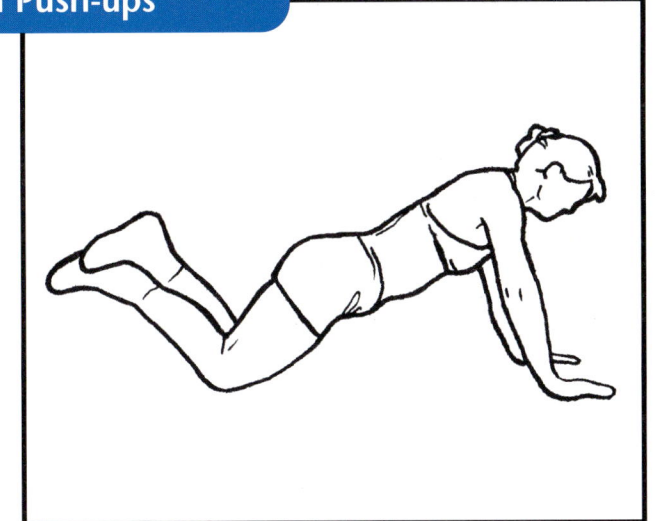

- Keep body rigid
- Push to straighten arms
- Keep knees on floor

Get UP&GO!

Seated Dips

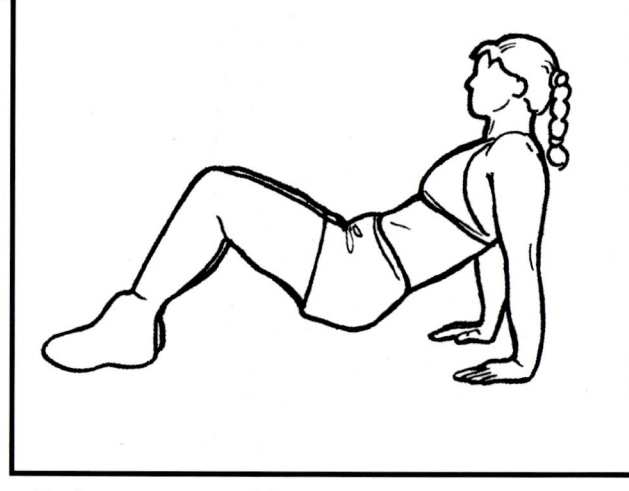

- Seated on bottom, knees bent
- Hands on floor, fingers towards bottom

- Push arms out straight
- Lifting bottom off the floor
- Keeps abs tight, shoulders back

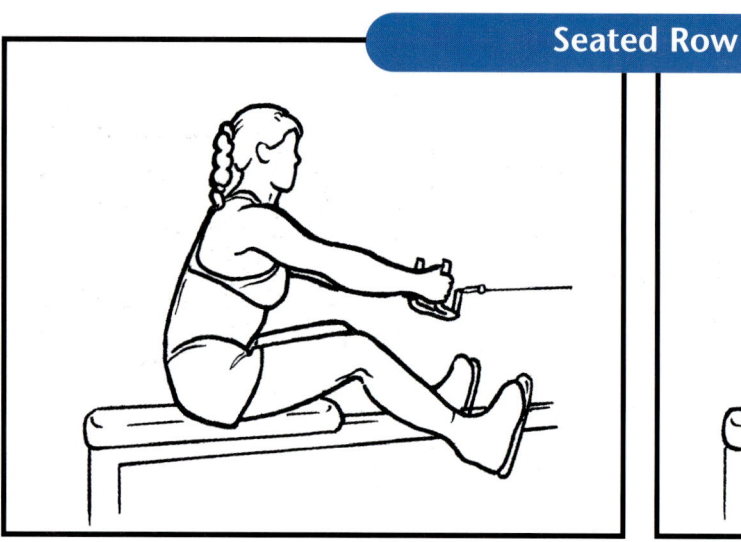

Seated Row

- Back slightly curved forwards
- Knees bent, arms straight

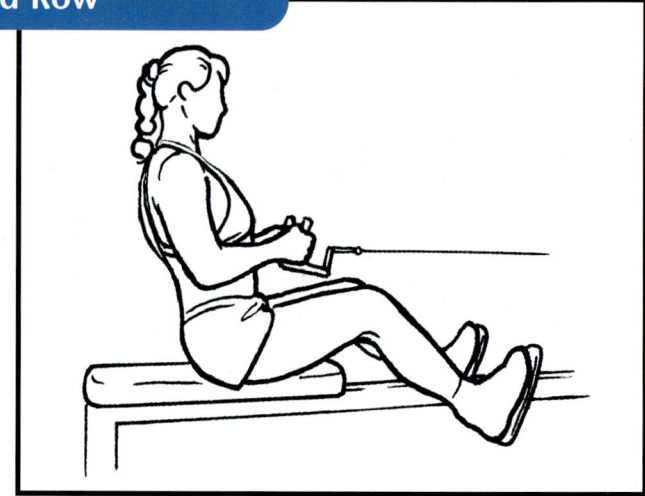

- Pull to a flat back position with shoulder blades held together
- Pull grip towards body
- Keep neck and shoulders relaxed
- Stop when elbows level with back

Appendix

Shoulder Press

- Back flat, abs tight and sucked in
- Bar set just above shoulder height
- Hands just wider than shoulders

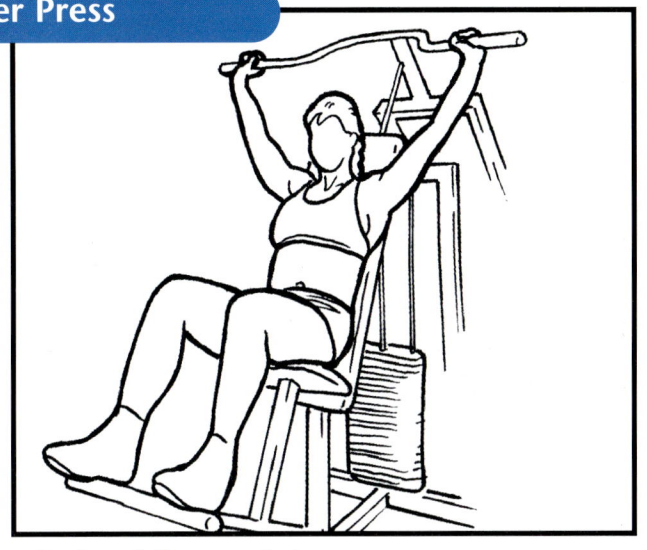

- Push to fully extended arms
- Keep back flat at all times
- hold abs tight

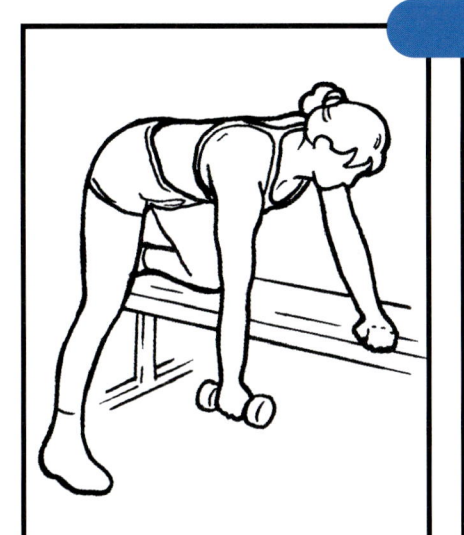

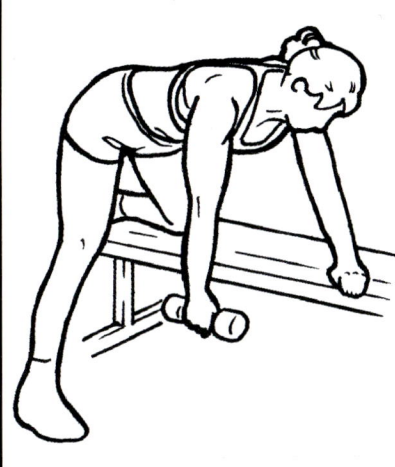

Single Arm Row

- Back flat
- Weight evenly on foot, knee, hand
- Arm straight

- Pull shoulder blades together and down toward hip
- Keep back flat

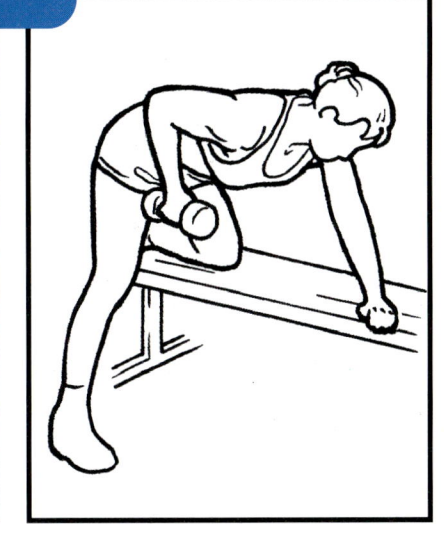

- Bring elbow up past hip
- Shoulder should lift slightly

Get UP&GO! 235

Appendix

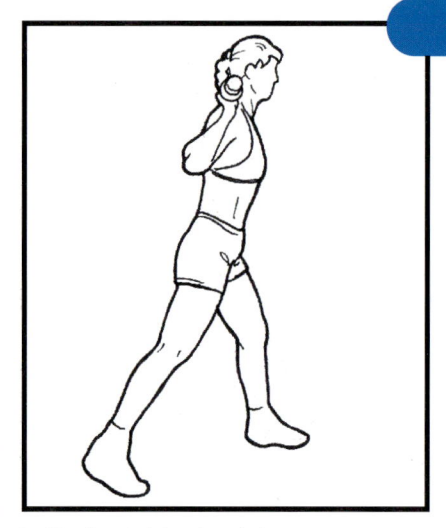

Split Squat

- Body rigid, abs tight
- Feet placed one foot forward and shoulder-width apart

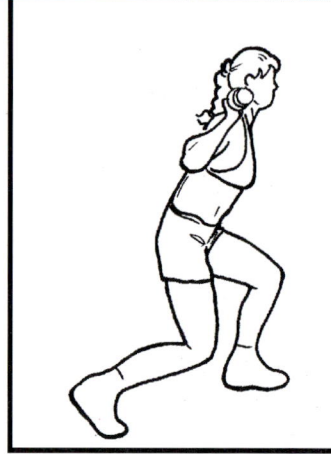

- Bend knees
- Lean slightly forward
- Abs tight

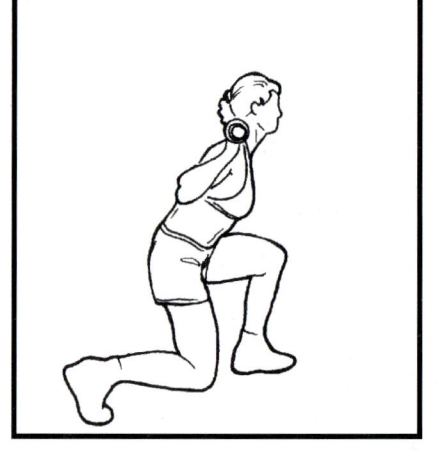

- Keep weight on front foot
- Lean slightly forward
- Push with bottom back to starting position

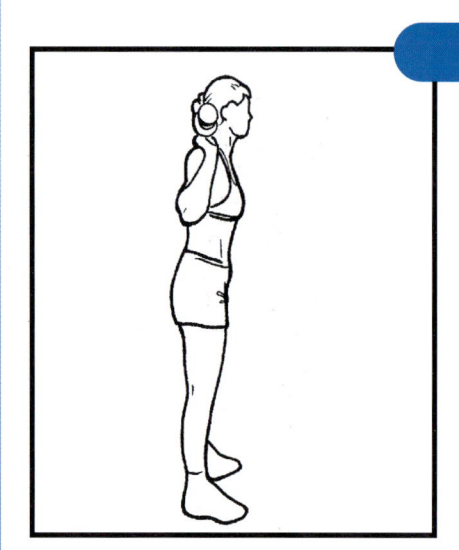

Squat

- Feet apart, body tall
- Hips tucked in, abs tight

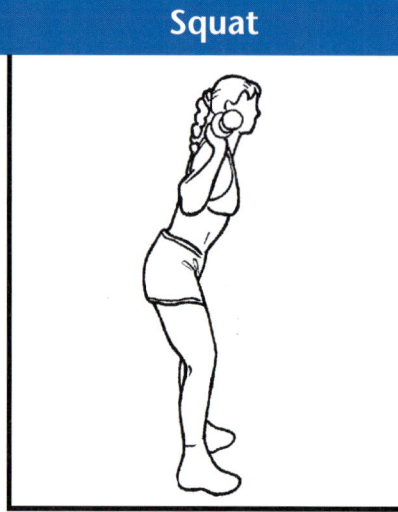

- Poke bottom out first
- Slight lean forward

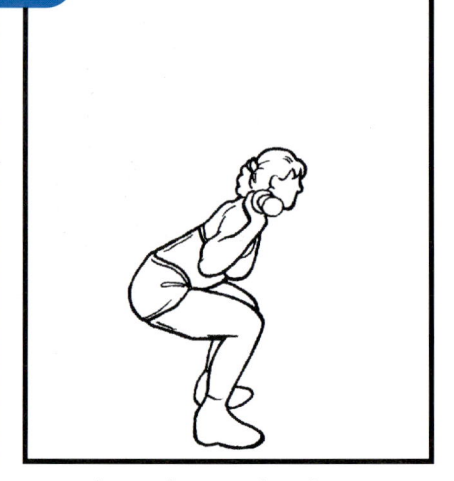

- Sit down, bottom level with knees
- Weight evenly on feet
- Shoulders above heels
- Squeeze bottom to push up

Appendix

Step-ups

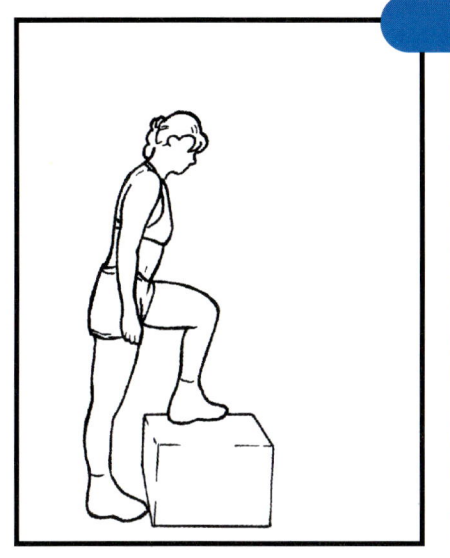

- Lean slightly forward
- Front foot on step box

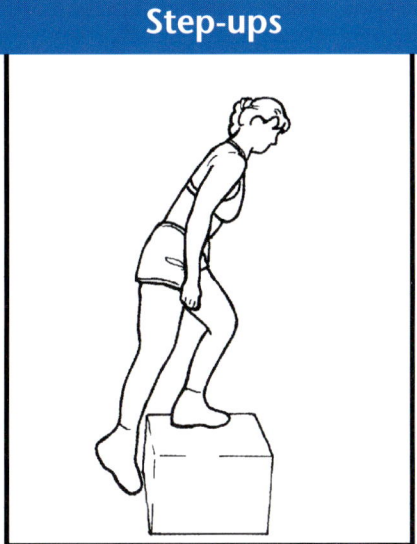

- Keep all weight on front foot
- Lift body

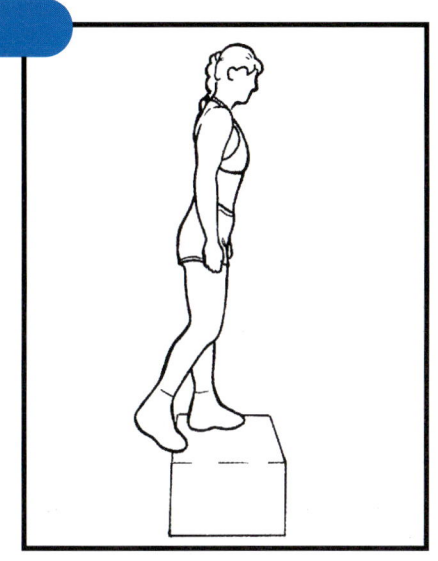

- Drag back foot up to top of box
- Push hips forward, body tall

Tricep Press-down

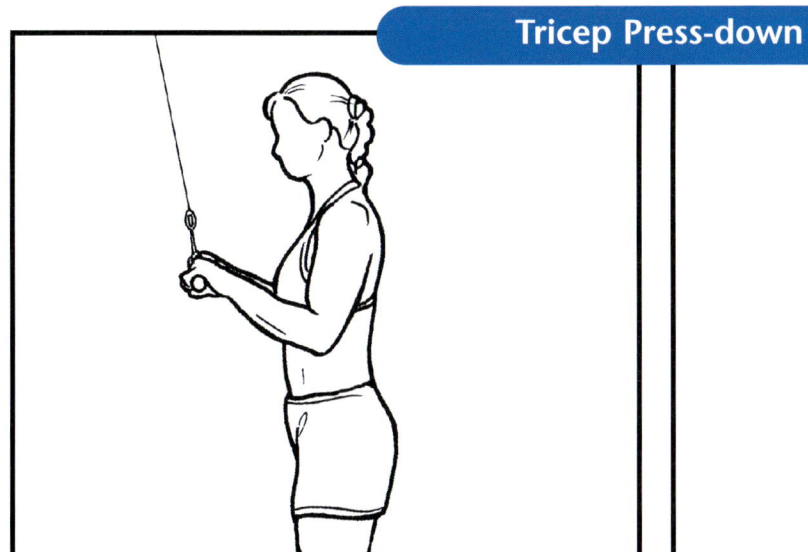

- Body straight, abs tight and sucked in
- Elbows tucked into side of body

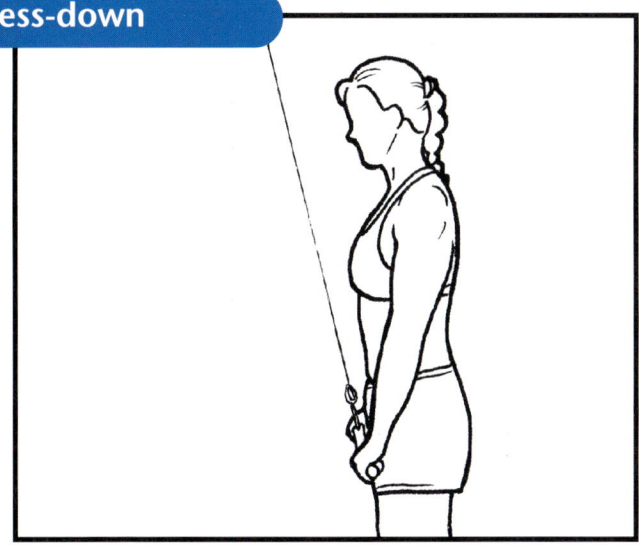

- Straighten arms until hands touch hips
- Keep shoulders back

Appendix

Overhead Tricep Extension

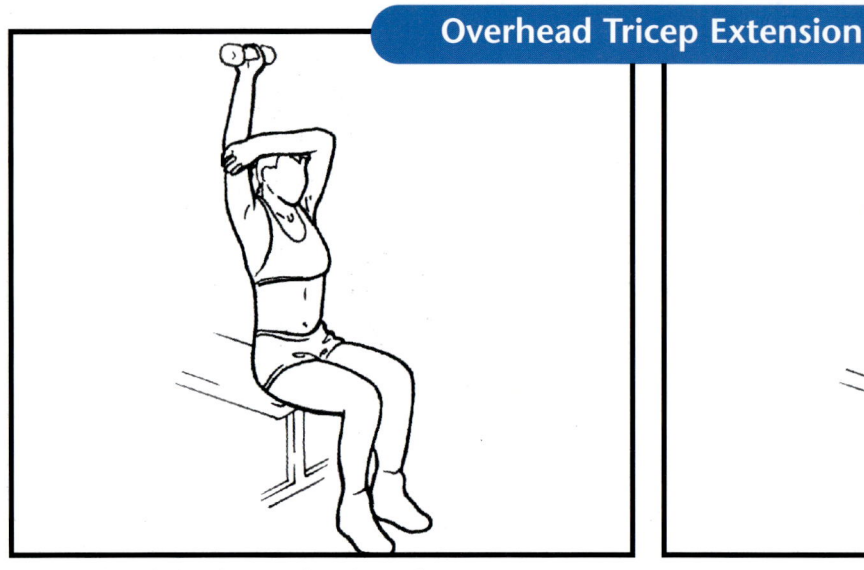

- Seated with back straight, abs tight
- One dumbbell held in your hand with arm extended above head
- Other hand placed on elbow of straight arm to keep it still, forearm can rest against your forehead to maintain stability

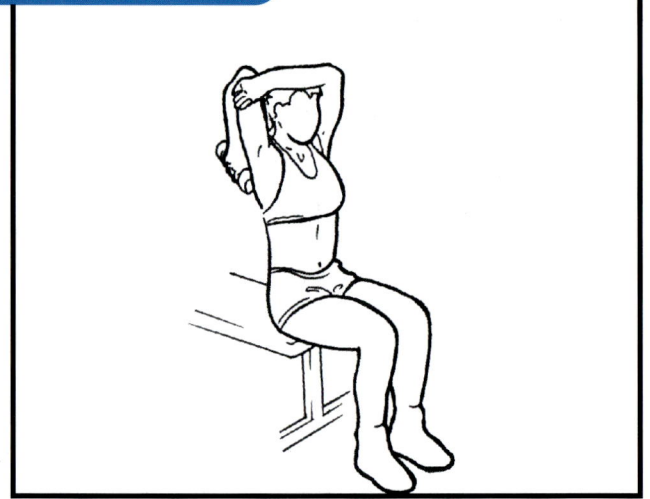

- Keeping your elbow still, lower dumbbell by bending elbow to back of shoulder
- Return dumbbell to top by straightening your elbow

Lying Tricep Extension

- Lying on a bench with your back flat, and abs tight
- Arms extended upwards with bar
- Hands held shoulder-width apart on bar

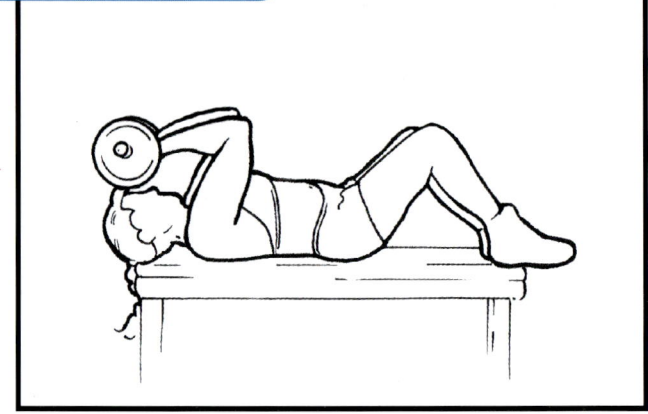

- Keep your elbows in the same position as you lower the bar towards your forehead
- Stop before your bar touches your forehead and straighten elbow to bring bar back to starting position

Wall Push-ups

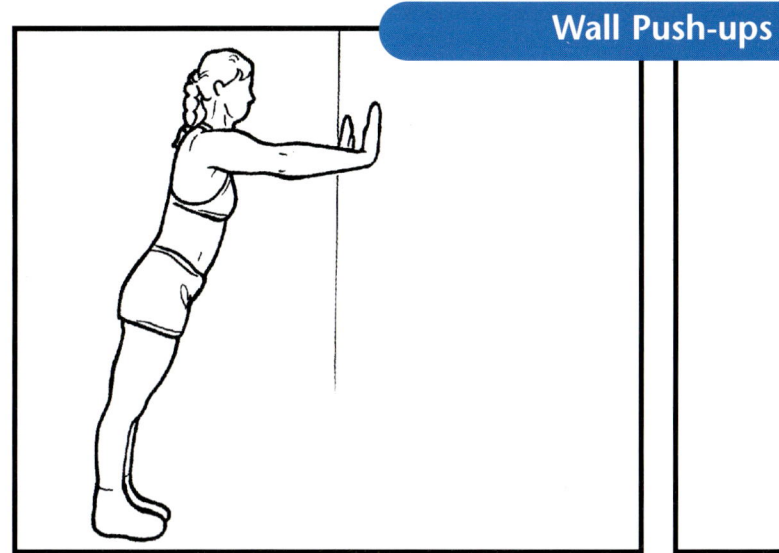

- Slight forward lean, body rigid
- Arms straight
- Hands wider than shoulders
- Weight on toes

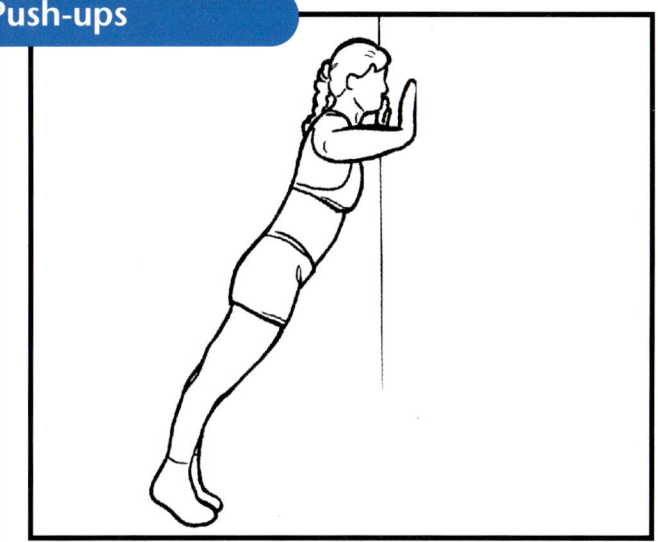

- Lean body into wall
- Body kept straight
- Stop with face almost on wall
- Push back to starting position

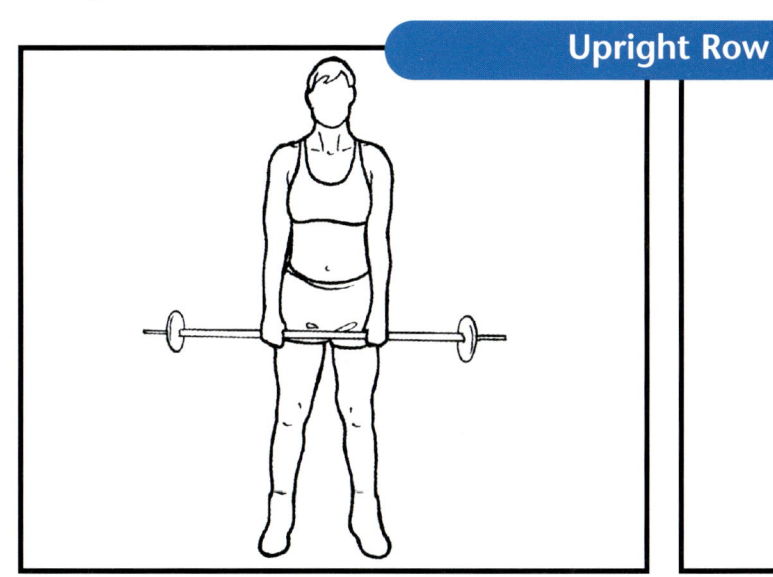

Upright Row

- Feet apart, shoulders back
- Hands shoulder-width apart

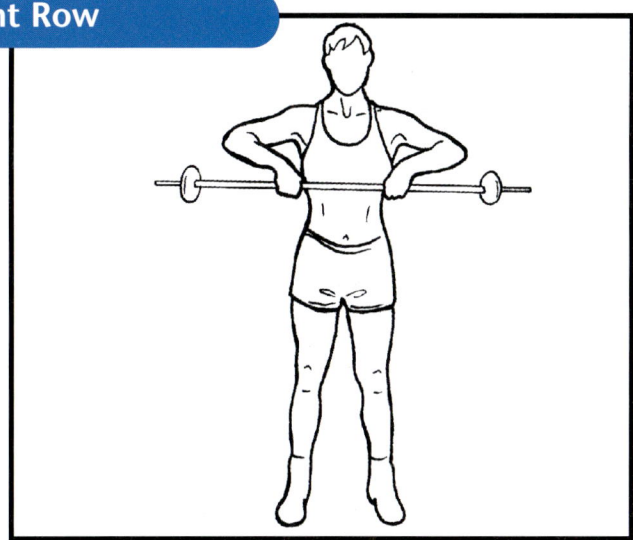

- Pull bar to chest height
- Keep elbows higher than wrists
- Neck relaxed

Index

Page numbers in italics refer to illustrations.

abdominal exercises 211, *212–13*
abdominal strength test 136–7, *136–7*
adenosine triphosphate 49, 50, 51–2, 53, 54–5
aerobic energy system 54
aerobic exercise
 as cardiovascular exercise 43
 combined with circuit classes *154*, 154–5
 for fat loss 168–79
 for muscle definition 202–4
aerobic fitness
 testing 130–2
 training for 183–91
age, and metabolic rate 56
agility drills *157*
alcohol 8, 45, 62, 77, 78
amino acids 46, 66
anaerobic energy system 52
antioxidants 76
arms, shaping of 210
ascorbic acid 73
athletes, types of 112–13
ATP 49, 50, 51–2, 53, 54–5
ATP-PC energy system 51–2, 54–5
back pain 116, 118
back, shaping of 209, *209*
beer 78
blood glucose 91
blood pressure 41–2
the body
 see also training; *specific parts of the body*
 accepting oneself 36
 body types 36–9, *37–9*
 cardiovascular system 41–2, 44
 digestive system 44–8
 energy systems 51–5
 listening to your body 57
 maintaining 35
 musculoskeletal system 48–50
 nervous system 50–1
 reactions to stress 27–8
 respiratory system 41, 43–5

body fat
 losing by eating well 100–1
 measuring 139, *140–1*
 relation to metabolic rate 56
 training for fat loss 168–82, 208
bodybuilding *see* training
the bottom, exercises for 211, *214–15*
the bowel 46–7
boxing 155, *156*
breakfast 56, 65
breathing rate 43
building up 98–9, *98–9*, 192–201, 208
bulking up *90*
caffeine 77
calciferous 73
calcium 74, 75–6
carbohydrate loading 102–4
carbohydrates
 after competition and training 107
 case study 94–5
 digestion of 46
 requirements 91–6
 sources 62, 62–5
 types 62–4
cardio equipment
 for aerobic fitness 185
 for fat loss 179
cardiovascular system 41–2, 44
champagne 78
children
 fat requirements 71
 making time for 21
chin-up test *134–5*, 135
cholesterol 68–9, 71
circuit classes 154–5
coffee 77
communication 24
competition, and diet 102–4
complex carbohydrates 62
cooling down 167, *167*
copper 74
cross-training 155–7, *156–7*, 203

cyanocobalamin 72
cycling
 as an exercise 152–3, *153*
 for aerobic fitness 185
 for fat loss 179
dehydration 77, 104
delayed muscle soreness 167
diet
 balance in 82, *83*, 84, 90
 carbohydrate loading 102–4
 carbohydrate requirements 91–6
 'dieting' 89
 eating in moderation 83
 fat requirements 71
 for building muscle mass 98–9, 193–4
 for competition 102–4, 114
 for endurance athletes 102–3, *105*
 keeping a diary 85–8
 losing body fat by eating well 100–1
 mineral requirements 74–6
 protein requirements 97–8
 relation to metabolic rate 56
 variety in 83, *84*
 vitamin requirements 72–3
 digestive system 44–8
 diuretics 77
 DMS 167
drinks
 Banana Soy Smoothie 64, *64*
 Lisa's Health Drink 100, *100*
 Pine Orange Blast 63, *63*
Endura Opti (drink) 103
energy systems 51–5
Ensure (drink) 103
exercise
 see also training
 catalogue of exercises 217–39
 contrasted with training 111
 effect on cardio-respiratory systems 44–5
 effect on digestive system 48
 effect on metabolic rate 56
 effect on muscles 50

effect on skeleton 48–9
fuel for 53
fat (body) *see* body fat
fatigue 65
fats (food) 46, 62, 68–71
fatty acids 46, 68–9
fibre, in diet 78–9
fight or flight syndrome 44
FIT principle 144–6
 fitness tests 124–37
 see also training
flexibility 118–20, *120–1*
fluid and food diaries 85–8
fluid replacement 104–6, *105*, 107, *107*
fluorine 74
folic acid 73, 76
food
 see also diet
 carbohydrates 62, 62–5, *63*, *64*
 energy from 61–2
 fats 68–9
 fibre 78–9
 minerals 74–6
 protein 66
 vitamins 72–3
 water 77–8
food and fluid diaries 85–8
fructose 46
fruit 63, *63*, 73
galactose 46
gender, and metabolic rate 56
GI index 94, 96
girth measurements 138, *138*
glucose 46, 96
Glycaemic Index 94, 96
glycogen 46, 53, 55, 91, 102, 103
goals and goal-setting 9–16, 162
haem iron 74, 76
heart rate 41–2, *42*, 130, 145, *145*
high-density lipoprotein 68
insoluble fibre 79
interval runs *157*

Index

iodine 74
iron 74, 76
kayaking 194, *194*
lactic acid 52
lactic tolerance training 184
lacto vegetarians 67
legs, shaping of 209–10
legumes 64, 66
linoleic acid 68–9
lipoproteins 68
liquid meals 103
liver 55
low-density lipoprotein 68
low-fat milk products 64
lungs 43
magnesium 75
massage 123
medicine ball drills *157*
metabolic rate 56
milk 64
minerals 74–6
mono-unsaturated fats 69
motivation 3–8
muscles
  abdominal muscles 118
  changing body shape 207–15
  delayed muscle soreness 167
  increasing muscle definition 50, *50*, 202–6
  increasing muscle size 98–9, *98–9*, 192–201, 208
  muscle balance 116–17, *117*, 163
  muscle mass and body type 37–9
  muscular endurance tests 132–7, *133–7*
  relation to protein intake 97
  musculoskeletal system 48–50
nervous system 50–1
netball 155
niacin 72
non-haem iron 74
nutrition *see* diet; food
Omega-3 fatty acids 68
Omega-6 fatty acids 68, 69
outrigger canoeing *144*
'overload' principle 146, 166
overtraining 120, 122–3, 166
ovo-lacto vegetarians 67
paperwork 23
PC 49, 51–2, 54–5
personal organisation 20
personal trainers *148*

phospho-creatine 49, 51–2, 53–4
phosphorus 75
phytochemicals 83, 84
planning
  time management 17–25, *19*
  to achieve goals 9–16
plyometric training *51*
polyunsaturated fats 68–9
port 78
posture 116, 117, 142, 163–5, *165*
potassium 75
potatoes 65
pre-event meals 103–4
pregnancy, training during 97, *97*
probiotics 48
processed foods 64
procrastination 18–19
progressive overload 166
protein
  digestion of 46
  energy from 62
  requirements 97–8
  sources 66
Pump classes 154, *154*
push-up test 132–3, *133*
pyridoxine 72
recovery
  avoiding overtraining 122, 123, 166
  food for 107
  importance of 169, 191
  stretching 119
  training for aerobic fitness 184–5
  training for fat loss 180
  training for muscle definition 203
relaxation 30–1
resistance training
  as an exercise *148*, 148–9
  effect on musculoskeletal system 48
  for aerobic fitness 191
  for fat loss 180–2
  for muscle definition 202, 204–6
  for older people 48, *49*
respiratory system 41, 43–5
rest *see* recovery; relaxation
resting metabolic rate 56
riboflavin 72

rock climbing *54*
running
  as an exercise 151, *151*
  for aerobic fitness 185
  for fat loss 169–72
  in cross-training 155
  12-minute walk test 130–1
saturated fats 68
selenium 75, 76
sex, and metabolic rate 56
shape (body) 207–15
shiftworkers 22–3
shoulders, shaping of 208–9
shuttle runs *157*
simple carbohydrates 62
skeleton 48–9
skinfold thickness measurements 139, *140–1*
slide Reebok 156, *156*
smoking 8
sodium 75
soluble fibre 79
soy milk 64
spirits 78
sport 158–9, *159*
sports drinks 103, 106, 107
strength tests 132–7, *133–7*
stress 25–31
stretching 119–20, *120–1*, 167, *167*
success 6–7
sugars 62, 64, 65
surf-lifesaving *125*
Sustagen (drink) 103
swimming
  as an exercise 152, *152*
  for aerobic fitness 186–91
  for fat loss 172–8, *177*
  in cross-training 155
  12-minute swim test 131–2
tea 77
thiamine 72
time management 17–25, *19*
tocopherols 73
training
  see also diet; exercise; recovery
  body control 118, *118–19*, 164–5
  catalogue of exercises 217–39
  contrasted with exercise 111
  example session 158
  FIT principle 144–6
  flexibility 118–20, *120–1*

  for aerobic fitness 183–91
  for competition 114–15
  for fat loss 168–82, 208
  for increased muscle size 98–9, *98–9*, 192–201, 208
  for muscle definition 202–6
  for shape 207–15
  importance of perserverance 143–4, 165
  making a start 7–8, 113
  overtraining 120, 122–3, 166
  phases of 113–14
  planning a program 11–13, 113, 115, 144–8, 162, 166
  posture and muscle balance 116–17, *117*, 162–5, *165*
  types of athletes 112–13
trans fatty acids 69
Transversus Abdominis muscle 118
travelling 24–5
treadmills *124*
triglycerides 46
12-minute run/walk test 130–1
12-minute swim test 131–2
unloading 169, 180, 184–5, 191
unsaturated fats 68–9
vegans 67
vegetables 63, 73
vegetarian diets 66–7
vitamins 48, 63, 72–3, 76
waist-hip ratio 139
walking
  as an exercise *150*, 150–1
  for aerobic fitness 185
  for fat loss 169–72
  on beaches *128*
  12-minute walk test 130–1
warming-up 119–20, *120–1*, 167, *167*
water 77–8, 106
weight training
  as an exercise 148–9, *149*
  combined with aerobic classes 154, *154–5*
  for fat loss 180–2
  for increased muscle size 194–201
  training smartly 166
wine 78
yoghurt 48
zinc 75, 76